A Textbook of

PHARMACOGNOSY

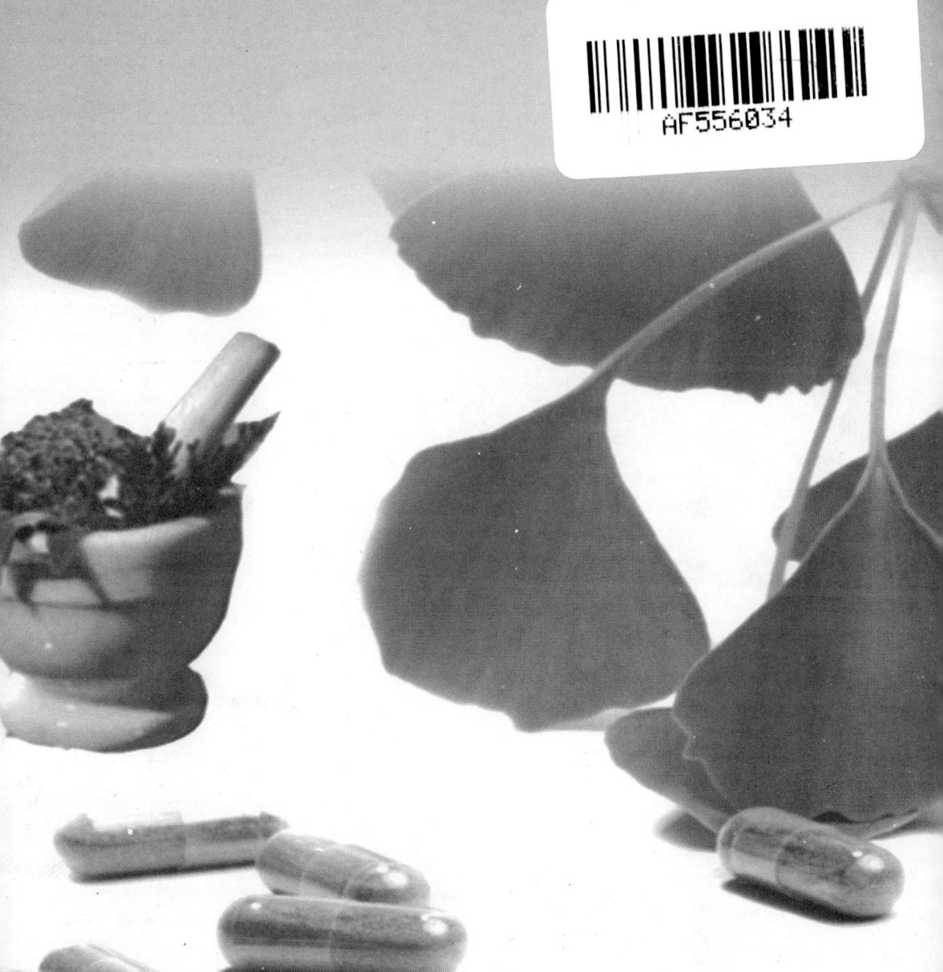

A Textbook of
PHARMACOGNOSY

N. KUMAR
B.Sc., M.Sc., Ph.D., PGDCA, PGDPM
Bangalore University, Karnataka

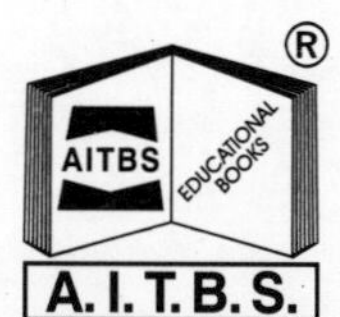

AITBS PUBLISHERS, INDIA
MEDICAL PUBLISHERS
J-5/6, Krishan Nagar, Delhi-110051 (INDIA)
Phone: 011-40167052, 49067602; Fax: 011-22009074
E-mail: aitbsindia@gmail.com & aitbsindia@hotmail.com

First Edition : 2010
Second Edition : 2015
Third Edition : 2024

ISBN: 978-93-7473-456-8

Published by:
Virender Kumar Arya for
AITBS Publishers, India
MEDICAL PUBLISHERS
J-5/6, Krishan Nagar, Delhi - 110051 (INDIA)
Phone: 011-40167052, 49067602; Fax: 011-22009074
E-mail: aitbsindia@gmail.com & aitbsindia@hotmail.com

Printed by AITBS, Delhi

PREFACE

Pharmacognosy is the study of drugs of natural origin obtained from our living environment. This includes: plants, animals, insects and microbes of both terrestrial and marine origin. Some medicinal products are also derived from mineral sources. The study of drugs from plants includes the subjects of botany, chemistry and pharmacology.

The American Society of Pharmacognosy defines pharmacognosy as "the study of the physical, chemical, biochemical, and biological properties of drugs, drug substances or potential drugs or drug substances of natural origin as well as the search for new drugs from natural sources".

"Pharmacognosy" is designed to help students develop a solid, basic understanding of basic concepts in Pharmacognosy without an encyclopedic presentation of detail. It is not possible to include all that is known into a book of this type. However, it is important that a textbook provide enough information to allow students to understand basic concepts and to make reasonable predictions and analyses. We have taken great care to select critically important information and present it in a way that maximizes understanding.

I extend my sincere and whole-heartly thanks to *Virender Kumar Arya,* the publisher of A.I.T.B.S. Publishers, India for his motivating guidance and cheerful co-operation of his staff members during preparation of this book.

—Author

Contents

■■■

CHAPTER 1

INTRODUCTION TO PHARMACOGNOSY

INTRODUCTION

Pharmacognosy is the scientific study of structural, physical, chemical and sensory characters of drugs from animal, vegetable and mineral sources. It has becomes an important interface among various branches of pharmaceutical sciences. It is now emerging as interdisciplinary science that incorporates inputs from chemistry, biology and biotechnology directed towards natural products based drug discovery. Undoubtedly plants have many molecules which have yet to be discovered. This has open many research opportunities to pharmacognosists ranging from characterizing biologically active principles, designing suitable analytical methods for quality control and standardization, activity based screening and drug development.

Thus to participate effectively in natural product drug discovery a pharmacognosist should have complete understanding of various disciplines including botany, organic and analytical chemistry, regulatory control, fundamentals of pharmacology, biochemistry, genetics, horticulture and commerce. Pharmaco-gnosist should be multifaceted to adopt rapidly changing scenario. To work more on herbal medicines one should not underestimate the subject.

MEANING OF PHARMACOGNOSY

The word Pharmacognosy is derived from two Greek words, 'Pharmakon' meaning 'drug' and 'gnosis' meaning 'knowledge'. Therefore, Pharmacognosy literally means knowledge of drugs. Pharmacognosy is one of the important branches of pharmacy. It deals with "the study of structural, physical, chemical and sensory characters of crude drugs of animal, vegetable and mineral origin and includes their history, cultivation, collection, storage and use." From a non-professional's point of view, Pharmacognosy is nothing but medicinal botany.

Though the term Pharmacognosy is a modern one, the knowledge of medicinal plants and their uses are as old as humankind is. It has developed from ancient civilizations, where plants or plants parts have been used to cure human diseases/ disorders. The healing power of certain herbs and plant parts such as leaves, barks, roots etc. were undoubtedly discovered by accident, but once discovered, knowledge of drugs was passed on from generation to generation.

Now-a-days, people are increasingly turning to indigenous systems of medicine, which are holistic and not only treat diseases but also prevent them. Further, they are free from side effects. With the rising popularity of traditional systems of medicine, there is a growing demand for professionals in this field. In order to become a medical practitioner in Indian system of medicine, a formal education is mandatory.

DEFINITION OF MATERIA MEDICA OR PHARMACOGNOSY

Materia Medica or Pharmacognosy, for the terms as used by pharmacists are synonymous, may be defined as that science which aims at a complete and systematic knowledge of crude drugs of animal or vegetable origin. The term drugs may be understood to include all parts of animals or vegetables used in medicine, or such of their products as have not undergone any material elaboration or separation into their constituents; it is, however, not susceptible of exact limitation, and hence substances may be included which are of dietetic or technical rather than medicinal use.

A complete knowledge of a drug must include a knowledge of the morphological nature and the structure, both macroscopic and microscopic, of such as are organised, of the botanical or zoological source, of the constituents both active and inactive, their nature, the amounts in which they are present, and the relation they bear to the constituents of other drugs. The geographical source, the cultivation, mode of collection, preparation for the market, the trade route, commercial varieties, history, uses, etc., must also be known. To attain this knowledge the aid of chemistry and of chemical methods of investigation, of botany and botanical methods, of physiology, geography, commerce, history, etc., must be sought, or at least the results of other investigators in these respects utilised, and the information thus obtained combined to form a complete knowledge of each drug, and these systematised to build up the science of pharmacognosy.

Pharmacognosy may be subdivided into *Scientific Pharmacognosy* and *Applied Pharmacognosy*. Applied Pharmacognosy is the application of scientific pharmacognosy to the solution of the pharmacognostical problems that are constantly arising in the daily work of the pharmacist. Thus, Scientific Pharmacognosy includes an intimate knowledge of the structure of vegetable drugs; Applied Pharmacognosy utilises this knowledge to identify the drug entire or in powder to determine its purity. Scientific Pharmacognosy treats of the constituents of drugs. Applied pharmacognosy ascertains the relative quality of a drug by determining the proportion in which one or more of these constituents is present.

HISTORY OF PHARMACOGNOSY

Although it is only within very recent years that pharmacognosy has substantiated its claim to rank as a science, the collection of herbs for medicinal use is of the remotest antiquity. Ancient Egyptian papyri, of which that of Ebers written about 1600 B.C. is the most important and most complete, prove that even at this early period the physicians were in possession of a very considerable number of drugs, including aloes, acacia gum, myrrh, Indian hemp, hemlock, opium, frankincense, cassia, cummin, coriander, castor seed, and many others. But as far as Western nations are concerned, Greece may be regarded as the cradle of medicine. About the middle of the twelfth century before the Christian era temples were built which served as centres for the exercise of the healing art. Most famous among these were the temples of the *deified Æsculapius* at Epidaurus, Cos, Trika, and Pergamos. At these temples, which were usually situated on high ground in pure air, cures were effected chiefly by hygienic means such as massage, baths, etc. Pythagoras (580 B.C.) added to this hygienic treatment the use of such drugs as squill and mustard. Hippocrates (466 B.C.), who placed the treatment of disease on a more rational basis, was familiar with numerous indigenous as well as exotic drugs, with many of which he doubtless became acquainted during his travels. Wormwood, acacia gum, chamomile, cinnamon, hemlock, gentian, henbane, myrrh, rhubarb, and many others were well known to him.

Theophrastus (about 370 B.C.) was a pupil of Aristotle, after whose death he became chief of the Aristotelian school. He enumerates some 500 plants which were known to him, distinguished cinnamon from cassia, and was acquainted with ergot. It was during this period (335-325 B.C.) that Alexander the Great undertook his expeditions to Persia, India, and Africa, as the result of which numerous treasures, and among them drugs, were brought back to Greece.

Alexander founded Alexandria, which he intended to become the seat of the learning and commerce of the world.

Although science in Egypt had fallen so low that the Greeks learnt but little from the Egyptians, the Alexandrian school was invaluable in preserving and transmitting to posterity the writings of Greek and other authors.

After the death of Alexander the Roman Empire rose. During this period Dioscorides, who was a Greek by birth, travelled in Egypt, Africa, Spain, Italy, and Syria, where he became acquainted with a great variety of plants and drugs. His observations and knowledge he placed on record in a compendious work on pharmacognosy which served for many centuries as an inexhaustible source of information. This remarkable work contains classified descriptions of a great number of vegetable, animal, and mineral drugs, no fewer than 500 medicinal plants, including many exotic ones, being discussed. To Dioscorides belongs the credit of being the first to separate pharmacognosy from medicine.

Pliny, who lived about the same time as Dioscorides and evidently made use to some extent of the same sources of information, studied natural history; his work on this subject consisted of forty-seven books, many of which have been unfortunately lost, Pliny himself perishing in the eruption of Vesuvius (A.D. 79). His 'Natural History,' in addition to books dealing with zoology, meteorology, astrology, etc., treats of as many as 1,000 plants.

Galen (A.D. 131 to 200) was a physician and studied chiefly the production of various 'galenical' preparations, dealing only incidentally with drugs. He recognised the adulteration of cinnamon, pepper, saffron, and myrrh, and points out that exhausted rhubarb was sold in place of the genuine. He wrote twenty books containing a large number of receipts for various preparations.

With the subsequent decline of the Roman Empire, a long period of scientific inactivity, or perhaps rather retrogression, took place. The Arabian Empire then rose, and seats of learning were established and encouraged at Bagdad, Cordova, Toledo, etc. The Arabians acted chiefly as the transmitters of Greek and Roman knowledge, adding comparatively little of their own. The most important of their writers were Geber, Rhazes, Avicenna, and Ibn Baitar.

Geber (A.D. 850), who studied at Cordova, wrote chiefly concerning salts of which a considerable number were known to him.

Rhazes (A.D. 875) studied medicine in Bagdad, and with him a period of independent investigation began. He was acquainted with asafetida, aloes, dandelion, henbane, stavesacre, and numerous other drugs; he prepared extracts by evaporating infusions and made them into pills, which he coated with psyllium mucilage in order to render them less unpleasant to take.

Avicenna (A.D. 980) was perhaps the most gifted of the Arabian physicians and a very prolific writer. His 'Canon Medicinae' served as the chief source of medical knowledge down to the fifteenth century.

Ibn Baitar (A.D. 1197-1248) devoted himself chiefly to botanical work in which he excelled, his 'Corpus Simplicium Medica-mentorum,' containing descriptions of about 2,000 drugs, of which 1,700 were of vegetable origin.

The Arabian school was followed by that of Salerno, near Naples, where a School of Medicine, established in the twelfth century or possibly earlier, was instrumental in continuing scientific work until the dawn of science in Europe in the fifteenth century. During this period the knowledge at least of indigenous medicinal plants was kept alive and added to in the gardens attached to the convents and monasteries of Central Europe.

The beginning of the sixteenth century witnessed a revival in the study of drugs, which was stimulated by the discovery of America, of the West Indies, and of the sea route to India. Matthiolus (1501-1577), who studied in Italy, published a commentary on Dioscorides, which enjoyed a great reputation;

he also collected and dried plants for pharmacognostical purposes and prepared careful illustrations. Monardes (1493-1578) collected drugs and other products brought from America, forming thus what was probably the first museum of materia medica. Clusius (1526-1609) also collected drugs from drug merchants and examined them; his 'Rarium Plantarum Historia' (1601) contains no fewer than 1,146 illustrations, many of which are of great excellence.

After the lapse of a considerable time, during which little of note was published, Pomet wrote his excellent and well-illustrated 'Histoire Generale des Drogues' (Paris, 1694), which was closely followed by Lemery's 'Traite Universel des Drogues Simples' (Paris, 1697) and 'Dictionnaire des Drogues Simples' (4th ed., Paris, 1727), and later by Geoffroy's 'Tractatus de Materia Medica' (Paris, 1741).

The period of modern pharmacognosy may be said to open with Guibourt's admirable 'Histoire Abregee des Drogues Simples' (Paris, 1820), of which several editions were published. Guibourt relied largely on his own observations, and treated the subject from a purely pharmacognostical point of view. This was not the case with Pereira, whose classical 'Elements of Materia Medica and Therapeutics' (London, 1839) embraced, as its title indicates, both pharmacognosy and therapeutics. Schleiden was the first to employ the microscope to distinguish drugs by differences in their structure, a departure which was rapidly advanced by Berg and Schmidt ('Anatomischer Atlas,' Berlin, 1865), Vogl, and Moeller. Hanbury studied chiefly the botany and commerce of drugs, while Fluckiger devoted himself chiefly to the chemistry and history, the collaboration of these two celebrated pharmacognosists resulting in the publication of the classical 'Pharmacographia' (London, 1874). Meyer ('Wissen-schaftliche Droguen-Kunde,' Berlin, 1891) followed the morphological development of drugs, Tschirch ('Anato-mischer Atlas,' Leipzig, 1900) their structural development, and E.M. Holmes their botanical origin.

By these and other workers a mass of material has been accumulated, the systematical arrangement of which has been attempted by Tschirch in his 'Handbuch der Pharmakognosie.'

COMMERCE

The oldest records of commercial intercourse between different peoples indicate that several thousand years before the Christian era a considerable trade existed in ancient Bactria, the modern Bokhara. At a very early period the Bactrians had undoubtedly made considerable progress in civilisation. The country was extremely fertile, and its position rendered it a convenient centre for the caravans that brought the spices and other products of India and China to Persia and Egypt. From Attock, near Peshawar, in the extreme North-West of India, caravan tracks led through Kabul to Bactria, and from China a northerly track had the same objective. From Attock similar routes passed through Assyria to the Black Sea, through Syria to the Mediterranean, and through Palestine to Egypt. During this period commerce was carried on almost entirely by caravans, the courses of the various routes being determined partly by the physical nature of the country to be traversed and partly by the presence of populous cities at which intermediate markets might be found; thus the routes from Bactria to Syria passed through Herat, Ecbatana, Nineveh, Babylon, and Palmyra.

During the rise of the Babylonian Empire (2000-1000 B.C.), at the time therefore at which the papyrus of Ebers was written, a considerable commerce existed between India, China, Syria (and the countries bordering on and even beyond the Mediterranean), and Egypt. In this commerce Arabia, favoured by its situation, took a very considerable part. Boats and rafts were used for descending the rivers, beasts of burden carrying the exchange back. Coasting vessels navigated the Persian Gulf, the Bed Sea, and the coasts of Arabia and India. Probably it was by one of these routes that cassia and other spices travelled from China to Egypt, and frankincense from Somaliland.

Towards the end of this period (Babylonian Empire) the Phoenicians developed their maritime commerce in the Mediterranean. Established at Tylos and Arados on the Bahrein Islands (near the western shore of the Persian Gulf) and navigating the Red Sea, the Persian Gulf, and the Indian Ocean, they practically controlled the trade between the East and the West, the outlets of the latter being their ports of Tyre and Sidon. Much of the extensive materia medica of the Greeks reached them through the Phoenicians, such as, for instance, gum acacia, cinnamon, cassia, indigo, etc. Rhubarb, on the other hand, probably travelled by caravan from Western China, passing South of the Caspian Sea to the Black Sea and the Bosphorus.

During the Persian Empire (600-400 B.C.) the caravan routes were carefully tended and repaired, and every effort made to divert the traffic through Persian territory. About this time Greece had risen to be an important country and carried on an extensive maritime commerce with the Black Sea countries, with Chios, Lesbos, and other islands of the Grecian Archipelago as well as with Egypt. The conquests of Alexander the Great gave a great impulse to this trade, as they brought the East into contact with the West. The foundation of Alexandria was destined to produce far-reaching results. Its situation made it the natural emporium for this commerce, and it rapidly drained the life-blood from Tyre and Sidon.

Shortly after the death of Alexander, Greece declined in importance, and the Romans, having overthrown the Carthaginians, who had succeeded the Phoenicians as the chief traders of the Western Mediterranean, rapidly extended their influence, which reached its zenith during the first two centuries of the Christian era. Rome became the centre of the world. The enormous wealth accumulated there attracted foreign merchants, who employed it as a central market for the distribution of the products from India, China, and other countries.

A trade had now sprung up between the seaports of Arabia and of the Persian Gulf with Ceylon(Sri Lanka), the Malay Archipelago, China, and Japan. Drugs and spices were landed in Arabia, and found their way thence by caravan to Alexandria, those reaching the Persian Gulf being conveyed by similar means to Syria. From Northern China the old caravan route passing South of the Caspian Sea and through Persia and Syria was still followed.

As Rome fell the Byzantine Empire rose. Byzantium, rebuilt by Constantine A.D. 330 and renamed after himself, occupied a most favoured site. When Alexandria fell to the Arabs (A.D. 640) the Alexandrian route was closed owing to the unwillingness of the Arabs to deal with Christians. The Indian trade was consequently diverted to the caravan routes to Greek colonies on the Black Sea, and thence to Constantinople. Drugs and spices from India and the East were then distributed from Constantinople, either by sea to the Mediterranean or by land to Germany.

Wars with the Mohammedans led, however, to the decline of Byzantine commerce. The Arabs established colonies on the African coast and obtained control of the Mediterranean coast traffic. Their empire rapidly spread from the Indus to the Pyrenees. The caravan routes were revived. At first Damascus and subsequently Bagdad became the centre of this trade and amassed enormous wealth. Their merchants penetrated to Nigeria, Medagascar, Siberia, India, and China. Canton was connected with the West by a caravan route which in northern Tibet divided into three branches, the most northern reaching the Black Sea, the middle Bagdad, and the most southern Daybal at the mouth of the Indus. Daybal was also the centre of the sea-trade from India, Ceylon, the East Indies, China, and Japan, to Bussorah and Bagdad, to Aden, Cairo, and Alexandria. Cairo received caravans from all parts of Africa bringing both African and Asiatic goods, and it soon rivalled Bagdad in magnificence. Centres of learning were simultaneously established in Bagdad, Cordova, Toledo, etc.

The Arabs became enervated and were gradually driven out of Europe during the fifteenth century. Towards the end of this period the carrying and distributing trade passed into the hands of the Italians. The Pisanese wrested Sardinia, Corsica, and the Balearic Islands from the Arabs, and, assisted by the Crusades, secured for Pisa a lucrative trade, which passed to Genoa and finally to Venice, the latter becoming the chief carrier of the world. She reopened the sea-trade of the Red Sea and Alexandria, which was safer and cheaper than the caravan routes; she received and distributed all the drugs and spices of the East, and thus acquired great power and great wealth, the zenith of her prosperity being reached towards the end of the fifteenth century.

About this time, however, Henry the Navigator, son of King John I of Portugal, eager to annex the Indian trade, and convinced by information obtained from the Arabs of the possibility of reaching India by sea, explored the west coast of Africa, discovering Madeira and establishing colonies on the mainland. The way was thus paved for Vasco da Gama, who in 1498 discovered the sea route to India, and landed on the Malabar Coast. The Portuguese established ports on the coasts of India, Goa being the chief, colonised Mozambique, the Spice Islands (1511), Ceylon (1518), Java, Sumatra, and Celebes. About the same time Spain became a colonial power. In 1492 Columbus discovered San Salvador, and on his subsequent voyage the West Indies. In 1519-1521, Mexico was conquered by Cortes, and immediately afterwards (1529-1535) Peru and Chili by Pizarro. The cities of Vera Cruz, Cartagena, and Caracas on the east, and of Acapulco, Panama, and Lima on the west, were founded.

The rich commerce of India was now soon diverted to Portugal, and Lisbon succeeded Venice as the emporium for Europe, a position which it occupied for nearly a century. To Lisbon or to Portuguese merchants in Antwerp the Dutch and English repaired to obtain their supplies of spices. Antwerp became the emporium of the north. When, however, in 1580 Philip II of Spain united Portugal with Spain, and soon afterwards declared war against England, he closed the ports of his empire to English merchants. This act was followed by the revolt of the Netherlands from Spanish dominion, and both the Dutch and the English found themselves compelled to engage in a direct trade with India.

They thus became rivals of the Portuguese and of one another. The Dutch were at first the more successful. They established themselves in India, in the East Indian Islands, the Moluccas and the Sunda Islands; they drove the Portuguese out, and took possession of the entire trade with India, the East Indies, Japan, and China. They also established colonies in the Cape, and in 1658 took Ceylon from the Portuguese. Several of the West Indian Islands, and part of the North-East of South America, fell into their hands. The commerce of all these colonies and countries flowed into Amsterdam, which thus supplanted Antwerp and Lisbon as the European emporium of Indian trade.

Meanwhile the English, who had met with less success, had nevertheless founded colonies in Calicut, Madras, Masulipatam, Calcutta, and Bencoolen, and had driven the Spaniards from Jamaica, Barbados, and other of the West Indian Islands. In 1600 the first English East Indian Company was formed which built forts in Java, Amboyna, and Banda. At first this company shared the spice trade, but eventually it was driven from the islands by the Dutch, who destroyed all spice trees but those on the island of Amboyna. The English were thus restricted to the coasts of India, where they competed successfully with the Portuguese. After the cessation of the Company's charter in 1833 trade rapidly increased. Cotton, sugar, tobacco, tea, coffee, and cinchona were introduced. Singapore, which had become a British possession in 1819, became, and still remains, the centre of East Indian trade. North America had already been colonised; here and in the West Indian Islands tobacco, all spice, cocoa, indigo, etc., had been introduced, and their cultivation had rapidly extended.

Drug Routes

Foreign drugs reach the London market chiefly by the following routes:

(1) **Central European.** From Reval and Riga (Russian); from Hamburg and Bremen (German); from Amsterdam and Rotterdam (Dutch and German); from Antwerp (Belgian and Dutch); from Dieppe, Boulogne, Havre, and Bordeaux (French); in all cases direct to London.

(2) **Mediterranean.** From Lisbon (Portuguese); from Vigo, Seville, Malaga, Valencia, and Barcelona (Spanish); from Marseilles (French); from Genoa, Leghorn, and Bari (Italian); from Messina, Palermo, and Catania (Sicilian); from Malta; from Salonica, Constantinople, Smyrna, Alexandretta, Jaffa, Beyrout (Turkish); from Suez, Tripoli, Tangiers, Algiers (African); either direct to London or often (from the Eastern Mediterranean) via Trieste or via Marseilles.

(3) **North-West African.** From Rabat, Mazagan, Saffi, Mogadore, Bathurst to London, Liverpool, or Southampton.

(4) **West-Central African.** From Sierra Leone, Bonny, Lagos, San Thome, and Benguela to Liverpool.

(5) **South African.** From Cape Town, Mossel Bay, Port Elizabeth, East London, Natal, and Delagoa Bay to Southampton and Liverpool.

(6) **East-Central African.** From Beira, Chinde, Quilimane, Mozambique, Zanzibar, Mombasa to London (often via Hamburg); from Mauritius, Reunion, Madagascar, and Seychelles to Liverpool.

(7) **Red Sea, Arabian, and Persian.** From Suakin, Massowah, Aden, Bunder-Abbas, Bushire, Bussorah, and Bagdad to London.

(8) **Indian.** From Karachi, Bombay, Mangalore, Calicut, Cochin, Aleppy, Colombo, Tuticorin, Madras, Calcutta, and Rangoon to London.

(9) **Malayan.** From the various islands via Singapore and Penang to London; from Batavia via Amsterdam to London; from Saigon via Marseilles to London.

(10) **Chinese.** From Shanghai and Hong Kong, often via Havre or Hamburg, to London.

(11) **Japanese.** From Nagasaki, Kobe, and Yokohama to London.

(12) **North American.** From Quebec, Montreal, Boston, New York, Baltimore, Newport, New Orleans, and San Francisco to Liverpool, London, and Southampton, sometimes via Havre and Cherbourg.

(13) **Central American.** From Greytown and Belize to Liverpool and London, sometimes via Hamburg.

(14) **West Indian.** From, the British islands to Liverpool Bristol, and Southampton; from the Dutch islands to London via Amsterdam.

(15) **South American.** From La Guayra, Savanilla, Cartagena, and Maranham to Liverpool; from Pernambuco, Bahia, Rio Janeiro, and Buenos Ayres to London and Liverpool; from Montevideo to Southampton; from Valparaiso, Santiago, Mollendo, Truxillo, and Guayaquil to Liverpool.

(16) **Australian.** From Brisbane, Sydney, Melbourne, Adelaide, and Perth to London; from Tasmania via Melbourne.

(17) **New Zealand.** From Auckland and Wellington to London.

SCOPE OF PHARMACOGNOSY

Pharmacognosy is one of the five major divisions of the pharmaceutical curriculum, represents the oldest branch of the profession of pharmacy. The ancients gathered herbs, animals, plants, and minerals and concocted them into ill-flavoured pungent mixtures. Innumerable remedies were known to the early practitioners of pharmacy and medicine, a fact indicated by the writings of Theophrastus, Pliny, Dioscorides, and their contemporaries. Thousands of plant and animal products used for the treatment of ills were described by Dioscorides in his book "Dc Materia Medica." Of these a surprisingly large number are still of importance in modern therapeutic practice: Aspidium, Cinnamon, Ergot, Ilyoscyamus, and Opium were used in much the same manner as today.

MATERIA MEDICA MEANING MEDICINAL MATERIALS

From this humble beginning medicine and pharmacy gradually emerged along separate paths: the physician diagnosing the ailment and prescribing the remedy and the apothecary or pharmacist specializing in the collection, preparation, and compounding of the substance. Thus, the term materia medica (meaning medicinal materials) was synonymous with the substances and products derived from natural sources and employed by the physicians of that era.

It was not until 1815 that the term Pharmacognosy was introduced by *Seydler*. This name is formed from two Greek words, pharmakon: drug, and gnosis: knowledge and literally means the "entire knowledge of drugs." The most comprehensive idea of the scope of pharmacognosy was presented by Fluckiger, who stated that it "is the simultaneous application of various scientific disciplines with the object of acquiring knowledge of drugs from every point of view."

PHARMACOGNOSY EMBRACES A KNOWLEDGE OF HISTORY

In a broad sense, pharmacognosy embraces a knowledge of the history, distribution, cultivation, collection, selection, preparation, commerce, identification, evaluation, preservation, and use of drugs and economic substances affecting the health of man and other animals. Such economic substances extend beyond the category of crude drugs and their derivatives and include a variety of commercial products: allergens, allergenic extracts, antibiotics, immunizing biologicals, flavouring agents, condiments, beverages, insecticides, rodenticides, and herbicides. In a restricted sense, the definition of pharmacognosy implies a particular knowledge of methods of identification and evaluation of drugs.

As a part of the pharmaceutical curriculum pharmacognosy plays an important role as liaison agent between pharmacology and pharmaceutical chemistry on one hand and between pharmacy and pharmacy administration on the other. Pharmacology, like pharmacognosy, is an outgrowth of the old-time materia medica; it is easy to see the correlation of these two sciences concerning drugs of biological origin. The pharmacology student has a more complete understanding of the action of belladonna leaf if he is aware of the physical nature of the drug and its chemical constituents. Some of the laboratory procedures in pharmaceutical chemistry have miniature counterparts in the extractions and microchemical tests essential for the identification and evaluation of certain drugs.

Methods of collection, curing, drying, and assaying affect the price of drugs and, insofar as economics are concerned, pharmacognosy is intimately associated with phases of pharmacy administration dealing with prescription pricing. The relationship of pharmacognosy to operative pharmacy and dispensing pharmacy is obvious when one considers the number of plant and animal products handled by the pharmacist in this synthetic age. Because of his knowledge of drug constituents and their physical and chemical properties, the pharmacist is able to predict incompatibilities in actual compounding. In dispensing non-compounded prescription specialties, he is conversant with a vast store of information permitting him to confer intelligently with his fellow colleagues in the medical, dental, and nursing professions.

SYSTEMS OF MEDICINE IN INDIA

The systems of medicine practised in India are: (1) Ayurveda, (2) Unanai and (3) Siddha. These systems are described below:

(1) AYURVEDA

History

"Ayurveda" literally means "the science of life". It is the oldest and most holistic medical system available on the planet today. It was placed in written form over 5,000 years ago in India, it was said to be a world medicine dealing with both body and the spirit. Before the advent of writing, the ancient wisdom of this healing system was a part of the spiritual tradition of the *Sanatana Dharma* (Universal Religion), or Vedic Religion.

VedaVyasa, the famous sage, shaktavesha avatar of Vishnu, put into writing the complete knowledge of Ayurveda, along with the more directly spiritual insights of self-realization into a body of scriptural literature called the Vedas and the Vedic literatures.

There were originally four main books of spirituality, which included among other topics, health, astrology, spiritual business, government, army, poetry and spiritual living and behaviour. These books are known as the four Vedas—*Rik, Sama, Yajur* and *Atharva*. The Rik Veda, a compilation of verse on the nature of existence, is the oldest surviving book of any Indo-European language (3000 B.C.). The Rik Veda (also known as *Rig Veda*) refers to the cosmology known as Sankhya which lies at the base of both Ayurveda and Yoga, contains verses on the nature of health and disease, pathogenesis and principles of treatment. Among the Rik Veda are found discussions of the three doshas—*Vayu or Vata, Pitta* and *Kapha,* and the use of herbs to heal the diseases of the mind and body and to foster longevity.

The Atharva Veda lists the *eight* divisions of Ayurveda—Internal Medicine, Surgery of Head and Neck, Opthamology and Otorinolaryngology, Surgery, Toxicology, Psychiatry, Pediatrics, Gerontology or Science of Rejuvenation, and the Science of Fertility.

The Vedic Sages took the passages from the Vedic Scriptures relating to Ayurveda and compiled separate books dealing only with Ayurveda. One of these books, called the *Atreya Samhita* is the oldest medical book in the world! The Vedic Brahmanas were not only priests performing religious rites and ceremonies, they also became Vaidyas (Physicians of Ayurveda).

The sage-physician-surgeons of the time were the same sages or seers, deeply devoted holy people, who saw health as an integral part of spiritual life. It is said that they received their training of Ayurveda through direct cognition during meditation.

In other words, the knowledge of the use of various methods of healing, prevention, longevity and surgery came through

Divine revelation; there was no guessing or testing and harming animals. These revelations were transcribed from the oral tradition into book form, interspersed with the other aspects of life and spirituality. What is fascinating is Ayurveda's use of herbs, foods, aromas, gems, colors, yoga, mantras, lifestyle and surgery. Consequently Ayurveda grew into a respected and widely used system of healing in India.

Around 1500 B.C., various authors took ayurvedic passages from the four scriptures and created ayurvedic texts for at least eight specific branches of medicine, divided into two main schools — *Atreya*, or physicians, and *Dhanvantari*, or surgeons. Through experimentation and research, these two schools transformed ayurveda from a primarily religious discipline to a scientific medical system.

Scholars from China, Tibet, Egypt, Persia, Greece and Rome flocked to India's Ayurvedic schools to learn about this holistic medicine.

Over 1,200 years ago, masters of the two schools assembled their knowledge into essential texts. Charak, a doctor of the Atreya school, compiled information on diagnosis and prevention of disease, internal and external causes of illness, herbal prescriptions and anatomy. He stated that all disease — *physical, mental* and *spiritual* — is fundamentally caused by a separation from Divine Oneness. He also gave strikingly detailed descriptions of human fetal development month-by-month.

Sushrut, from the Dhanvantari school, classified functions of organs, nerves and joints, catalogued various kinds of wounds and described sophisticated surgical equipment used in technical procedures like amputation and plastic surgery. His text also includes the first mention of the science of massage using MARMA points, vital nerve intersections like those used in Chinese acupuncture.

After the flowering of ayurvedic knowledge came hard times. First, schools began splitting over technical interpretations. In the 1600s, the British East India Company took control over the subcontinent. By 1833, it had sufficient authority to ban all ayurvedic colleges and opened the first Western-style medical university. Ayurvedic medicine survived only in rural areas where local doctors treated those who could not afford Western medicine.

Only in 1920 did the discipline of ayurveda begin to regain its former respect. When India established independence in 1947, ayurvedic medical schools were once more officially accepted and allowed to open.

Today, well over 100 ayurvedic colleges in India grant degrees after a five-year program. More than 300,000 ayurvedic physicians belong to the All-India Ayurveda Congress, making it the largest medical organization in the world.

Branches of Ayurveda

Ayurveda has eight specialized branches, namely internal medicine including gynaecology, surgery, the treatment of diseases of the head and neck, toxicology, paediatrics, psychiatry and rejuvenation therapy.

In India, Ayurvedic spas can be found all over the country. The most famous Ayurveda Shalas are found in Kerala.

Kerala's equable climate, natural abundance of forests (with a wealth of herbs and medicinal plants), and the cool monsoon season (June-November) are best suited for Ayurveda's curative and restorative packages. Kerala is the only State in India, which practises this system of medicine with absolute dedication.

Today, it's a unique, indispensable branch of medicine — a complete naturalistic system that depends on the diagnosis of your body's *vata, pitta* and *kapha* — to achieve the right balance. Ayurveda believes in the treatment of not just the affected part, but also the individual as a whole. Making it the natural way to refresh yourself, eliminate all toxic imbalances from the body and thus regain resistance and good health.

Benefits of Ayurveda

When alternative lifestyles and stressful schedules are talking points in the cosmopolitan circuits, Ayurveda, the art of ancient

Indian healing cannot be far behind. The inability of modern allopathy to allay all sicknesses and diseases has made an increasing number of people turn to Ayurveda, which has a cornucopia of ancient secret cures for stubborn diseases. Along with yoga, Ayurveda is the new balm for fevered souls. It uses natural herbs and their oils to treat ailments and ensure a healthy life. Most of the centres for Ayurveda, called Ayurveda Shalas, are in Kerala on the South Coast. This is beach country as well, so bring along your sunscreens and hats. In fact many westerners have made Ayurvedic spas their annual treat, combining a relaxing holiday with cleansing for their bodies.

Ayurvedic Manufacture Control

The manufacture of Ayurvedic medicines is being regulated by the Government of India through the Drugs and Cosmetics Act 1940.

(2) UNANI

Origin and Development

The Unani system of medicine owes, as its name suggests, its origin to Greece. It was the Greek Philosopher-physician Hippocrates (460-377 B.C.) who freed Medicine from the realm of superstition and magic, and gave it the status of Science. The theoretical framework of Unani Medicine is based on the teachings of Hippocrates. After Hippocrates a number of other Greek scholars enriched the system considerably.

Of them Galen (131-210 A.D.) stands out as the one who stabilised its foundation, on which Arab physicians like Rhazes (850-925 A.D.) and Avicenna (980-1037 A.D.) constructed an imposing edifice. Unani medicine got enriched by imbibing what was best in the contemporary system of traditional medicine in Egypt, Syria, Iraq, Persia, India, China and other Middle East and Far East countries.

In India, the Unani system of medicine was introduced by the Arabs. Soon it took firm roots in the soil. The Delhi Sultans, the Khiljis, the Tughlaqus and the Mughal Emperors provided state patronage to the scholars and even enrolled some as state employees and court physicians. The system found immediate favour with the masses and soon spread all over the country.

During the British rule, Unani Medicine suffered a setback and its development was hampered due to withdrawal of governmental patronage. But since the system enjoyed faith among the masses it continued to be practised. An outstanding physician and scholar of Unani Medicine, Hakim Ajmal Khan (1868-1927) championed the cause of the Unani system in India.

The development of Unani Medicine as well as other Indian systems of Medicine gained considerable momentum after independence. Even prior to independence a Health Survey and Development Committee was appointed in the Year 1943. The Committee underscored the future role to be played by the indigenous systems of medicine of India.

At present the Unani system of medicine, with its own recognized practitioners, hospitals and educational and research institutions, forms an integral part of the national health care delivery systems and is the world leader.

Fundamentals

Unani Medicine, is based on the principles put forward by Hippocrates. He was the first person to establish that disease was a natural process, that its symptoms were the reactions of the body to the disease, and that the chief function of the physician was to aid the natural forces of the body. He was the first physician to introduce the method of taking medical histories. His chief contribution to the medical realm is the humoral theory.

The Humors

The humoral theory presupposes the presence of four humors — Dam (blood), Balgham (phlegm), Safra (yellow bile) and Sauda (Black bile) — in the body. The temperaments of persons are expressed by the words sanguine, phlegmatic, choleric and melancholic according to the preponderance in them of humors — blood, phlegm, yellow bile and black bile, respectively. The humors themselves are assigned temperaments — blood is hot and moist, phlegm cold and moist, yellow bile hot and dry, and black bile cold and dry. Every person is supposed to have a unique humoral constitution which represents his healthy state. To maintain the correct humoral balance there is a power of self-preservation or adjustment called quwwat-e-Mudabbira (medicatrix naturae) in the body. If this power weakens, imbalance in the humoral composition is bound to occur which causes disease. In Unani Medicine, great reliance is placed on this power. The medicines used in this system, in fact, help the body to regain this power to an optimum level and thereby restore humoral balance, thus restoring health. Also, correct diet and digestion are considered necessary to maintain humoral balance.

Distinctive Characteristics

1. Existence of Pneumas;
2. Holistic Approach;
3. Herbal Treatment;
4. Psychological Dimensions; and
5. Qualitative action of weather and seasonal requirement.

Diagnosis

Another distinctive feature of the Unani system of medicine is its emphasis on diagnosing a disease through *"Nabz"* (pulse), a rhythmic expansion of arteries which is felt by fingers. The reading of the pulse permits a rather straightforward assessment of several factors:

(i) Which humor is out of balance?;

(ii) What is the nature of the imbalance; that is, excess of heat or coldness, wetness or dryness?; and

(iii) Which of the primary organs are effected? Other methods of diagnosis include examination of Baul (urine), Baraz (stool), etc.

Prevention of Disease

Unani system of medicine recognizes the influence of surroundings and ecological conditions on the state of health of human beings. The system aims at restoring the equilibrium of various elements and faculties of the human body. It has laid down six essential prerequisites for the prevention of diseases and places great emphasis, on the one hand, on the maintenance of proper ecological balance and, on the other, on keeping water, food and air free from pollution. These essentials, known as 'Asbab-e-Sitta Zarooriya', are air, food and drinks, bodily movement and repose, psychic movement and repose, sleep and wakefulness, and excretion and retention.

Therapeutics

In Unani system of medicine various types of treatment are employed, such as *Ilaj bit-Tadbeer* (regimental therapy), *Ilaj bil-Ghiza* (dietotherapy), *Ilaj bid-Dawa* (pharmacotherapy) and *jarahat* (surgery).

The *regimental therapy* includes venesection, cupping, diaphoresis, diuresis, Turkish bath, massage, cauterization, purgin and emesis, exercise, leeching etc. *Dietotherapy* aims at treating certain ailments by administration of specific diets or by regulating the quantity and quality of food, whereas pharmacotherapy deals with the use of naturally occurring drugs, mostly herbal, though drugs of animal and mineral origin are also used. Similarly, surgery has also been in use in this system for quite long. In fact, the ancient physicians of Unani medicine were pioneers in this field and had developed their own instruments and techniques. In Unani medicine, single drugs or their combinations in raw form are preferred over compound formulations. Further, the materia medica of Unani medicine being vast, the medicines are easy to get for most of them are available locally. The naturally occurring drugs used in this system are symbolic of life and are generally free from side-effects, and such drugs as are toxic in crude form are processed and purified in many ways before use. Some Unani single drugs drawn from nature.

In Unani medicine, although general preference is for single drugs, compound formulations are also used in the treatment of various complex and chronic disorders. The medicines administered go well with the temperament of the patient, thus accelerating the process of recovery and also eliminating the risk of drug reaction.

Difference between Ayurvedic and Unani Medicine

Most of the herbal drugs are common in Ayurvedic and Unani medicine. In the Ayurvedic system, names are in Sanskrit, whereas in Unani system, in Arabic or Persian. In fact both the systems have practically emerged as one integrated system.

(3) SIDDHA

Siddha system is one of the oldest systems of medicine in India. The term 'Siddha' means achievement and the 'Siddhars' were saintly figures who achieved results in medicine through the practice of Yoga. Eighteen 'Siddhars' seem to have contributed towards the development of this medical system. Siddha system's literature is in Tamil and it is practiced in Tamil speaking parts of India. The system is also called Agasthyar system in the name of its famous exponent sage Agasthya. A number of medical works of this system are ascribed to him but it may be difficult at this time to say the exact number that can be credited to him. This system of medicine developed within the Dravidian culture, which is of the pre-vedic period. The Siddha system is largely therapeutic in nature.

The original Home allotted to mankind by the Creator was in the temparate and fertile region of the East and pointedly in India. It is from here that the human race began its culture and career. India may, therefore, be safely stated as that the first country from which human culture and civilization originated and spread. According to Indian history prior to Aryans migration, the Dravidian was the first inhabitant of India of whom the Tamilians were the most prominent. The Tamilians were not only the earliest civilized but also those who may more considerable progress in civilization than any other early people. The languages of India were divided into two great classes, the northern with Sanskrit as the pre-pondering element and the southern with Dravidian language as independent bases. The science of medicine is of fundamental importance to man's well being be and his survival and so it must have originated with man and developed as civilization. It is, therefore rather pointless to try to determine the exact point of time to which the beginning of these systems could be traced. They are eternal, they began with man and may end with him. The Siddha was flouriest in south and Ayurveda prevalent in the north. Instead of giving the name of any of individual as the founder of these systems our ancestors attributed their origin to the creator. According to the tradition it was Shiva who unfolded the knowledge of Siddha system of medicine to his concert Parvati who handed it down to Nandi Deva and he the Siddhars. The Siddhars were great scientists in ancient times.

According to tradition, the origin of Siddha system of medicine is attributed to the great Siddha Ayastiyar. Some of his works are still standard books of medicine and surgery in daily use among the Siddha medical practitioners.

This principles and doctrines of this system, both fundamental and applied, have a close similarity to Ayurveda, with specialization in Iatro-chemistry. According to this system the human body is the replica of the universe and so are the food and drugs irrespective of their origin.

Like Ayurveda, this system believes that all objects in the universe including human body are composed of five basic elements namely, earth, water, fire, air and sky. The food, which the human body takes and the drugs it uses are all, made of these five elements. The proportion of the elements present in the drugs vary and their preponderance or otherwise is responsible for certain actions and therapeutic results.

As in Ayurveda, this system also considers the human body as a conglomeration of three humours, seven basic tissues and the waste products of the body such as faeces, urine and sweat. The food is considered to be basic building material of human body which gets processed into humours, body tissues and waste products. The equilibrium of humours is considered as health and its disturbance or imbalance leads to disease or sickness.

This system also deals with the concept of salvation in life. The exponents of this system consider achievement of this state is possible by medicines and meditation.

Materia Medica in Siddha Medicine System

The system has developed a rich and unique treasure of drug knowledge in which use of metals and minerals is very much advocated. Some idea about the depth of knowledge the system possesses in the field of mineral, materia medica can be formed from the detailed drug classification, briefly described below:

(i) There are 25 varieties of water-soluble inorganic compounds called 'UPPU'. These are different types of alkalies and salts.

(ii) There are 64 varities of mineral drugs that do not dissolve in water but emit, vapours when put in fire. Thirty-two of these are natural and remaining are artificial.

(iii) There are seven drugs that do not dissolve in water but emit vapour on heating.

The system has classified separately classes of metals and alloys, which melt when, heated and solidifies on cooling. These include items like gold, silver, copper, tin, lead and iron. These are incinerated by special processes and used in medicine.

There is a group of drugs that exhibit sublimation on heating and includes mercury and its different forms like red sulphide of mercury, mercuric chloride and red oxide of mercury etc.

Sulphur, which is insoluble in water, finds a crucial place in Siddha materia medica along with mercury for use in therapeutics and in maintenance of health.

The above classification shows detailed knowledge and study of minerals that this system has evolved for treatment. In addition, there are drugs obtained from animal sources. The system has published and handbook on Siddha treatment for common diseases and ailments.

Chemistry in Siddha Medicine System

In Siddha system chemistry had been found well developed into a science auxiliary to medicine and alchemy. It was found useful in the preparation of medicine as well as in transmutation of basic metals into gold. The knowledge of plants and mineral were of very high order and they were fully acquainted with almost all the branches of science. The Siddhars were also aware of several alchemical operations divided into several processes such as – calcinations, sublimation, distillation, fusion, separation conjunction or combination, congelation, cibation, fermentation, exaltation, i.e., the action or process of refining gold, fixation, i.e., bringing to the condition of being non-volatile, i.e., to the state of resisting the action of fire, purification, incineration of metals, liquifaction, extraction and so on.

Even cupellation of gold and silver which is an essential process in Alchemy in which is claimed to have been discovered by the Arabs, was known to the Siddhars long long before.

They were even polypharmacists and as such were engaged in boiling, dissolving, precipitating and coagulating chemical substances. Some of their secret methods, especially those in fixing and consolidating certain volatile substances that could not resist the action of fire, such as Mercury, Sulphur, Orpiment, Vermilion, Arsenic etc. continue still a mystery.

Strength in Siddha Medicine System

The Siddha system is capable of treating all types of disease other than emergency cases. In general this system is effective in treating all types of skin problems particularly Psoriasis, STD, urinary tract infections, diseases of liver and gastro intestinal tract, general debility, postpartum anaemia, diarrhoea and general fevers in addition to arthritis and allergic disorders.

Basic Diagnosis and Treatment in Siddha Medicine System

The diagnosis of disease involves identifying its causes. Identification of causative factors is done through the examination of pulse reading, urine examination, examination of eyes, study of voice, colour of body, examination of the tongue and status of the digestive system of human body. The system has worked out detailed procedure of urine examination, which includes study of its colour, smell, density, quantity and oil drop-spreading pattern. Diagnosis involves the study of person as a whole as well as his disease.

This Siddha system of medicine emphasis's that the medical treatment shall be oriented not merely to disease but has to take into account the patient, his environment, the meteorological consideration, age, sex race, habits, mental frame, habitat, diet, appetite, physical condition, physiological constitution etc. This means the treatment has to be individualized with far less chances of committing mistakes in diagnosis of treatment.

(4) OTHER SYSTEMS

(i) Yoga

Yoga is a system of exercises for physical and mental well being. It combines stylised poses with deep breathing and meditation. The term Yoga is itself derived from a Sanskrit word meaning to join together. The ultimate aim in yoga is to unite the human soul with the universal spirit.

Yoga was developed about five thousand years ago. The first written description was found in 'Yoga Sutras', attributed to Patanjali. According to Patanjali, within the human body there are channels called Nadi and centres called Chakra. If these channels and centres are tapped, energy hidden in the body can be released. This energy is called Kundalini.

Patanjali stated eight stages of Yoga, the Yama (universal moral commandments), Niyama (self-purification through discipline), Asana (posture), Pranayama (breath-control), Pratyahara (withdrawal of mind from external objects), Dharana (concentration), Dhyana (meditation) and Samadhi (state of super-consciousness). Besides the different stages present in Yoga, there are various forms of discipline touching different aspects of human life. These disciplines include Hathayoga (physical exercise), Gyanyoga or Dhyanyoga (exercise for the mind and intellect) and Karmayoga (disciplined actions in daily life).

Benefits of Yoga

This ancient health and fitness practice provides both *physical* and *mental therapy*. It considers ageing as largely an artificial condition, caused mainly by autointoxication or self-poisoning. By keeping the body parts clean and well-lubricated, cell deterioration can be greatly reduced. To get the maximum benefits of yoga one has to follow three main guidelines, i.e., practice of Asanas, Pranayama and Yoga Nidra.

With the regular practice of asanas, we can control our cholesterol level, reduce weight, normalise blood pressure and improve cardiac performance. Asanas harmonize our mental energy flow by clearing any blockages in the subtle body, leading to mental equilibrium and calmness.

The practice of pranayama, the correct breathing technique, helps to manipulate our energies. Most of us breathe incorrectly (only thoracically not using our abdomen, thereby utilizing only half of our lung capacity). Pranayama is a technique wherein it re-educates our breathing process, helps to release tensions and develop a relaxed state of mind. It balances our nervous system, reduces the need for sleep and encourages creative thinking. Increasing oxygen to our brain, improves mental clarity, alertness and physical well-being.

Yoga Nidra is a form of meditation. Performed while lying on the back in the Shavasana pose, it relaxes the physiological and psychological systems. This technique completely rejuvenates the body and mind, giving a sense of well-being.

(ii) Meditation

More and more doctors are prescribing meditation as a way to lower blood pressure, improve exercise performance in people with angina, help asthmatics breathe easier, relieve insomnia and generally ease the everyday stresses of life. Meditation is a safe and simple way to balance a person's physical, emotional and mental states. The concept of meditation works on the principle that when the mind is calm and focused on the present, it is neither reacting to memories from the past nor being preoccupied with plans for the future, two major sources of chronic stress known to impact health.

Several techniques of meditation but they all have one thing in common — focus on quietening the busy mind. The concept is not to remove stimulation but rather to direct concentration to one healing element: one sound, one word, one image, or one's breath.

All forms of meditation can be broadly classified into concentrative meditation and mindful meditation.

Concentrative meditation focuses attention on a breath, an image, or a sound (mantra), in order to still the mind and allow greater awareness and clarity to emerge. The simplest form of concentrative meditation is to sit quietly and focus attention on the breath. Yoga and meditation practitioners believe that there is a direct correlation between one's breath and one's state of the mind. For example, when a person is anxious, frightened, agitated or distracted, the breath will tend to be shallow, rapid and uneven. On the other hand, when the mind is calm, focused and composed, the breath will tend to be slow, deep and regular.

As one focuses one's awareness on the breath, the mind becomes absorbed in the rhythm of inhalation and exhalation. As a result, breathing will become slower and deeper, and the mind will become more tranquil and aware.

Mindful meditation, involves becoming aware of the continuously passing parade of sensations and feelings, images, thoughts, sounds, smells, and so forth without becoming involved in thinking about them. The person sits quietly and simply witnesses whatever goes through the mind, not reacting or becoming involved with thoughts, memories, worries or images. This helps to gain a more calm, clear and non-reactive state of mind.

Studies show that after meditation, reactions are faster, creativity greater and comprehension broader. In addition, by silencing the mind, meditation can also put one in touch with the self, allowing the body's own inner wisdom to be heard.

(iii) Aromatherapy

Aromatherapy has been around for over 6000 years. In India and other ancient civilizations of the East, plant essences were used for their fragrance to purify the air. Agarbatis and dhoop (incense sticks) are still in use as they were in ancient times in India.

The modern era of aromatherapy dawned in 1930 when the French chemist Rene Maurice Gattefosse coined the term 'aromatherapy' for the therapeutic use of essential oils. He was fascinated by the benefits of lavender oil in healing his burnt hand without leaving any scars. He started investigating the effect of other essential oils for healing and for their psychotherapeutic benefits.

Our sense of smell works at a subconscious level. Olfactory nerves conduct smell sensations to a part of the brain which also regulates and controls our moods, emotions, memory and learning. Studies with brain wave frequency have shown that smelling lavender increases alpha waves which are associated with relaxation in the back of the head. Fragrance of jasmine increases beta waves, which are associated with a more alert state in the front of the head.

Essential oils are contained in plant materials like leaves, flowers, roots, seeds, bark and resin. Each essential oil contains as much as 100 chemical components, which together exert a strong effect on the whole person.

Depending on which component is predominating in an oil, the oils act differently. For example, some oils are relaxing, some soothing and some pain relieving. They leave no harmful residues.

Aromatherapy is particularly effective for stress, anxiety, and psychosomatic induced problems, muscular and rheumatic pains, digestive disorders and gynaecological problems, such as PMS, menopausal complaints and postnatal depression.

(iv) Homeopathy

Dissatisfied with the common medical practices of the time, Dr. Samuel Hahnemann sought to create a system of gender healing. He began creating a new system using plants, minerals and animal substances, combining them into energetic compounds. With these substances, he stimulated and encouraged the body's natural healing forces of recovery.

The word 'Homoeopathy' is derived from two Greek words, homoeo meaning similar, and pathos meaning suffering. Homoeopathy simply means treating diseases with remedies, prescribed in minute doses, which produce symptoms similar to the disease when taken by healthy people. It is based on the natural law of healing — 'Similia Similibus Curantur' which means 'like is cured by like'. For example, the effects of peeling an onion are very similar to the symptoms of acute cold. The remedy prepared from the red onion, Allium cepa, is used to treat that type of cold.

Conventional medicine believes that symptoms are caused by the illness of the body whereas homeopathy views the symptoms as the body's natural reaction to fighting illness, and seeks to stimulate the symptoms rather than suppress them. Homeopathy is concerned with the treatment of the whole person, as an individual, rather than the disease alone. A homoeopath does not concentrate his therapy on, say arthritis or bronchitis or cancer. Rather, he treats the mental, emotional and physical aspects of the patient. The physicians interest is not only to alleviate the patient's present symptoms but also his long-term well being.

Homeopathic medicines contain extremely small quantities of substances called potencies, prepared in a special way by diluting, shaking and pounding the mixture. These high dilutions not only enhance their curative properties, but also avoid undesirable side effects. Homeopathy has been serving humanity for over two centuries and has emerged as a time-tested therapy.

Homoeopathy came to India in 1859 when Dr. John Martin Honigberger was called to treat Maharaja Ranjit Singh, the ruler of Punjab, for paralysis of vocal cords and oedema. The Maharaja was relieved of his complaints and in return Dr. Honigberger received valuable rewards and was made the officer-in-charge of a hospital. This royal patronage gave Homoeopathy its roots in India. Homoeopathy has blended so well into the traditions of the country that it has been recognised as one of the National Systems of Medicine and plays an important role in providing health care to a large number of people.

(v) Tibetan Medicine

Two thousand years ago the indigenous people of Tibet had a traditional medical system which was closely connected to their native spiritual system. They use an ancient form of medicine known as Gso-wa Rig-pa or 'The Knowledge of Healing' whose origins are believed to be based on the teachings of the Buddha.

Tibetan medicine has existed in its present form for over one thousand years. Over several centuries, medical knowledge was incorporated from the Indian Ayurveda, the Chinese system, and the medical systems of Hellenic Greece and Persia. In addition, this system incorporated the Buddhist thought.

In Buddhist thought, all suffering and hence all illness, is caused by attachment, anger and ignorance, known as the 'Three Interior Poisons'. The physical manifestation of the 'Three Poisons' assume the form of three humors which are Lung (pronounced loong), mKhris-pa and Bad-kan. In English these are generally translated as wind, bile and phlegm. When they are in harmony, they maintain well-being, but when they are disturbed or out of harmony, they are the cause of illness. Desire corresponds to disharmony of rlung (wind). Some symptoms of rlung disorder are frothy urine, a rough, dry tongue or a 'jumpy' pulse.

Hatred corresponds to disharmony of bile. Some symptoms of bile disorder include the presence of thick or yellowish-red urine, thick, yellowish fur on the tongue or a 'full' pulse.

Ignorance causes phlegm disorders. The urine is odorless, thin and whitish, and the pulse is 'sluggish or heavy'. Furthermore, the Tibetan Buddhist believes that karma (the law of cause and effect) from one's previous incarnations can also be responsible for our illnesses in our present experience.

Ignorance generates other negative states of mind such as desire, hatred, jealousy and pride, which also contribute to our suffering. Understanding one's emotions is an essential part of the Buddhist journey to full awakening and freedom from unwanted conditions of all sorts. However, since most of us have very little ability to work with our emotional energies, medicines and other remedies are required. Treatment can include consultations on lifestyle and diet, recommendations of mantras and meditation, moxibustion (burning of the herb mugwort), the use of supplements and massage with specially formulated herbal oils and occasionally, accupuncture.

The ideal image of a healer in Tibetan medicine, is that of "a man of noble character, capable of immediately making the right diagnosis of a patient's illness, without any examination or the least assistance" (Burang). Needless to say, such physicians are quite rare. Consequently, before a physician acquires credibility, he must train at least twenty years in the tradition.

Tibetan medicine is a holistic tradition, and a lasting cure can only take place when the whole psychosocial environment of the patient is accounted for, superficial methods which consider only the outward symptoms of illness are frowned upon. Consequently, Tibetan medicine is increasingly gaining recognition in the West as particularly effective for patients with chronic diseases such as hepatitis, certain kinds of mental illness, ulcers, paralysis, gall stones, kidney stones, and arthritis. Tibetans look at well-being as a consequence of three integrated types of medical practices: secular therapies, such as medicine, diet, surgery, spiritual cures where Buddha is the Absolute healer and the Dharma, or teachings of Sakyamuni, the "King of Medicine."

The Tibetan physician focuses his attention on spiritual factors even in the treatment of the simplest illnesses and regards medicine and medical instruments as holy objects. Even the pharmaceuticals, which are mixtures of vegetable, animal and mineral compounds, are prepared with meticulous attention to religious ritual. For example, after the Tibetan physician gathers dozens of different ingredients that go into the making of the single small pill, he performs a meditative ritual.

(vi) Naturopathy

The nature cure movement started in Germany with the "water cure" (Hydrotherapy). The credit of making water cure famous goes to Vincent Priessnitz (1799-1851), who was a farmer. The nature cure movement gained momentum in India as Mahatma Gandhi, "Father of the Nation", became interested in this system and included it in his programmes. He also established a nature cure Hospital in Uruli Kanchan in Pune, Maharashtra which is still functioning.

Naturopathy believes that nature is the greatest healer and the body has the capacity to prevent itself from diseases and regain health. The treatment can include consultations on lifestyle and diet, recommendations of mantras and meditation, *moxibustion* (burning of the herb mugwort), use of supple-ments and massage with specially formulated herbal oil, and occasionally, *acupuncture*.

The practice of nature cure is based on the three principles; accumulation of morbid matter, abnormal composition of blood and lymph and lowered vitality. The system of nature cure states that the basic cause of disease is not bacteria. Bacteria develop after the accumulation of morbid matter when a favourable atmosphere for their growth develops in body. All diseases arise due to this morbid matter in the body, and if latitude is given for its removal, the body provides a cure. It also believed that the human body possesses inherent self-constructing and self-healing powers. Nature cure takes into account the totality of factors responsible for diseases such as habits in living, thinking, working, sleeping, relaxation, sexual indulgence, and considers the environmental factors involved, which on the whole disturbs the normal functioning of the body and leads it to a morbid, weak and toxic state.

A Nature cure physician helps in nature's effort to overcome disease by controlling the natural forces to work within safe limits. The five main modalities of treatment are air, water, heat, mud and space.

The recent development of nature cure advocates the practice of drugless therapies like massage, electrotherapy, physiotherapy, acupuncture, acupressure and magnetotherapy.

(vii) Acupuncture

Acupuncture is based on an ancient Chinese theory. This theory states that life force flows through the human body via fourteen invisible channels regulating the mental and physical processes. The 'puncture' in the world acupuncture, refers to the insertion of tiny needles in specific points on the surface of the body. The use of this therapy has been widely successful of easing withdrawal from the addiction to drugs and alcohol, and is used in many detoxification clinics in the United States. Although it has been practiced for many years as a method of traditional healings, Indians have only recently started to embrace this method.

(viii) Acupressure

This science deals with the human body and the flow of natural energy within the body. It is practiced with the use of only one tool, the human thumb. Pressure is applied on different pressure points on the body that stimulate the corresponding glands of the body. It has been around for many years, and flourishes in countries like China and India.

(ix) Gem Therapy

Crystals, gems and minerals are solidified reflections of properties that are already within the human body. Gems and precious metals are used to balance planetary influences and to act directly on a life force. Having the capacity to both attract and dispel positive or negative energies, their healing properties are applied by wearing them in or having them in some way close to the body. The healing effect of gems can be experienced even by placing them in water overnight and drinking the water the next day, drinking water from vessels made of specific metals such as gold, silver, or copper. Precious stones and metals are also oxidized and purified in medicines in India called "bhasma", these substances go deep into the body and can help in the healing of deep-seated illness or in rejuvenation.

Healing using quartz crystals is among the most ancient of all known therapies. Due to their perfect molecular structure, crystals vibrate at a constant rate. It is this quality of crystals that make them ideal tools for harmonizing and balancing the body. All crystals and gemstones vibrate at their own unique frequencies. By selecting the crystal with the correct vibration to counter an individual's malady, the body's natural rhythm is restored.

If gems are to be used for healing they should be purified. Immersing gems in salt water for two days purifies them. Their power can also be enhanced by chanting sacred syllables (mantra) over them. Gems are most effective when they weigh more than two carats and are worn in contact with the skin. If a precious stone of two carats or more is not available, it is better to use a semi precious stone that is larger. To allow direct contact with the skin, all rings and pendants should have an open backed setting and the preferred metal is gold.

Individual stones have properties that influence the "doshas" in individuals and increase the well-being of the wearer. Some of the commonly worn stones include the Topaz, which is said to help overcome fear. A yellow Sapphire is worn to enhance energy and vitality and is generally considered good for health. Opal is considered to have a positive influence on the wearer, promoting friendship, compassion, creativity and understanding. Precious stones like Diamond, Sapphires, Rubies and semi precious stones like Lapis Lazuli, Coral, Beryl and Moonstone, have their own attributes and are recommended to correct various imbalances in the body.

(x) Pranic Healing

Pranic healing is based on the principle that the body has the capacity to heal itself, and a catalyst is used to accelerate the healing process. This catalyst is called the Prana (vital source of life that is all around us). It is a non-touch, non-invasive process. This system of medicine believes that all living beings have two selves, the physical self and the energy that forms the exterior cover. The two are said to be intertwined and intrinsic, so much so that the energy is often referred to as the "etheric twin". According to Pranic healing, the requirement for being healthy is when both the energy and the physical self are in harmony.

Healers try to cure disease by clearing or cleaning energy systems. The system comprises of 11 major *chakras* (corresponding to vital organs), or power centres in the body. These are the Basic chakra (located at the base of the spine), Sex chakra, Meng Mein chakra (located approximately at the back of the navel), Navel chakra. Spleen chakra, Solar Plexus chakra, Heart chakra, Throat chakra, Ajna chakra, Forehead chakra and the Crown chakra. Each chakra has its own position and it controls a set of organs.

The healers use their hands to detect malfunctioning in the body (called scanning). They clean the used up or diseased energy with sweeping movements of their hands and dispose this waste energy in a bowl of salt and water (water dissolves the diseased energy and salt disintegrates it). Then, they receive the Prana from the atmosphere with one hand and project it to the diseased chakras of the patient with the other hand.

This system can be used to alleviate a large number of ailments ranging from brain tumours, stomach disorders, ulcers, skin diseases to mental diseases like depression, schizophrenia, and mental retardation.

(xi) Reiki

Allowing energy to flow through people and directing the excess energy either to ourselves or to others is the essence of Reiki. 'Re' means 'universal' and 'ki' means 'vital like force'. Disease, according to Reiki is caused by an energy imbalance, the depletion or congestion of energy. The treatment in this system of medicine consists of correcting this imbalance. Reiki is similar to Pranic healing, as it also uses Prana or energy to affect a cure, but the techniques of Reiki vary from Pranic healing. Here, the healer draws the Prana or energy through his or her crown (chakra), and allows the energy to flow through the hands or the chakra. The healer or therapist is the energy channel.

The history of magnetism dates before the birth of Christ. The earliest mention of the magnet being used as a healing agent is in the Atharvaveda, the ancient Indian treatise on medicine and a part of one of the four Vedas.

The ancient Egyptians were also familiar with the properties of magnetic forces, as they utilized it to preserve mummies. Their legendary queen, Cleopatra, was said to have worn a tiny magnet on her forehead in order to preserve her charm.

It was only in the beginning of the 16th century that magnets became an object of scientific research. A Swiss alchemist and physician, Paracelsus, discovered magnets healing powers, and was soon followed by other researchers. Dr. Samuel Hahneman, the father of homeopathy, was convinced of the magnet's healing powers and recommended its use. Today, Magnetotherapy is widely recognized and has scientific support.

Magnetotherapy is very effective in drawing out pain and relieving stiffness. When the body comes into contact with magnets, the magnetic waves pass through the tissues and induce secondary currents, which produce heat, thus reducing pains and swellings. Magnets also promote the growth of cells and increase the number of healthy red blood corpuscles. The red corpuscles contain hemoglobin, which in turn contain iron. The magnets influence the iron in the blood, thereby removing calcium, cholesterol and other deposits. It cleanses, purifies and ionises the blood. The ionised blood flows easily, resulting in ease in the activity of the heart and normalization of blood pressure. The secretion of hormones is also regulated, and this improves the lustre of the skin.

Magnets of various shapes, sizes and strengths are used to regulate and strengthen the natural system and preserve the balance of magnetic field in the body. Two types of artificial magnets are used — electromagnets and permanent magnets. For most treatments, disc shaped magnets of medium to high potency are generally used.

(xii) Chakra Therapy

Chakras are centres of psychic energy located at points along the spinal cord. They are associated with the five elements: earth, water, fire, air and ether.Each chakra corresponds to a specific mantra (sound) and geometric pattern (yantra). Through meditation on these chakras we can gain mastery over our body and each corresponding element.

TRADITIONAL MEDICINE AND GLOBALIZATION

Traditional medicines are and will indomitable arena of pharmacognosy. To integrate and work with globalization, traditional medicine must reassess and open itself to the requirements of scientific rationality, convert itself in its diagnostic and therapeutic approach methods as well as in its deontology. It will thus ensure its influence, productivity, and progress as well as enhance its therapeutic efficiency and competitiveness. This requires the use of modern medicine's diagnostic means and therapeutic control—namely, laboratory analysis, various diagnostic tests, conventional radiography and tomography, tomodensiometry (scanner), magnetic resonance, and all current and future medical techniques.

Secondly it should involve chemical and pharmacological study of medicines in order to determine their components, its active principles, its toxicity, and posology. This will lead to their commercialization nationally as well as internationally. An introduction to light and heavy pharmaceutical industries, which will give the medicines a rational galenic form for their conservation, use and large scale production. The public authorities should be involved in —

1. Setting-up traditional medicine and traditional pharmacopoeia institutes for chemical, pharmacopoeia and clinical research.
2. Setting-up the national organization of traditional health practitioners.
3. A regular evaluation of the abilities of these organizations through joint (both systems) bodies to ascertain the real impact of their action on people's health.
4. Providing legal recognition of this type of medicine.
5. Action at the grass root level to protect traditional knowledge.
6. The creation and upkeep of protected ethno-botanic gardens to perpetuate vegetal species used in African pharmacopoeia.

TRADITIONAL MEDICINE: FUTURE NEED

WHO has been promoting traditional medicines as a source of less expensive, comprehensive medical care, especially in developing countries. Eighty percent of the world's population relies on medicinal plants for their primary health care. Such herbal medicines are easily available, cheaper, time tested and considered safer than some of modern synthetic drugs. Recently WHO introduced guidelines on research and evaluation of traditional medicine and practice.

This guideline has a major objective of developing traditional medicine leads into standardized and scientifically validated drugs. This guideline aims to ensure quality and safety of botanicals before being evaluated for its efficacy. On this background pharmacognosy is playing paramount role in evolution of novel medicines taking lead from natural products.

STUDY QUESTIONS

1. Explain the meaning of Pharmacogonosy.
2. Discuss the system of medicine in India.

■■■

2

CHAPTER

Drugs, Natural/Technical Products and Pharmaceutical Aids Derived from Plants and Animals

INTRODUCTION

Drug is a pure substance or combination of pure substances (isolated from natural sources, semi-synthetic, or purely chemical in origin) intended to mitigate, treat, cure or prevent a disease in humans (and other animals).

In other words, any chemical compound used in the *diagnosis, treatment,* or *prevention* of disease or other abnormal condition is *drugs.*

Crude Drug. Natural products, which are not pure compounds (i.e., plants or parts of plants, extracts, or exudes).

Allopathy. Also known as "conventional medicine" in Western societies. Allopathy focuses on treating the symptoms of diseases primarily through prescription drugs. This approach utilizes a process of reductionism (focusing on the symptoms exhibited in a part of the organism rather than focusing on the organism as a whole.)

Ayurvedic Medicine. Literally meaning the "science of life." A 5,000 year-old system of medicine originating in India that combines natural therapies with a highly personalized, holistic approach to the treatment of disease.

Homeopathy. A system of medicine founded in the late 18th century in which remedies consist of diluted substances from plants, minerals and animals. It is based on a theory that "like cures like." Remedies specifically match different symptom pattern profiles of illness to stimulate the body's natural healing process.

Naturopathy. A holistic medical system that treats health conditions by utilizing what is believed to be the body's innate ability to heal. Naturopathic physicians aid healing processes by incorporating a variety of natural methods based on the patient's individual needs.

Indigenous or Tribal Medicine. A health care system that tends to incorporate various methods of botanical and animal medicines as well as specific ceremonial rituals of the culture to cure disease. The medicinal knowledge is passed from generation to generation primarily through oral traditions. The system tends to be unique to each tribe.

Traditional Chinese Medicine. A 3,000-year-old holistic system of medicine combining the use of medicinal herbs, acupuncture, food therapy, massage, and therapeutic exercise. Chinese physicians look for the underlying causes of imbalance in the "yin" and "yang" which lead to disharmony in the "qi" energy in the body. Traditional Chinese Medicine addresses how illness manifests itself in a patient and treats the patient, not the ailment or disease.

APPROACHES

Aromatherapy. This approach uses essential oils extracted from medicinal plants to treat various health conditions. The oils are generally diluted, then used topically, internally, or to stimulate olfactory senses.

Flower Essences. In the 1930s, Dr. Edward Bach developed an approach to healing using "flower essences." Flower essences are made by infusing flowers or other plant parts in spring water and then adding alcohol as a preservative. The essences are used internally or topically to balance emotional states. The underlying philosophy focuses on stabilizing emotions in order to dissipate illness and stimulate internal healing processes.

Herbal Medicine. An approach to healing which uses plant or plant-derived preparations to treat, prevent, or cure various health conditions and ailments. This approach is incorporated into various medical systems. Although herbal medicine does not have a specific point of conception, at present an estimated 80% of the world's population rely on medicinal plant preparations for their primary healthcare needs, according to the World Health Organization. Despite the extensive use which can be attributed to the use of plants in traditional medical systems, our knowledge of the plants and their values remain largely unexplored.

DRUGS OBTAINED FROM PLANTS

Many pharmaceutical drugs used in western medicine are made from plants or the properties of plants have inspired their development. Among the early isolates were morphine from *Papaver somniferum*, strychnine from *Strychnos nux-vomica*, quinine from *Cinchona* and codeine from *Papaver somniferum*.

In some cases, chemicals extracted from plants are used directly as medicines, for example reserpine (lowers blood pressure, extracted from *serpent-root Rauvolfia serpentina*), ephedrin (a *decongestant*, from the shrub *Ephedra*), *digitalin* (used to treat irregularities in heart rhythm, from *Foxglove Digitalis sp.*), and *vinblastine* and *vincristine* (for treating childhood leukaemia and Hodgkin's disease, from the rosy periwinkle *Catharanthus roseus*).

In other cases, chemicals are extracted from plants and used as chemical building-blocks to create new compounds which are then used as drugs. The drugs *etoposide* and *teniposide* (used for treating skin cancers and warts) are manufactured from epipodophyllotoxin, a chemical found in May apple *Podophyllum sp. Progesterone* (used as an oral contraceptive) is manufactured from diosgenin, found in certain species of *yam Dioscorea sp.*

Some drugs, including some that are synthesised today from inorganic sources, were inspired in their historical development by the physiological activities of chemicals found in plants. Aspirin, which is today synthesized inorganically, was inspired in its development by folk uses of the bark of *willow Salix* to treat *fever*.

Although drugs extracted from or inspired by plants are used very extensively, the actual number of plant species that has contributed to western medicine. Apart from plants sensu stricto, fungi play major roles in western medicine, notably through the use of genera such as *Penicillium* and *Streptomyces* as sources of antibiotics.

PLANT PARTS (CRUDE DRUG TERMINOLOGY)

Aetheroleum. Refers to the essential or volatile oil as a distinct aromatic product obtained from the plant.

- **Balsamum.** Refers to a solution of resin and volatile oil usually produced by special cells in some plants.
- **Bulbus.**Refers to the bulb or an underground bud (specialized stem structure) of a plant, from which both a shoot and roots may extend.
- **Cortex.** Refers to the bark of the plant. Bark can be collected from the root, stem, or branches.
- **Flos.** Refers to the flowers of plant usually consisting of a single flower or the entire inflorescences (i.e., head, umbel, panicle, spike, etc.).
- **Folium.** Refers to the leaf of plant. Usually the middle leaves of plants are collected.
- **Fructus.** Refers to the fruit (the ripened ovary of the flower-bearing seeds) or berry of the plant. In pharmacognosy,

fructus is not always synonymous with the botanical definition.

- **Herba.** Refers to the aerial parts or the aboveground parts of plants which may include the flower, leaf, and the stem of the plant, and occasionally fruits too.
- **Lignum.** Refers to the wood or the secondary thickening of the stem. This may or may not contain the bark as well.
- **Oleum.** Refers to the fixed oil preparation pressed or squeezed from the plant material.
- **Pericarpium.** Refers to the peel or rind of fruit.
- **Pyroleum.** Refers to the tar from dry distilled plant material.
- **Radix.** Refers to the root of a plant, though radix is sometimes synonomous with rhizome.
- **Resina.** Refers to the resin that is secreted by the plant or by distillation of the balsamum.
- **Rhizoma.** Refers to the rhizome or a creeping horizontal stem, generally bearing roots on its underside.
- **Semen.** Refers to the seed of a plant, usually removed from the fruit, and may or may not contain the seed coat.

DRUGS OBTAINED FROM ANIMALS

When drugs derived from raw materials of animal origin including human are used, it is important to take into account any possibility that communicable disease agents such as virus may cause infectious disease or any possible hazards to patients. In such case, it goes without saying that the primary subject that has to be considered is the absence of any infectious agents such as virus in the raw materials of animal origin including human as the source of the drug. More important points are whether the drugs derived from such raw materials are free of such infectious agents and whether there is any possibility of transmission of infectious agents when the drugs are administered to patient.

The eligibility of animals including human, as the source of raw materials of drugs, in other words "the subject which is free from any disease or transmission of infectious agents that is infectious to human being at an appropriate production process and use of the drug product" is that "The drug should be entirely free from any risk of infections by means of whole procedures which include evaluation of appropriateness of the animals including human as the source of their raw materials, establish-ment of appropriate production processes and their appropriate control, and strict adherence to the clinical indications of the final product."

HORMONES OBTAINED FROM ANIMALS

Hormones are chemical messengers produced by glands in the endocrine system. Endocrine tissues are specialised to produce such hormones, which have genes switched on according the hormones they were designed to produce. The pituitary gland and hypothalamus are the most important in regards to control and development.

Hormone	Obtained from	Animals
Thyroid	Thyroid gland	Sheep, Pig
Insuiin	Pancrease	Cattle, Pig
Oxytocin	Pituitary gland	Cattle, Pig
Vasopressin	Posterior pituitary gland	Cattle, Pig
Gonadotrpin	Anterior	Horse serum or pituitary gland urine of pregnant women.

ENZYMES

Enzymes are very efficient catalysts for biochemical reactions. They speed up reactions by providing an alternative reaction pathway of lower activation energy. Like all catalysts, enzymes take part in the reaction - that is how they provide an alternative reaction pathway. But they do not undergo permanent changes and so remain unchanged at the end of the reaction. They can only alter the rate of reaction, not the position of the equilibrium.

Enzymes	Obtained from	Animals
Pepsin	Glandular layer of stomach	Pig
Pancretin	Pancrease	Pig
Renin	Glandular layer of stomach	Calf
Urokinage	Urine	Human
Hyalurodinage	Testes	Mammalian

EXTRACTS OF ANIMAL ORGANS

An extract is a substance made by extracting a part of a raw material, often by using a solvent such as ethanol or water. Extracts may be sold as tinctures or in powder form.

Hormone	Obtained from	Animals
Cod liver oil	Fresh liver	Cod fish
Liver extract concentrate	Liver Stomach Mucosal cells of stomach	Mammalian Porcoine

NATURAL/TECHNICAL PRODUCTS

Natural products, including plants, animals and minerals have been the basis of treatment of human diseases. History of medicine dates back practically to the existence of human civilization. The current accepted modern medicine or allopathy has gradually developed over the years by scientific and observational efforts of scientists. However, the basis of its development remains rooted in traditional medicine and therapies.

Herbal drug development includes various steps, starting from a passport data on raw materials, correct identification, pharma-cognostic and chemical quality standardization, safety and pre-clinical pharmacology, clinical pharmacology and randomized, controlled clinical trials.

Addressing standardization is vital and needs broader consideration. Ayurvedic medicine was developed at times of limited access to technologically variable norms of standardization.

The dynamic process of evolution could alter and affect the identity and structure of natural materials. For commercialization, correct identification and supply of raw material to avoid adulteration has become a challenge.

Additionally, some botanical species might have been extinct. Lastly, the properties of botanicals as recorded in classics may have undergone change due to time and environmental factors.

Standardization of ayurvedic botanicals and medicines is required, although one cannot readily apply the typical modern pharmaceutical pharmacopoeial standards. The concept of active markers in the process of standardization needs a flexible approach in favour of the complex nature of these materials.

PHARMACEUTICAL AIDS

A pharmaceutical drug, also referred to as medicine, medication or medicament, can be loosely defined as any chemical substance intended for use in the medical diagnosis, cure, treatment, or prevention of disease. Medications can be classified in various ways, such as by chemical properties, mode or route of administration, biological system affected, or therapeutic effects. An elaborate and widely used classification system is the Anatomical Therapeutic Chemical Classification System (ATCCS). A sampling of classes of medicine includes:

1. *Antipyretics*: reducing fever (pyrexia/pyresis)
2. *Analgesics*: reducing pain (painkillers)
3. *Antimalarial* : treating malaria
4. *Antibiotics*: inhibiting germ growth
5. *Antiseptics*: prevention of germ growth near burns, cuts and wounds.

Table 2.1: Hindi, Botanical Names and Medicinal Uses

Hindi Name	Botanical Name	Medicinal Uses/ Pharmaceutical Action
1. Amalaki	*Phyllanthus emblica*	Rasayana
2. Ashwagandha	*Withania somnifera*	Immunomodulatory
3. Bhallataka	*Semecarpus anacardium*	Antiarthritc
4. Bilva	*Aegle mermelos*	Antidiarrhoeal
5. Chandan	*Santalum album*	Antiviral
6. Chitraka	*Plumbago zeylanica*	Antitumour
7. Dadima	*Punica granatum*	Antidiarrhoeal
8. Eranda	*Ricinus communis*	Hepatoprotective
9. Guduchi	*Tinospora cordifolia*	Immunomodulatory
10. Haridra	*Curcuma longa*	Antimicrobial
11. Haritaki	*Terminalia chebula*	Hypolipidemic
12. Manjishtha	*Rubia cordifolia*	Antioxidant
13. Maricha	*Piper nigrum*	Bioenhancer
14. Nimba/Neem	*Azadirachta indica*	Antidiabetic
15. Pippali	*Piper longum*	Bioenhancer
16. Sariva	*Hemeidesmus indicus*	Antiulcer
17. Shunthi	*Zingiber officinale*	Antiemetic
18. Vacha	*Acorus calamus*	Psychotropic
19. Vidanga	*Embelia ribes*	Antifertility
20. Yashtimadhu	*Glycyrrhiza glabra*	Antiulcer

Medications may be divided into over-the-counter drugs (OTC) which may be available without special restrictions, and prescription only medicine (POM), which must be prescribed by a licensed medical practitioner. The precise distinction between OTC and prescription depends on the legal jurisdiction. A third category, behind-the-counter medications (BTMs), is implemented in some jurisdictions. BTMs do not require a prescription, but must be kept in the dispensary, not visible to the public, and only be sold by a pharmacist or pharmacy technician.

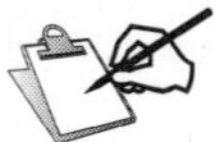

STUDY QUESTIONS

1. Which are the drugs that obtained from plants?
2. Which are the drugs obtained from animals?

3 CHAPTER

SYSTEMS OF CLASSIFICATION OF DRUGS FROM NATURAL ORIGIN

INTRODUCTION

Crude drugs of vegetable, animal and mineral sources form the subject matter of pharmacognosy. Although pharmacognosy is concerned mainly with naturally occurring substance of medicinal importance, it is not entirely limited to such substances. Thus, surgical dressings prepared from natural fibres, flavouring and suspending agents, disintegrants, filtering and support media etc. are included within the subject along with poisonous and hallucinogenic plants and raw materials for oral contraceptives.

The term *crude drug* generally applies to the products from plant and animal origin found in a raw form. However, the term is also applied to include pharmaceutical products from mineral kingdom in original form and not necessarily only of organic origin such as kaolin, bentonite etc. Crude drugs can thus be defined as to the natural products that has not been advanced in value or improved in condition by any process or treatment beyond that which is essential for its proper packing and prevention from deterioration.

CLASSIFICATION OF CRUDE DRUGS

The most important natural sources of drugs are higher plant, microbes and animals and marine organisms. Some useful products are obtained from minerals that are both organic and inorganic in nature. In order to pursue (or to follow) the study of the individual drugs, one must adopt some particular sequence of arrangement and this is referred to a system of classification of drugs. A method of classification should be

(i) Simple
(ii) Easy to use
(iii) Free from confusion and ambiguities.

Because of their wide distribution, each arrangement of classification has its own merits and demerits, but for the purpose of study the drugs are classified in the following different ways:

1. Alphabetical classification
2. Morphological classification
3. Taxonomic classification
4. Pharmacological classification
5. Chemical classification
6. Chemotaxonomical classification.

1. ALPHABETICAL CLASSIFICATION

Alphabetical classification is the simplest way of classification of any disconnected items. Crude drugs are arranged in alphabetical order of their Latin and English names (common names) or sometimes local language names (vernacular names).

Some of the pharmacopoeias, dictionaries and reference books which classify crude drugs according to this system are as follows.

1. Indian Pharmacopoeia
2. British Pharmacopoeia
3. British Herbal Pharmacopoeia

4. United States Pharmacopoeia and National Formulary
5. British Pharmaceutical Codex
6. European Pharmacopoeia.

In European Pharmacopoeia these are arranged according to their names in Latin where in U.S.P. and B.P.C., these are arranged in English.

MERITS

- It is easy and quick to use.
- There is no repetition of entries and is devoid of confusion.
- In this system location, tracing and addition of drug entries is easy.

DEMERITS

There is no relationship between previous and successive drug entries.

Examples: Acacia, Benzoin, Cinchona, Dill, Ergot, Fennel, Gentian, Hyoscyamus, Ipecacuanha, Jalap, Kurchi, Liquorice, Mints, Nuxvomica, Opium, Podophyllum, Quassia, Rauwolfia, Senna, Vasaka, Wool fat, Yellow bees wax, Zeodary.

2. MORPHOLOGICAL CLASSIFICATION

In this system, the drugs are arranged according to the morphological or external characters of the plant parts or animal parts, i.e., which part of the plant is used as a drug, e.g., leaves, roots, stem etc. The drugs obtained from the direct parts of the plants and containing cellular tissues are called as organized drugs, e.g., Rhizomes, barks, leaves, fruits, entire plants, hairs and fibres. The drugs which are prepared from plants by some intermediate physical processes such as incision, drying or extraction with a solvent and not containing any cellular plant tissues are called as unorganized drugs. Aloe juice, opium latex, agar, gambir, gelatin, tragacanth, benzoin, honey, bees wax, lemon grass oil etc. are examples of unorganized drugs.

Organised Drugs

- **Woods.** Quassia, Sandalwood, Red Sandalwood.
- **Leaves.** Digitalis, Eucalyptus, Gymnema, Mint, Senna, Spearmint, Squill, Tulsi, Vasaka, Coca, Buchu, Hamamelis, Hyoscyamus, Belladonna, Tea.

— **Barks.** Arjuna, Ashoka, Cascara, Cassia, Cinchona, Cinnamon, Kurchi, Quillia, Wild cherry.
— **Flowering Parts.** Clove, Pyrethrum, Saffron, Santonica, Chamomile.
— **Fruits.** Amla, Anise, Bael, Bahera, Bitter Orange peel, Capsicum, Caraway, Cardamom, Colocynth, Coriander, Cumin, Dill, Fennel, Gokhru, Hirda, Lemon peel, Senna pod, Star anise, Tamarind, Vidang.
— **Seeds.** Bitter almond, Black mustard, Cardamom, Colchicum, Ispaghula, Kaladana, Linseed, Nutmeg, Nux vomica, Physo-stigma, Psyllium, Strophanthus, White mustard.
— **Roots and Rhizomes.** Aconite, Ashwagandha, Calamus, Calumba, Colchicum corm, Dioscorea, Galanga, Garlic, Gention, Ginger, Ginseng, Glycyrrhiza, Podophyllum, Ipecac, Ipomoea, Jalap, Jatamansi, Rauwolfia, Rhubarb, Sassurea, Senega, Shatavari, Turmeric, Valerian, Squill.
— **Plants and Herbs.** Ergot, Ephedra, Bacopa, Andrographis, Kalmegh, Yeast, Vinca, Datura, Centella.
— **Hair and Fibres.** Cotton, Hemp, Jute, Silk, Flax.

Unorganised Drugs

— **Dried Latex.** Opium, Papain.
— **Dried Juice.** Aloe, Kino.
— **Dried Extracts.** Agar, Alginate, Black catechu, Pale catechu, Pectin.
— **Waxes.** Bees wax, Spermaceti, Carnauba wax.
— **Gums.** Acacia, Guar Gum, Indian Gum, Sterculia, Tragacenth.
— **Resins.** Asafoetida, Benzoin, Colophony, copaiba Guaiacum, Guggul, Mastic, Coal tar, Tar, Tolu balsam, Storax, Sandarac.
— **Volatile Oil.** Turpentine, Anise, Coriander, Peppermint, Rosemary, Sandalwood, Cinnamon, Lemon, Caraway, Dill, Clove, Eucalyptus, Nutmeg, Camphor.

- **Fixed Oils and Fats.** Arachis, Castor, Chalmoogra, Coconut, Cotton seed, Linseed, Olive, Sesame, Almond, Theobroma, Cod-liver, Halibut liver, Kokum butter.
- **Animal Products.** Bees wax, Cantharides, Cod-liver oil, Gelatin, Halibut liver oil, Honey, Shark liver oil, shellac, Spermaceti wax, wool fat, musk, Lactose.

MERITS

Morphological classification is more helpful to identify and detect adulteration. This system of classification is more convenient for practical study especially when the chemical nature of the drug is not clearly understood.

DEMERITS

- The main drawback of morphological classification is that there is no co-relation of chemical constituents with the therapeutic actions.
- Repetition of drugs or plants occurs.

3. TAXONOMICAL CLASSIFICATION

Taxonomical classification is purely a botanical classification and is based on principles of natural relationship and evolutionary developments. They are grouped in Kingdom, phylum, order, family genus and species. As all the entire plants are not used as drugs, part of the plant is used as a drug, for example, cinnamon bark. Thus it is of no significance from identification point of view to put plants in a taxonomic order.

MERITS

Taxonomical classification is helpful for studying evolutionary developments.

DEMERITS

This system also does not co-relate in between the chemical constituents and biological activity of the drugs.

4. PHARMACOLOGICAL CLASSIFICATION

Grouping of drug according to their pharmacological action or of most important constituent or their therapeutic use is termed as pharmacological or therapeutic classification of drug.

This classification is more relevant and is mostly followed method. Drugs like digitalis, squill and strophanthus having cardiotonic action are grouped together irrespective of their parts used or phylogenetic relationship or the nature of phytoconstituents they contain. Table 3.1 gives an outline of pharmacological classification of drugs.

MERITS

This system of classification can be used for suggesting substitutes of drugs if they are not available at a particular place or point of time.

DEMERITS

Drugs having different action on the body gets classified separately in more than one group that causes ambiguity and confusion. Cinchona is antimalarial drug because of presence of quinine but can be put under the group of drug affecting heart because of antiarrythymic action of quinidine.

Classification of Drugs based on Pharmacological Action

Table 3.1: Pharmacological Classification of Drugs

Pharmacological Action	Drugs
Anticancer	Vinca, Podophyllum, Taxus
Anti-inflammatory	Colchicum, Turmeric
Antiamoebic	Ipecac root, Kurchi bark
Antiasthmatic	Ephedra, Lobelia
Anthelminthic	Male fern, Quassia wood
Antispasmodic	Datura, Hyoscyamus
Astringent	Catechu
Analgesic	Opium, poppy
Bitter tonic	Quassia wood, Nux-vomica, Gentian
Carminatives	Coriander, fennel, clove, peppermint
Purgatives	Senna, Rhubarb
Expectorant	Tulsi, Balsam of Tolu, Vasaka
Cardiotonic	Digitalis, Squill, Strophanthus
Tranquilizers	Rauwolfia Roots

5. CHEMICAL CLASSIFICATION

The crude drugs are divided into different groups according to the chemical nature of their most important constituent. Since the pharmacological activity and therapeutic significance of crude drugs are based on the nature of their chemical constituents. The chemical classification of drugs is dependent upon the grouping of drugs with identical constituents. An out of this classification is as follows:

1. **Carbohydrates.** Carbohydrates are polyhydroxy aldehydes or ketones containing an unbroken chain of carbon atoms.
   - *Gums*: Acacia, Tragacanth, Guargum.
   - *Mucilages*: Plantago seed.
   - *Others*: Starch, Honey, Agar, Pectin, Cotton.
2. **Glycosides.** Glycosides are compounds which upon hydrolysis give rise to one or more sugars (glycone) and non-sugar (aglycone).
   - *Anthraquinone Glycosides*: Aloe, Cascara, Rhubarb, Senna.
   - *Saponins Glycosides*: Quillaia, Arjuna, Glycyrrhiza.
   - *Cyanophore Glycosides*: Wild cherry bark.
   - *Isothiocyanate*: Glycosides Mustard.
   - *Cardiac Glycosides*: Digitalis, Strophantus.
   - *Bitter Glycosides*: Gentian, Calumba, Quassia, Chirata, Kalmegh.
3. **Tannins.** Tannins are complex organic, non-nitrogenous derivatives of polyhydroxy benzoic acids.
   - *Examples*: Pale catechu, Black catechu, Ashoka bark, Galls, Myrobalan, Bahera, Amla.
4. **Volatile Oils.** Monoterpenes and sesquiterpenes obtained from plants.
   - *Examples*: Cinnamon, Fennel, Dill, Caraway, Coriander, Cardamom, Orange peel, Mint, Clove, valerian.
5. **Lipids.**
   - *Fixed oils*: Castor, Olive, Almond, Shark liver oil.

— *Fats*: Theobroma, Lanolin.

— *Waxes*: Beeswax, Spermaceti.

6. **Resins.** Complex mixture of compounds like resinols, resin acids, resinotannols, resenes.

— *Examples*: Colophony, Podophyllum, Cannabis, Jalap, Capsicum, Turmeric, Balsam of Tolu and Peru, Asafoetida, Myrrh, Ginger.

7. **Alkaloids.** Nitrogenous substance of plant origin.
   - *Pyridine and Piperidine*: Lobelia, Nicotiana.
   - *Tropane*: Coca, Belladonna, Datura, Stramonium, Hyoscyamus, Henbane.
   - *Quinoline*: Cinchona.
   - *Isoquinoline*: Opium, Ipecac, Calumba.
   - *Indole*: Ergot, Rauwolfia.
   - *Amines*: Ephedra.
   - *Purina*: Tea, Coffee.
8. **Protein.** Gelatin, Ficin, Papain.
9. **Vitamins.** Yeast.
10. **Triterpenes.** Rasna, Colocynth.

MERITS

It is a popular approach for phytochemical studies

DEMERITS

Ambiguities arise when particular drugs possess a number of compounds belonging to different groups of compounds.

6. CHEMOTAXONOMICAL CLASSIFICATION

This system of classification relies on the chemical similarity of a taxon, i.e., it is based on the existence of relationship between constituents in various plants.

There are certain types of chemical constituents that characterize certain classes of plants. This gives birth to entirely new concept of chemotaxonomy that utilizes chemical facts/characters for understanding the taxonomical status, relationships and the evolution of the plants. For example, tropane alkaloids generally occur among the members of *Solanaceae* thereby, serving as a chemotaxonomic marker.

Similarly other secondary plant metabolites can serve as the basis of classification of crude drugs. The berberine alkaloid in Berberis and Argemone; Rutin in Rutaceae members, ranunculaceous alkaloids among its members etc. are other examples.

It is the latest system of classification and gives more scope for understanding the relationship between chemical constituents, their biosynthesis and their possible action.

STUDY QUESTIONS

1. Explain the classification of crude drugs.
2. Discuss the classification of drugs based on pharmacological action.
3. Write a short note on chemical classification of drugs.

■■■

4 CHAPTER

ADULTERATION, DRUG EVALUATION AND PHARMACOPOEIAL STANDARDS

ADULTERATION

Anyone who adulterates any drug or medical preparation in such a manner as to lessen its efficacy or change the operation, or makes it noxious, knowing that it shall be sold or used for any medicinal purpose, as if it had not gone undergone any adulteration, is said to cause *adulteration*. It is sufficient if the efficacy of a drug is lessened, it need not necessarily become noxious to life.

METHODS OF DRUG EVALUATION

ORGANOLEPTIC EVALUATION

The freshly (just after collection) peeled stem bark of the plant were spreaded on a clean dry plastic sheet and investigated different organoleptic features by repeated observations using magnifying glass and ruler (where required) and recorded.

Similarly the dried stem bark and root were also subjected to organoleptic evaluation.

The characters recorded are described below:

Fresh Bark

- **Condition.** Moist.
- **Shape of pieces.** Flat strips.
- **Dimensions.** Varies, 8-12 cm long, 1-2.5 cm wide and 0.2-0.4 cm thick.
- **Colour.** Outer surface pale greenish brown, inner surface dull greenish yellow.
- **Odour.** Aromatic, characteristic.
- **Taste.** Aromatic and bitter. Proper chewing leads to typical pungent and worm sensation of tongue lasting for 10-15 minutes.
- **Fracture.** Fibrous.

The outer surface of the bark had scattered lenticels and small and large scars left by the prickles and branches. Outer surface was marked by wavy longitudinal striations; inner surface also had longitudinal striations. The cork was found frequently exfoliated.

Dried Bark

- **Condition.** Hard and contracted.
- **Shape of pieces.** Recurved and channeled quills.
- **Dimensions.** Varies, 6-8 cm long and 0.4-0.8 cm wide.
- **Colour.** Outer surface blackish brown, inner surface brownish buff coloured.
- **Odour.** Slight.
- **Taste.** Same as fresh bark.
- **Fracture.** Splintery.

MICROSCOPIC STUDIES

The transverse sections (TS) of stem bark were obtained by usual techniques. Good sections were collected and placed on a grease free microscopic slide along with a drop of glycerine water (1:1). The sections were covered with clean cover slip and observed under the compound microscope at 40x magnification. A camera lucida was attached with the microscope and the sections were suitably traced out.

The transverse section exhibited a cork consisting of narrow cells. The cortex contained small starch grains, crystals of calcium oxalate, but no sclereids. After cortex there was a narrow band of pericyclic sclerenchyma. The medullary rays were numerous, mainly one cell wide. Calcium oxalate crystals were also found in the phloem.

PHYSICO-CHEMICAL EVALUATIONS

Physico-chemical parameters such as the percentage of loss on drying (LOD), total ash, acid insoluble ash, water soluble ash were determined as per the Indian Pharmacopoeia. Water and alcohol soluble extractives were estimated by hot extraction and cold maceration according to the method prescribed by WHO. All determinations were performed in triplicate and the results are presented as mean ± standard error of mean (SEM).

Water soluble ash was found to be quite greater than acid insoluble ash value. The results showed greater extractive values (almost double) in hot extraction method. In both methods alcohol yielded higher extractives.

PHYTOCHEMICAL SCREENING

The dried and powdered stem bark was subjected to preliminary phytochemical screening for qualitative detection of phytoconstituents. The dried and coarsely powdered stem bark (100 g) was extracted successively with petroleum ether (40-60°C), chloroform (59.5-60°C), ethyl acetate (76.5-77.5°C), and ethanol (90%) in a soxhlet extractor by continuous hot percolation.

Finally the marc was macerated with chloroform water. Each time before extracting with the next solvent of higher polarity the powdered drug (marc) was dried in a hot air oven below

50°C for 10 minutes. Each extract was concentrated by distilling off the solvent, which was recovered subsequently. The concentrated extracts were evaporated to dryness and the extracts obtained with each solvent were weighed. Their percentages were calculated in terms of initial air dried plant material. The colours of extracts were observed. The successive extracts were subjected to various qualitative phytochemical tests for the identification of chemical constituents present in the plant material.

The results demonstrated presence of true alkaloids, carbohydrates, flavonoids and amino acids in the stem bark of *Z. nitidum*.

THIN LAYER CHROMATOGRAPHIC STUDIES

Preparation of bark extract (test solution). Approximately 1 gm of dried coarsely powdered stem bark was taken in a 100 ml glass beaker and moistened with little amount (sufficient to moisten) of 25% liq. NH_3 with occasional stirring for 20 mins. Then the beaker was kept on boiling hot water bath to dry the contents for a few minutes. The beaker was cooled at room temperature and added 10-15 ml of chloroform and extracted on boiling hot water bath for 10 mins. Then the extract (1-2 ml) was collected in clean stoppered glass test tube and used for spotting the chromatographic plates.

Reference solution. A minute quantity of brucine (reference alkaloid) was dissolved in minimum amount (around 1 ml) of chloroform and kept in clean stoppered glass test tube and used as reference.

Stationary phase. Silica gel G, particle size 10-40 μ, applied as a thin layer on a clean glass plate support and activated just before use.

Mobile phase. The mobile phase chosen was, Toluene : Ethyl acetate : Diethylamine = 70 : 20 : 10.

Development method. One dimensional ascending method by using standard protocol as per Indian Pharmacopoeia was followed. The stem bark extract, prepared by above said method along with the reference alkaloid brucine solution, were chromatographed in the same plate.

Visualization. After development no visible spots were found. No spots were observed under UV light (short and long). Visua-lization was attempted by spraying with Dragendorff's reagent.

Documentation. After visualization by spraying with Dragen-dorff's reagent, dark and light orange brown spots were found. The Rf values of the spots were recorded carefully and the chromatogram was documented by graphical copying.

Result. The stem bark extract yielded four orange brown spots of different intensity, and the reference brucine showed one distinct spot.

PHARMACOPOEIA STANDARDS

Pharmacopoeia is a reference work for pharmaceutical drug specifications. Its containing directions for the identification of samples and the preparation of compound medicines. The name has also been applied to similar *compendia* issued by private individuals. The word compendium comes from the Latin word "compenso", meaning "to weigh together or balance".

The term 'drug' has become something of a misnomer. Strictly, a drug is a chemical substance used to treat disease in animals, including man. Today, a drug is a pure chemical substance whose structure is known and is formulated, by mixing it with other materials, into a preparation suitable for administration. This results in the familiar tablets, pills, injections, liquid mixtures, emulsions, and syrups; ointments, creams, and salves; infusions and tinctures; drops for eyes, ears, and noses; sprays for inhalation, gases delivered by machine, supositories. and the like.

In earlier times drugs were not always pure, single substances, but mixtures of substances together with many unknown constituents, and were derived from medicinal plants. Here the dried leaves, roots, stems, bark, or rhizomes of plants were ground into powders or used to prepare infusions, tinctures, syrups etc. For example, malaria was treated with infusions made from cinchona bark, and constipation by extracts of casacara sagrada bark.

Approved drugs are those which have passed all the stringent tests for safety and efficacy granted by organizations such as the Committee on the Safety of Drugs (in the U.K.) and the *Federal Drugs Administration* (FDA) (in the U.S.). Approved drugs then become listed in National Formularies and pharmacopoeias of various countries. The designation BP, USP, or EP after the name of a drug implies it conforms to the standards described in the British, U.S., or European Pharmacopoeias. Even crude drugs, made from medicinal plants, were standardized during preparation to give galenicals having the same potency from batch to batch and as given in the pharmacopoeias.

With the advances in science and medicine it became appropriate to extract and purify drugs of plant origin, separating them from other plant constituents so that they could be formulated as with pure drugs. As the chemical structures of drugs were discovered it became clear that it could be economically sound to synthesize the compound chemically, rather than to rely on its synthesis by plants, together with all the attendant problems of extraction and purification. The commonly-held view that drugs produced naturally are good while synthetics are bad is a myth. The same substance produced by nature or by chemical synthesis is identical in its actions. The idea of vital force, believed to be locked away in molecules of natural origin, was destroyed in 1828 when Wohler produced the naturally-occuring substance urea from inorganic starting materials.

Chemical modification of a drug can be made without necessarily affecting either its biological effects or its potency.

In this way, a new substance is produced which is not covered by any legislation. So-called designer drugs produced from drugs used for their abuse potential thus enter the illicit marketplace. In these situations rapid actions are necessary to prevent the rapid spread of their use.

Indian Pharmacopeia (I.P.)

The Indian Pharmacopeia is an official drug compendium of the Indian sub-continent and is the sole authority for all prescription and over-the-countre medicines and other health care products manufactured or sold in India.

British Pharmacopoeia (B.P.)

The British Pharmacopoeia (B.P.) is the official collection of standards for U.K. medicinal products and pharmaceutical substances.

United States Pharmacopeia (U.S.P.)

The United States Pharmacopeia is an official public standards-setting authority for all prescription and over-the-counter medicines and other health care products manufactured or sold in the United States. U.S.P. also sets recognized standards for food ingredients and dietary supplements. These standards help to ensure the quality, purity, strength, and consistency of products made for public consumption.

TYPES OF STANDARDS

The three types of standards in pharmacopoeial are—

(i) Analytical standards;

(ii) Structural standards; and

(iii) Physical constants.

(i) Analytical standards require the presence of minimum quantity of desire constituents in the form of total ash, acid-insoluble ash, yield to alcohol, water soluble extract etc.

(ii) Structural standards prescribe limitation for foreing material added for substitution. The standard prescribed for this kind of impurity is 2 per cent. So it is better that drugs are free from such materials, e.g., fungus, insects, hair rodents and other pests.

(iii) **Physical standards** are very useful for fats, oil, resins and waxes. Physical constants include average mass of plant members, density and refractive index.

STUDY QUESTIONS

1. Explain the meaning of adulteration.
2. Discuss the methods of drug evaluation.

■■■

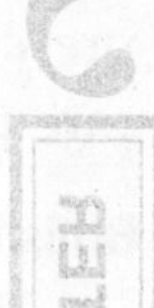

CHAPTER 5

CHEMICAL NATURE OF DRUGS OBTAINED FROM PLANTS

CARBOHYDRATE

A carbohydrate is any member of a widespread class of natural organic substances that includes sugars, starch and cellulose. The chemical composition of carbohydrates — as analysed in the nineteenth century — is a combination of carbon (C), hydrogen (H) and water (H_2O). Many carbohydrates have the general chemical formula $Cx(H_2O)x$, but the class is too large to fit into a simple chemical formula. Carbohydrates are often isomers — meaning, they have the same atomic composition but different structures. Fructose, galactose and glucose are isomers with the chemical formula $C_6H_{12}O_6$. There are many classification schemes for carbohydrates. The most common one separates them into four major groups: *mono-saccharides, disaccharides, oligosaccharides* and *poly-saccharides*.

TYPES OF CARBOHYDRATES

Carbohydrates, also known as *saccharides,* are classified according to the number of single carbohydrate molecules in each chemical structure. Carbohydrate compounds having just one carbohydrate molecule are called *monosaccharides*; compounds with two carbohydrate molecules are called *dissarcharides*; and those compounds containing more than two carbohydrate molecules are named *polysaccharides*. All carbohydrates either are monosaccharides or can be hydrolyzed (broken down) into two or more monosaccharides.

1. MONOSACCHARIDES

These are the only sugars that can be absorbed and utilized by the body. Disaccharides and polysaccharides must be ultimately broken down into monosaccharides in the digestive process known as *hydrolysis*.

(i) Glucose (also known as Dextrose or Grape Sugar)

This monosaccharide is the most important carbohydrate in human nutrition because it is the one that the body fuses directly to supply its energy needs. Glucose is formed from the hydrolysis of di- and polysaccharides, including starch, dextrin, maltose, sucrose and lactose; from the monosaccharide fructose largely during absorption; and from both fructose and galactose in the liver during metabolism.

Glucose is the carbohydrate found in the bloodstream, and it provides an immediate source of energy for the body's cells and tissues. Glucose is also formed when stored body carbohydrate (glycogen) is broken down for use.

Fruits and vegetables are wholesome food sources of glucose. It is also present in such unwholesome (to humans) substances as *molasses, honey* and *corn syrup*.

(ii) Fructose (also known as Levulose or Fruit Sugar)

Fructose, a monosaccharide, is very similar to another monosaccharide, galactose. These two simple sugars share the same chemical formula; however, the arrangements of their chemical groups along the chemical chain differ. Fructose is the sweetest of all the sugars and is found in fruits, vegetables and the nectar of flowers, as well as in the unwholesome (to humans) sweeteners, molasses and honey. In humans, fructose is produced during the hydrolysis of the disaccharide, sucrose.

(iii) Galactose

Galactose differs from the other simple sugars, glucose and fructose, in that it does not occur free in nature. It is produced in the body in the digestion of lactose, a disaccharide.

2. DISACCHARIDES

Disaccharides, on hydrolysis, yield two monosaccharide molecules. Three particular disaccharides warrant discussion in a lesson on nutritional science: sucrose, maltose and lactose.

(i) Sucrose

The disaccharide, sucrose, consists of one molecule of each of two monosaccharides-glucose and fructose. Sucrose is found in fruits and vegetables and is particularly plentiful in sugar beets (roots) and sugarcane (a grass). Refined white and brown sugars are close to 100% sucrose because almost everything else (including the other kinds of sugars present, the vitamins, the minerals and the proteins) have been removed in the refining process. Maple syrup and molasses are, like refined sugars, unwholesome sweeteners; both contain over 50% sucrose. It almost goes without saying that any foods, so-called, containing significant amounts of refined sugar are high in sucrose.

(ii) Maltose (also known as Malt Sugar)

This disaccharide, unlike sucrose, is not consumed in large amounts in the average American diet. It is found in malted cereals, malted milks and sprouted grains. Also, corn syrup is 26 percent maltose and corn sugar is 4 percent maltose. None of these "foods" is wholesome, with perhaps, the exception of sprouted grains.

Maltose occurs in the body as an intermediate product of starch digestion. (Starch is a polysaccharide.) When maltose is hydrolyzed, it yields two molecules of glucose.

(iii) Lactose (also known as Milk Sugar)

This disaccharide is found only in milk. Human milk contains about 4.8 g per 100 ml and cow's milk contains approximately 6.8 g per 100 ml. When lactose is hydrolyzed it yields one unit of the monosaccharide glucose and one unit of the monosaccharide galactose. The enzyme lactase is needed to digest lactose, and this enzyme is not present in most, if any, people over age three. This is one of the many reasons why milk is an unwholesome food for people over three years of age.

3. POLYSACCHARIDES

Like the disaccharides, the polysaccharides cannot be directly utilized by the body. They must first be broken down into monosaccharides, the only sugar form the body can use.

Polysaccharides contain up to 60,000 simple carbohydrate molecules. These carbohydrate molecules are arranged in long chains in either a straight or in a branched structure. There are four polysaccharides that are important in the study of nutritional science: starch, dextrin, glycogen and cellulose.

(i) Starch

Starch is abundant in the plant world and is found in granular form in the cells of plants. Starch granules can be seen under a microscope and they differ in size, shape and markings in various plants. The starch granules of wheat, for example, are oval-shaped; whereas the starch granules of corn are small, rounded and angular.

These starch granules are laid down in the storage organs of plants-in the seeds, tubers, roots and stem pith. They provide a reserve food supply for the plant, sustain the root or tuber through the winter and nourish the growing embryo during germination.

Most starches are a mix of two different molecular structures, amylose and amylopectin. The former has a linear structure and the latter has a branched or bushy structure. The proportion of the two fractions varies according to the species of plant. For example, potato starch and most cereal starches have approximately 15-30% amylose. But the waxy cereal grains, including some varieties of corn plus rice and grain sorghum, have their starch most entirely as amylopectin. The starches in green peas and in some sweet corn varieties are mainly amylose.

The polysaccharides, as mentioned earlier, are not water soluble as are the mono- and disaccharides. Though not water soluble, starches can be dispersed in water heated to a certain temperature. The granules swell and gelatinize. When cooled, this gelatin sets to a paste. The jelling characteristics of starches are considered to result from the amylose present, while amylopectin is considered to be responsible for the gummy and cohesive properties of the paste.

(ii) Dextrin

There are several "varieties" of this polysaccharide. Dextrins are most commonly consumed in cooked starch foods, as they are obtained from starch by the action of heat. Dextrins are intermediary products of starch digestion, also, and are formed by the action of amylases on starches. They render the disaccharide maltose on hydrolysis.

(iii) Glycogen

Glycogen is the reserve carbohydrate in humans. It is to animals as starch is to plants. Glycogen is very similar to amylopectin, having a high molecular weight and branched-chain structures made up of thousands of glucose molecules. The main difference between glycogen and amylopectin is that glycogen has more and shorter branches, resulting in a more compact, bushlike molecule with greater solubility and lower viscosity (less stickiness or gumminess).

Glycogen is stored primarily in the liver and muscles of animals. About two-thirds of total body glycogen is stored in the muscles and about one-third is stored in the liver.

(iv) Cellulose

Like starch and glycogen, cellulose is composed of thousands of glucose molecules. It comprises over 50% of the carbon in vegetation and is the structural constituent of the cell walls of plants. Cellulose is, therefore, the most abundant naturally-occurring organic substance. It is characterized by its insolubility, its chemical inertness and its physical rigidity. This polysaccharide can be digested only by herbivores such as cows, sheep, horses, etc., as these animals have bacteria in their rumens (stomachs) whose enzyme systems breakdown cellulose molecules. Humans do not have the enzyme needed to digest cellulose, so it is passed through the digestive tract unchanged.

NUMBER OF CARBONS

Monosaccharides can be further classified by the number of carbons present.

Hexoses (6-carbons) are by far the most prevalent.

Number of Carbons		
Six = Hexose	**Five = Pentose**	**Three = Triose**
Glucose	Ribose	Glyceraldehyde
Galactose		
Fructose		

FUNCTIONAL GROUPS

Aldoses contain the *aldehyde group*. Monosaccharides in this group are glucose, galactose, ribose, and glyceraldehyde.

Ketoses contain the *ketone group*. The major sugar in this group is fructose.

Reducing contain a *hemiacetal* or *hemiketal group*. Sugars include, glucose, galactose, fructose, maltose, lactose.

Non-reducing contain *no hemiacetal groups*. Sucrose and all polysaccharides are in this group.

FUNCTION

The primary function of carbohydrates is to provide energy for the body, especially the brain and the nervous system. An enzyme called amylase helps break down carbohydrates into glucose (blood sugar), which is used for energy by the body.

FOOD SOURCES

Carbohydrates are classified as simple or complex. The classification depends on the chemical structure of the food, and how quickly the sugar is digested and absorbed. Simple carbohydrates have one (single) or two (double) sugars. Complex carbohydrates have three or more sugars.

TESTS FROM DRUGS CONTAINING CARBOHYDRATES

OSAZONE FORMATION

An aqueous solution of phenylhydrazine hydrochloride buffered with sodium acetate is added to each of glucose, fructose, and sucrose. They are heated.

Narrative. An aqueous solution of phenylhydrazine hydrochloride buffered with sodium acetate is added to three test tubes containing glucose, fructose, and sucrose. The solutions are heated in a boiling water bath. Reducing sugars do not form simple phenylhydrazone derivatives. Instead two molecules of phenylhydrazine condense with each molecule of sugar to produce a solid derivative called an *osazone*. A yellow solid rapidly forms with fructose and a short time later with glucose. Sucrose does not react for at least 30 minutes when it begins to hydrolyze.

SELIWANOFF'S TEST

Seliwanoff's test is a chemical test which distinguishes between aldose and ketose sugars. Ketoses are distinguished from aldoses via their ketone/aldehyde functionality. If the sugar contains a ketone group, it is a ketose and if it contains an aldehyde group, it is an aldose. This test is based on the fact that, when heated, ketoses are more rapidly dehydrated than aldoses.

MOLISCH'S TEST

Molisch's test is a colour test for sugar, which condenses with α-naphthol or thymol in the presence of strong sulfuric acid, which converts the sugar to furfural derivatives.

A positive reaction is characterized by the appearance of a purple ring at the interface of the test tube. All carbohydrates, whether monosaccharide, disaccharide, and polysaccharide should react positively to this test.

FEHLING'S TEST

Blue copper sulfate is mixed with a solution of potassium hydroxide and potassium sodium tartrate to form a deep blue solution of *Fehling's reagent*. The solution is heated on a hot plate. Later, sucrose is added and no change is observed. On the other hand, glucose, a reducing sugar, reacts with Fehling's reagent to form a brick red precipitate of copper (I) oxide.

ALKALOIDS

Alkaloids are the natural compounds found in all vegetables that include nitrogen and are considered to be disintegration of substances that comprise proteins. They are exuded in particular cells or tubes and can be of great use in safeguard against normal enemies as they have a bitter flavour.

Generally, alkaloids are amalgams that do not have any scent and boast of a distinctive outcome on the animals' body mechanism or function. Owing to these properties, alkaloids have significant therapeutic value and form the ingredients of many important medicines. The alkaloids also comprise strong vegetable toxics and sedatives. Substances like caffeine and theobromine that are closely associated with natural purine (substance that can be converted to uric acid in the body) compounds are normally categorized as alkaloids.

CLASSIFICATION OF ALKALOIDS

PYRROLIDINE ALKALOIDS

Alkaloids are basically derived from the amino acid called ornithine. This cluster of amino acid comprises the tropane alkaloids, atropine, hyoscine and hyoscyamine from the family of nightshade. For instance, the nightshade family includes henbane, belladonna, datura (thornapple), and bittersweet.

Acting as a cluster these alkaloids impede the activities of parasympathetic nerve (originates in the lower part of the spinal cord and brain stem, stimulates digestive secretions, opposes physiological effects of the sympathetic nervous system, constricts the pupils; slows the heart, dilates blood vessels). Incidentally, the pyrrolidine alkaloids also comprise the 'truth medication' scopolamine (also known as hyoscine) and cocaine.

PYRIDINE AND PIPERIDINE ALKALOIDS

Pyridine and piperidine alkaloids are a mono carbon hoop including one nitrogen atom and this group of alkaloids comprises numerous species of toxic plants that include *venomous hemlock* (Conium maculatum), *tobacco* (Nicotiana tobacum) and *lobelia*. Incidentally, while tobacco is a member of the nightshade family, scientifically known as *Solanaceae*, poison hemlock is a constituent of the carrot family or *Apiaceae*. Coniine, a single ring compound produced in the plant from octanoic acid is a toxic alkaloid present in poison hemlock that is responsible for paralysis, asphyxia (suffocation) and ultimately death.

PYRROLIZIDINE AND QUINOLIZIDINE ALKALOIDS

Pyrrolizidine and quinolizidine are a complicated group. Incidentally, this group of alkaloids has always proved to be of immense pharmacological interest for researchers and clinical examiners. All these alkaloids are known to have lethal features and may prove to be fatal. While pyrrolizidine is obtained from ornithine and is known to be injurious for the liver, quinolizidine is obtained from amino acid called *lysine*.

Pyrrolizidine is generally found in ragworts, which is a problem for the grazing animals, comfrey, borage and coltsfoot. In the last instance, the evidence for toxicity is smaller and still unclear.

INDOLE ALKALOIDS

Indole alkaloids comprise serotonin chemically know as 5-hydroxyltryptamine or 5-HT and others of their kind. These comprise the anesthetizing alkaloids of the passion flower, ophthalmic alkaloids associated with the physostigmine derived from the calabar bean as well as the uterine tonics such as ergotamine. This variety of alkaloids also comprises the Indian snakeroot or the *Rauwolfia serpentaria* that consist of reserpine. It may be mentioned here that reserpine contains potent hypotensive and when isolated from the entire plant possess depressive consequences. Among the numerous central nervous stimulants such as strychnine, psilocybin and johimbine, indole alkaloids comprise indole carbon-nitrogen loop. Indole carbon-nitrogen ring is also present in the fungal alkaloids ergine and psilocybin, the neurotransmitter serotonin as well as the mind jerking medication LSD.

QUINOLINE ALKALOIDS

Quinoline alkaloids include twofold carbon rings comprising one nitrogen atom (N) and they enclose quinine from the bark of *Cinchona ledgeriana*. Incidentally, Cinchona ledgeriana is a South American tree in the coffee family (Rubiaceae). The alkaloid quinine is poisonous to *Plasmodium vivax* and three supplementary classes, including the single-celled organisms or protozoans that cause malaria.

The microbes attack the red blood cells where they multiply, finally escaping from the split cells. The ailment is differentiated by interludes of high temperature and chills, linked with the concurrent break of red blood cells. Malaria is certainly one of the most widespread ailments all over the humid expanses of the globe, and it is spread through the bite or blood meal of the female *Anopheles mosquito*.

ISOQUINOLINE ALKALOIDS

Isoquinoline alkaloids are associated with quinoline alkaloids and constitute an important division of the alkaloid family. Isoquinoline alkaloids can be divided into several sub-classes and among others, comprise elements such as simple isoquinolines, benzylisoquinolines, phthalideisoquinolines, protopines, morphine alkaloids, protoberberines as well as ipecac alkaloids.

Simple isoquinolines are the alkaloids of mescaline cactus or Lopophora willamsii such as mescaline, while benzylisoquinolines are antecedents of many alkaloids that comprise opium poppy's papaverine. On the other hand, *phthalideisoquinolines* encompass all narcotine, protopines are restricted to the poppy family comprising protopine and protoberberines include berberine, hydrastine, canadine among others. Protoberberines are derived from *Berberis* sp., as well as golden seal.

Morphine alkaloids include morphine, codeine and thebaine all from the opium poppy family, whereas ipecac alkaloids comprise emetic alkaloid emetine obtained from ipecacuanha.

Isoquinoline alkaloids comprise two-fold carbon loop that contains one nitrogen atom (N). This form of alkaloid comprises the narcotic alkaloids generally present in particular members of the poppy family or *Papaveraceae* like the opium poppy or *Papaver somniferum.*

In fact, when we use the term narcotic, it is generally points to the pain-relieving and sleep-inducing qualities of these intensely addictive alkaloids that include substances like *morphine, codeine* and *thebaine.*

A major source of a powerful isoquinoline alkaloid utilized in curing deadly poisons is *Chondodendron tomentosum,* a member of the *Menispermaceae* family, which is an extract from the barks and stem of a vine indigenous to South America. Indians in the Amazon area use this sticky derivative to cover the venomous nips of their blowguns - their amour against enemies as well as for hunting. Alkaloid D-tubocurarine possess a special healing power as it actively obstructs the acetylcholine receptor spots at the neuromuscular intersections enabling muscles to unwind as well as protect them from paralysis. This variety of alkaloid is also effective in relaxing as well as preventing the paralysis of the muscles in the respiratory tract as well as the heart.

Significantly, D-tubocurarine alkaloids have been extensively used to unwind the muscles of the heart during open heart surgeries.

In addition, this variety of alkaloid has also been used by medicos in curing spastic or convulsive paralysis of tetanus venom that causes unmanageable retrenchment of muscle all over the body.

PURINE ALKALOIDS

Purine alkaloids normally include caffeine, theophylline, theobromine and aminophyline which are obtained from cocoa, tea and coffee. These substances are collectively named xanthines as they are obtained from the purine nucleotides adenine and guanine. They are medicinally beneficial as they are active in extending the effectual life of a number of hormones such as adrenaline.

By the by, purine alkaloids contain a molecular arrangement amazingly analogous to the nitrogenous purine base adenine that is generally present in DNA, RNA and ATP. Purine alkaloids comprise a two-fold carbon sphere containing four nitrogen atoms (N). Predominantly among the purine alkaloids are moderate invigorators like coffee or *Coffea Arabica* in the coffee species or *Rubiaceae*. Tea or Camellia sinensis in the tea family or Theaceae, yerba mate or Ilex paraguariensis a member of the holly species or Aquifoliaeae, guarana or Paullinia cupana in the soapberry species or *Sapindaceae* and cola or Cola nitida in the chocolate species scientifically known as *Sterculiaceae*.

Incidentally, the most important origin of theobromine is from the seeds or beans of cacao scientifically known as Theobroma cacao. In fact, Theobroma cacao is one more member of the chocolate family that is scientifically called Sterculiaceae.

TERPENOID ALKALOIDS

Generally speaking, terpenoid alkaloids are an assortment of amalgams or compounds that are obtained biosynthetically through different procedures that produce a number of group of terpenes like sesquiterpenoids, montoterpenoids, diterpenoids as well as steroids. Incidentally, this variety of alkaloids is found in an irregular manner in the plant kingdom.

For instance, the monoterpenoid alkaloids like gentianine are usually found in the plant family *Gentianaceae*. *Sesquiterpenoids,* for instance, dendrobine are generally found in the *Orchidaceae* or cassinine in the *Celastraceae,* diterpenoids like aconitine are found in the *Ranunculaceae* family and steroidal alkaloids. Similarly, buxamine is found in discrete plant families like Buxaceae, protoverine is located in the Liliacea and solanidine in the Solanaceae. Interestingly, a number of terpenoid alkaloids also display anti-feedant and anti-fungal features. And most importantly, the fascinating alkaloids in this sub-group are present in the genus Veratrum and they are normally beneficial for curing hypertension (high blood pressure), neuralgia as well as rheumatism.

EXTRACTION OF ALKALOIDS

The extraction of alkaloids from plants was one of the major activities of people studying alchemy. Alkaloids were considered to be the secret of any particular plant. They were commonly used in medicine as well as for recreational uses. Opium extracted from the Opium poppy though very controversial today due to its use in the manufacture of heroin was in an earlier time used to control pain. Digitalis out of the Foxglove plant was used to fight heart disease and reduce the risk of heart attack.

These days the medicinal use of alkaloids from plants is overshadowed by the great media attention given to recreational drugs. Alkaloids were used for recreational purposes for a long time before some of them were classified as illegal. Funnily enough the motives behind their sudden illegal status were not related to the well being of the population. *Cannabis/Marijuana* was forced into illegal status by the powerful lobby of the owners of plantations who feared that the apparently very versatile and useful hemp plant would be used to force them out of business.

ADVANCED TECHNIQUES

The basic principle of drug manufacture is to extract the alkaloid from the plant matter for further use. A lot of plants contain very interesting substances known as alkaloids, these alkaloids are what recreational drugs are made of. To extract this alkaloid from the plant an extraction technique is used based on the solubility properties of the substance in different liquids that have different levels of acidity. This is a lot more complicated than the techniques discussed above but yields a very potent product. Examples of products by this technique are *Opium, DMT* and *Ephedrine*. It requires additional equipment such as a vacuum filtration funnel to perform the extraction process.

METHODS OF ISOLATE ALKALOIDS FROM PLANTS

To isolate alkaloids from plants, the dried and powdered plant material is extracted with pet ether (or hexane, colemans etc.) first. This removes fats, oils, terpenes, waxes etc. This extract is discarded.

The material is now subjected to an alcohol extraction, e.g., with methanol or ethanol. The extract is evaporated to leave the crude alkaloids mixture.

This extract is partitioned between an diluted aq. tartaric acid solution and ethyl acetate. Other acids like citric acid can be used, and other solvents may substitute here. The ethyl acetate layer contains neutral and weakly basic alkaloids. Evaporate the solvent to isolate them.

The aqeous layer is neutralised with NH_3 or Na_2CO_3 and again extracted with ethyl acetate. The organic layer now contains basic alkaloids, while the aqeous layer contains quarternary ammonium ions.

Many alkaloids can be isolated directly from the alkoholic extract by chromatographic methods. This is a separation which works well for tropane alkaloids (atropine, cocaine, scopolamine).

The alcohol extract is fractionated by column chromatography on SiO_2, solvent chloroform followed by chloroform with rising methanol content. This separates lipids and terpenes from the crude alkaloid fraction. The alkaloid fraction is again chromatographed (SiO_2; $CHCl_3$: MeOH = 10:1) to isolate the pure alkaloids.

VOLATILE OILS

Volatile oils are a class of Volatile Organic Compounds derived from plants through distillation. It takes many kg of a plant to produce a tiny amount of the essential oils. For example, almost 8 kg of peppermint goes into making an ounce of the essential oil.

The oils are called "volatile" because they evaporate (become airborne) at low temperatures - room temperature for many. Care must be taken in the distillation process to preserve the key components (hydrocarbons or terpenes); overheating, for instance, will release the oils into the atmosphere and render the remaining substance impotent.

Essential oils that retain the volatile component have many uses. Some have antibacterial, antimutagenic and even antitumour effects.

Generally speaking volatile oils are mixtures of hydrocarbons and oxygenated compounds derived there from. As the oxygenated form is more soluble in both water and alcohol, it is this form that on the whole determines the taste and smell of the mixture. The most common hydrocarbon is the terpene, built up by the successive accumulation of isoprene molecules (CsHs).

PROPERTIES OF VOLATILE OILS

1. Chemicals that evaporate at room temperature.
2. Oil having the odour or flavour of the plant from which it comes; used in perfume and flavourings
3. Highly concentrated aromatic extracts which are distilled from a variety of aromatic plant material including grasses, leaves, flowers, needles and twigs, peel of fruit, wood and roots.

These are the substances to which many plants owe their characteristic or essential odours. On this account they are often spoken of as "essential oils," or as the "essences" of plants.

They *differ* from the *fixed oils* in that –

1. They are volatile, therefore can be distilled and do not leave a permanent grease stain.
2. They do not form soaps with alkalies.
3. They are soluble enough in water to impart to it their odour and taste.
4. They do not become rancid, but on exposure to light and air tend to oxidize and resinify.

They mix freely in any proportions with chloroform, ether, and the fixed oils, and are all soluble in absolute alcohol. Some, like oil of turpentine, require several times their own weight of official alcohol for complete solution. They are all mixtures, some of them quite complex.

METHODS OF PREPARATION OF VOLATILE OILS

The majority of volatile oils are produced by distillation. With certain oils, chiefly those valued for their aroma (e.g., oil of lemon), a distillation process would promote oxidation or other changes in the constituents of the oil, and impair its flavouring power. For these oils a process not involving the use of heat is adopted.

Preparation by Distillation

The boiling-point of many volatile oils is above 200° and at this high temperature chemical changes, e.g., oxidation, would in some instances take place.

Distillation of a volatile oil with water follows the law governing the distillation of immiscible liquids, namely that distillation takes place when the sum of the vapour pressures is equal to the atmospheric pressure. Hence the boiling-point of such a "mixture" would be lower than that of the constituent with the lower boiling-point. In other words, below the boiling-point of water (100°). The process of distillation after admixture with water therefore provides a means of separating a volatile oil from the drug in which it occurs, at a much lower temperature than would be possible without the addition of water. Further, if water were not added, considerable carbonisation of the drug would take place, and the resultant volatile decomposition products would distil over with the oil and render it useless.

Direct heating of a mixture of drug and water by a naked flame would, similarly, cause partial carbonisation: of the layer of drug resting on the bottom of the still, and again volatile decomposition products would give an empyreumatic odour to the volatile oil, and impair its value. Consequently some forms of still for the production of volatile oils are provided with a false, perforated bottom, below which is placed the water. Upon heating, steam rises through the perforations, passes through the drug and on to the condenser, carrying with it the volatile oil.

In the more modern stills the admixture is heated by means of a steam coil.

PREPARATION BY SCARIFICATION

This method is used for the preparation of oil of lemon, oil of orange, and oil of bergamot. These oils are found in large oil-glands just below the surface in the peel of the fruit. The two principal methods of scarification are the "sponge," and the ecuelle a piquer. The "sponge" process is used almost exclusively for the production of oil of lemon and oil of bergamot in Sicily and Southern Italy, whence the bulk of the world's supply is obtained. The *ecuelle* a *piquer method* is used in Southern France for the preparation of oil of lemon.

(a) Sponge Process

In the sponge process the lemons are halved transversely, or longitudinally when the peel is required for candied peel. The contents of the fruit are then removed, and after the peel has been immersed in water for a short time it is ready for expression. The operator takes a sponge in one hand, and with the other presses the softener! peel against the sponge, so that the oil-glands burst open and the sponge absorbs the exuded oil, which is transferred to a collecting vessel. The turbid liquid consisting of oil and water is allowed to stand for a short time, whereupon the oil separates as an upper layer which is poured off. It still contains a small proportion of water and suspended matter, which is removed by repeated decantation after suitable periods for sedimentation. The whole of the above process is carried out in cool darkened rooms in order to minimize the harmful effects of heat and light on the oil.

(b) Ecuelle a Piquer Process

For the ecuelle a piquer process the apparatus is made of pewter, and takes the form of a cup-shaped funnel about 25 cm. across. It is provided with a lip and short, closed stem, which serves both as a handle and as a reservoir for the exuded oil. Projecting from the inner surface of the cup are numerous brass pins across which the softened peel is drawn with a rotary movement. The liquid exuding from the ruptured oil glands collects in the stem, whence it is transferred to a collecting vessel and treated.

HYDROCARBONS IN ESSENTIAL OILS

Terpenes (unsaturated hydrocarbons; a phytochemical) can take the following forms:

Monoterpenes (primary alcohols containing 10 carbon atoms). The most common grouping of volatile oils. Examples of this class include—*camphor, menthol, Thujone, Thymol, Nerol, Linalool, Limonene, Geraniol, perillyl alcohol,* found in such plant matter as *citrus peels, mint leaves, lavender,* and *thyme*. These phytochemicals are known to *trigger apoptosis* ('suicide' in defective cells) and to inhibit the synthesis of cholesterol in the liver.

Sesquiterpenes (contain 15 carbon atoms). Found mainly in higher plants, sesquiterpene volatile oils are not as commonly found as monoterpines. Examples include *Nerolidol, Farnesol,*

Ylangene, found in Neroli, *mints, sandalwood, ginger*, and *German chamomile*. These phytochemicals have anti-allergen and anti-inflammatory properties.

USE

As a rule, do not use volatile oils undiluted on skin. Mix with carrier oils, creams, or lotions. You can decide which option to use depending on the area of the body being massaged and the specific properties of the volatile/essential oil.

OCCURRENCE

Most of them are found in plants, and each in a definite part of the plant from which it is derived, e.g., oil of orange in the rind of the fruit; oil of cinnamon in the bark; oil of rose in the petals. From these parts they are obtained either by distillation or by means of a suitable solvent, such as benzin, which is afterward removed. Some of the delicate essential oils used in perfumery, as violet and heliotrope, are obtained by spreading the petals or flowers between wax plates, and afterward separating the absorbed oil from the wax.

A few of the volatile oils do not exist in the living plant, and are formed either by the action of ferments on glucosides in the presence of water, as the oil of bitter almonds, or by destructive distillation. These latter are known as empyreumatic oils.

For convenience, the volatile oils preexisting in the plant may be grouped according to their nature, and those developed in the plant part by artificial means may be grouped according to their method of production.

For convenience, the ***volatile oils*** preexisting in the plant may be grouped according to their nature, and those developed in the plant part by artificial means may be grouped according to their ***method of production***.

A. Existing in Plant as Such

1. Terpenes, Cxhx (oils of turpentine, juniper, etc.).
2. Terpenes + stearoptens (oils of lemon, peppermint, etc.).

B. Not Existing in Plant as such, but Developed from Plant Constituents

3. From enzyme action (oils of mustard and bitter almond).
4. Empyreumatic (oil of cade, oil of tar, creosote).

Group 1 is composed of oils which are mixtures of terpenes (hemiterpenes, terpenes, sesquiterpenes, diterpenes, pinene, etc., $C_{10}H_{16}$), the simplest hydrocarbon oils of the aromatic series. Of all the volatile oils, they are the least soluble in water and the most ready to resinify and deteriorate. Examples are: the oils of copaiba, cubebs, erigeron, juniper, and turpentine. The last named consists almost wholly of dextrorotary pinene.

Group 2 includes the mixtures of terpenes which are holding in solution one or more oxygenated bodies (of variable chemic nature, as aldehydes, ketones, ethers, acids, etc.). The terpene portion is known as the eleopten, and the oxygenated portion as the stearopten. The latter is usually solid, though sometimes liquid. It can be separated from the eleopten by cold (as the menthol of peppermint oil) or by fractional distillation. It is not always readily soluble in 95 per cent alcohol. Examples of stearoptens which are separated and used by themselves are camphor and menthol. It is to the stearopten that the characteristic odour of these oils is chiefly due, but the amount of stearopten present varies with the different oils. For example, the oils of orange or lemon contain only a small percentage of their peculiar stearopten and are nearly all eleopten, while the oils of winter-green and birch are almost entirely composed of a liquid stearopten, which chemically is methyl salicylate.

The oils of this group are for the most part more soluble in water, and, because of the stearopten, more agreeable in flavour than those of Group 1, so they are largely used in the manufacture of the medicated waters and spirits. Some of them are heavier than water, as the oil of cinnamon.

Group 3 contains those oils which do not preexist in the living plant, but result from ferment action in the presence of water. The official ones are the oil of bitter almond and the volatile oil of mustard.

Group 4 contains the empyreumatic oils, those which do not preexist in the plant, but result from its destructive distillation. The official ones are: *Oil of cade* (oleum cadinum), from juniper wood, and *oil of tar* (oleum picis liquidae), from the wood of *Pinus palustris* and other species of pine. Both have a tarry odour, and are added to ointments for the treatment of *chronic skin diseases*.

OILS CONSISTING CHIELFY HYDROCARBONS

Terpenes. These are isomeric substances of the formula $C_{10}H_{16}$ but they vary considerably in structure. In volatile oils almost all the terpenes, and similarly the sesquiterpenes, occur in an optically active form. In common with all substances containing an asymmetric carbon atom, they are able to rotate the plane of polarized light either to the right (*dextro-rotatory*), or to the left (*Levo-rotatory*). The more important terpenes are:

Pinene. This is widely distributed in volatile oils, d-pinene being the principal constituent of American oil of turpentine, and l-pinene of French oil of turpentine.

Limonene. The d-form (also known as *citrene*, and *carvene*) is the principal terpene in oils of lemon, caraway, and dill; L-limonene is present in small proportion in oil of lemon; dl-limonene, a mixture containing equal proportions of both, and therefore optically inactive, occurs in oils of nutmeg, and Siberian fir. It is also known as *dipentene*. Terebene, an artificial terpene prepared from oil of turpentine, consists almost wholly of dipentene.

Phellandrene. This terpene occurs in oil of Siberian fir, and is present to a considerable extent in the oil obtained from species of Eucalyptus, e.g., *Eucalyptus amygdalina*. Its presence in substantial proportion in eucalyptus oil used for medicinal purposes is undesirable, and therefore the Pharmacopoeia prescribes a test which excludes oils containing an undue proportion.

Camphene. This terpene is exceptional in being solid at room temperature. It occurs in small quantities in oils of rosemary and Siberian fir .

Sesquiterpenes. These also are isomeric, their general formula being $C_{15}H_{24}$. As earlier stated, they are usually the highest-boiling fraction of the oils in which they occur. The principal sesquiterpenes occurring in official volatile oils are *Oaryophyllene*. This is the main constituent of oil of copaiba, and is present in oil of clove.

Oadinene. This is found in oils of cubebs, cade, and lemon. With the terpene pinene, it comprises almost the whole of oil of juniper. Other constituents, occurring in small proportions, are azulene, to which is due the blue tint of freshly distilled oil of chamomile, santalene, present in oil of sandal wood, and bisabolene, in oil of lemon.

Polyterpenes. These substances have the same empirical formula, C_5H_8, as the terpenes and sesquiterpenes, but they are more complex. The only official volatile oil which consists principally of terpenes is Oil of Turpentine.

GLYCOSIDES

Glycosides are molecules in which a sugar is bound to a non-carbohydrate moiety, usually a small organic molecule. Glycosides play numerous important roles in living organisms. Many plants store chemicals in the form of inactive glycosides; which can be activated by enzyme hydrolysis. This causes the sugar part to be broken off, making the chemical available for use. Many such plant glycosides are used as medications. In animals (including humans), poisons are often bound to sugar molecules as part of their elimination from the body.

Formally, a glycoside is any molecule in which a sugar group is bonded through its anomeric carbon to another group via a glycosidic bond. Glycosides can be linked by an O- (an O-glycoside), N- (a glycosylamine), S- (a thioglycoside) or C- (a C-glycosyl) glycosidic bond. The given definition is the one used by IUPAC.

The sugar group is then known as the ***glycone*** and the non-sugar group as the ***aglycone*** or genin part of the glycoside. The glycone can consist of a single sugar group (monosaccharide) or several sugar groups (oligosaccharide).

Alcoholic Glycosides

An example of an alcoholic glycoside is salicin which is found in the genus salix. Salicin is converted in the body into salicylic acid, which is closely related to aspirin and has analgesic, antipyretic and anti-inflammatory effects.

Anthraquinone Glycosides

These glycosides contain an aglycone group that is a derivative of anthraquinone. They are present in senna, rhubarb and aloes; they have a laxative effect.

Coumarin Glycosides

Here the aglycone is coumarin. An example is apterin which is reported to dilate the coronary arteries as well as block calcium channels. Those obtained from dried leaves of Psoralia corylifolia have main glycosides psoralin and corylifolin.

Cyanogenic Glycosides

In this case, the aglycone contains a cyanide group, and the glycoside can release the poisonous hydrogen cyanide if acted upon by some enzyme. They are stored in the vacuole but if the plant is attacked they are released and become activated by enzymes in the cytoplasm. These remove the sugar part of the molecule and release toxic hydrogen cyanide. Storing them in inactive forms in the cytoplasm prevents them from damaging the plant under normal conditions.

An example of these is *amygdalin* from almonds. They can also be found in the fruits (and wilting leaves) of the rose family (including cherries, apples, plums, almonds, peaches, apricots, raspberries, and crabapples). Cassava, an important food plant in Africa and South America, contains cyanogenic glycosides and therefore has to be washed and ground under running water prior to consumption. Sorghum (Sorghum bicolour) expresses cyanogenic glycosides in its roots and thus is resistant to pests such as rootworms (Diabrotica spp.) that plague its cousin maize (Zea mays L.). Some cyanogenic glycosides may have anti-cancer properties.

Flavonoid Glycosides

Here the aglycone is a flavonoid. This is a large group of flavonoid glycosides. Examples include:

— Hesperidin (aglycone : Hesperetin, glycone: Rutinose)
— Naringin (aglycone : Naringenin, glycone: Rutinose)
— Rutin (aglycone : Quercetin, glycone: Rutinose)
— Quercitrin (aglycone : Quercetin, glycone: Rhamnose)

Among the important effects of flavonoids are their antioxidant effect. They are also known to *decrease capillary fragility*.

Phenolic Glycosides (Simple)

The *aglycone* is a simple phenolic structure. An example is arbutin found in the Common Bearberry Arctostaphylos uva-ursi. It has a urinary antiseptic effect. Rutin found in rooibos tea.

Saponins

These compounds give a permanent froth when shaken with water. They also cause hemolysis of red blood cells. Saponin glycosides are found in liquorice. Their medicinal value is due to their expectorant effect.

Steroidal Glycosides or Cardiac Glycosides

Here the aglycone part is a steroidal nucleus. These glycosides are found in the plant genera Digitalis, Scilla, and Strophanthus. They are used in the treatment of heart diseases, e.g., congestive heart failure (historically as now recognised does not improve survivability; other agents are now preferred) and arrhythmia.

Steviol Glycosides

These sweet glycosides found in the stevia plant Stevia rebaudiana bertoni have 40-300 times the sweetness of sucrose. The two primary glycosides, stevioside and rebaudioside A, are used as natural sweeteners in many countries. These glycosides have steviol as the aglycone part. Glucose or rhamnose-glucose combinations are bound to the ends of the aglycone to form the different compounds.

Thioglycosides

As the name implies (q.v. thio-), these compounds contain sulfur. Examples include sinigrin, found in black mustard, and sinalbin, found in white mustard.

TANNINS

Tannins are astringent, bitter plant polyphenols that either bind and precipitate or shrink proteins. The astringency from the tannins is what causes the dry and puckery feeling in the mouth following the consumption of unripened fruit or red wine. Likewise, the destruction or modification of tannins with time plays an important role in the ripening of fruit and the aging of wine.

The term *tannin* refers to the use of wood tannins from oak in tanning animal hides into leather; however, the term is widely applied to any large polyphenolic compound containing sufficient hydroxyls and other suitable groups (such as carboxyls) to form strong complexes with proteins and other macromolecules. The compounds are widely distributed in many species of plants, where they play a role in protection from predation and perhaps also in growth regulation.

Tannins are incompatible with alkalis, gelatin, heavy metals, iron, lime water, metallic salts, strong oxidizing agents and zinc sulfate.

OCCURRENCE

Tannins are distributed in species throughout the plant kingdom. They are commonly found in both gymnosperms as well as angiosperms. Histologically tannins are mainly physically located in the vacuoles or surface wax of plants. These storage sites keep tannins active against plant predators, but also keep some tannins from affecting plant metabolism while the plant tissue is alive; it is only after cell breakdown and death that the tannins are active in metabolic effects.

Tannins are found in leaf tissues, bud tissues, seed tissues, root tissues and stem tissues. An example of the location of the tannins in stem tissue is that they are often found in the growth areas of trees, such as the secondary phloem and xylem and the layer between the cortex and epidermis. Tannins may help regulate the growth of these tissues.

They are also found in the heartwood of conifers and may play a role in inhibiting microbial activity, thus resulting in the natural durability of the wood.

There may be a loss in the bioavailability of still other tannins in plants due to birds, pests, and other pathogens.

The leaching of tannins from the decaying leaves of vegetation adjoining a stream may produce what is known as a blackwater river.

HYDROLYSABLE TANNINS

At the center of a hydrolysable tannin molecule, there is a carbohydrate (usually D-glucose). The hydroxyl groups of the carbohydrate are partially or totally esterified with phenolic groups such as gallic acid (in gallotannins) or ellagic acid (in ellagitannins). Hydrolyzable tannins are hydrolyzed by weak acids or weak bases to produce carbohydrate and phenolic acids.

Examples of gallotannins are the gallic acid esters of glucose in tannic acid ($C_{76}H_{52}O_{46}$), found in the leaves and bark of many plant species.

CONDENSED TANNINS

Condensed tannins, also known as proanthocyanidins, are polymers of 2 to 50 (or more) flavonoid units that are joined by carbon-carbon bonds, which are not susceptible to being cleaved by hydrolysis. While hydrolyzable tannins and most condensed tannins are water soluble, some very large condensed tannins are insoluble.

USES

Tannins may be employed medicinally in antidiarrheal, hemostatic, and antihemorrhoidal compounds.

The anti-inflammatory effect of tannins help control all indications of gastritis, esophagitis, enteritis, and irritating bowel disorders. Diarrhoea is also treated with an effective astringent medicine that does not stop the flow of the disturbing substance in the stomach; rather, it controls the irritation in the small intestine.

Tannins not only heal burns and stop bleeding, but they also stop infection while they continue to heal the wound internally. The ability of tannins to form a protective layer over the exposed tissue keeps the wound from being infected even more. Tannins are also beneficial when applied to the mucosal lining of the mouth.

Tannins can also be effective in protecting the kidneys. Tannins have been used for immediate relief of sore throats, diarrhea, dysentery, hemorrhaging, fatigue, skin ulcers and as a cicatrizant on gangrenous wounds. Tannins can cause regression of tumors that are already present in tissue, but if used excessively over time, they can cause tumors in healthy tissue. Tannins are used indirectly as molluscicides to interrupt the transmission cycle of schistosomiasis. They have also been reported to have anti-viral effects. When incubated with red grape juice and red wines with a high content of condensed tannins, the poliovirus, herpes simplex virus, and various enteric viruses are inactivated.

LIPIDS

Lipids are a broad group of naturally-occurring molecules which includes fats, waxes, sterols, fat-soluble vitamins (such as vitamins A, D, E and K), monoglycerides, diglycerides, phospholipids, and others. The main biological functions of lipids include energy storage, as structural components of cell membranes, and as important signaling molecules.

Lipids may be broadly defined as hydrophobic or amphiphilic small molecules; the amphiphilic nature of some lipids allows them to form structures such as vesicles, liposomes, or membranes in an aqueous environment. Biological lipids originate entirely or in part from two distinct types of biochemical subunits or "building blocks"– *ketoacyl* and *isoprene* groups.

Using this approach, lipids may be divided into eight categories: *fatty acyls, glycerolipids, glycerophospholipids, sphingolipids, saccharolipids* and *polyketides* (derived from condensation of ketoacyl subunits); and *sterol lipids* and *prenol lipids* (derived from condensation of isoprene subunits).

Although the term lipid is sometimes used as a synonym for fats, fats are a subgroup of lipids called *triglycerides*. Lipids also encompass molecules such as fatty acids and their derivatives (including tri-, di-, and monoglycerides and phospholipids), as well as other sterol-containing metabolites such as cholesterol. Although humans and other mammals use various biosynthetic pathways to both breakdown and synthesize lipids, some essential lipids cannot be made this way and must be obtained from the diet.

SAPONIFICATION

Saponification is the hydrolysis of an ester under basic conditions to form an alcohol and the salt of a carboxylic acid (carboxylates). Saponification is commonly used to refer to the reaction of a metallic alkali (base) with a fat or oil to form soap. Saponifiable substances are those that can be converted into soap.

Sodium hydroxide (NaOH) is a caustic base. If NaOH is used a hard soap is formed, whereas when potassium hydroxide (KOH) is used, a soft soap is formed. Vegetable oils and animal fats are fatty esters in the form of triglycerides. The alkali breaks the ester bond and releases the fatty acid salt and glycerol. If necessary, soaps may be precipitated by salting it out with saturated sodium chloride. The saponification value is the amount of base required to saponify a fat sample.

In a classic laboratory procedure the triglyceride trimyristin is obtained by extracting nutmeg with diethyl ether. Saponification to the sodium salt of myristic acid takes place with NaOH in water. The acid itself can be obtained by adding dilute hydrochloric acid.

WAXES AND OTHER ESTERS

Waxes is a general term used to refer to the mixture of long-chain a polar lipids forming a protective coating (cutin in the cuticle) on plant leaves and fruits but also in animals (wax of honeybee, cuticular lipids of insects, spermaceti of the sperm whale, skin lipids, uropygial glands of birds, depot fat of planktonic crustacea), algae, fungi and bacteria. Some waxes are of mineral origin. Montan wax originates from mob or lignite, that fossilized compound representing a late step of the transformation of vegetal into hydrocarbons.

The various materials named waxes do not form a chemically homogeneous group. All waxes are water-resistant materials made up of various substances including hydrocarbons (normal or branched alkanes and alkenes), ketones, diketones, primary and secondary alcohols, aldehydes, sterol esters, alkanoic acids, terpenes (squalene) and monoesters (wax esters), all with long or very long carbon chains (from 12 up to about 38 carbon atoms) and solid in a large range of temperature (fusion point between 60 and 100°C).

More commonly, waxes are esters of an alcohol other than glycerol (long chain alcohol, sterol, hydroxycarotenoids, vitamin A) and a long chain acid (wax esters). Wax esters are saponified by hot alkaline solutions and give a fatty acid and an alcohol. They are soluble in aromatic solvents, chloroform, ethers, esters and ketones.

In plants the outer covering consists of an hydroxy fatty acid polymer called cutin. The underground parts and healed wound surfaces of plants are covered with an analogous substance, suberin. These substances are frequently mixed with other lipids and form a complex mixture called epicuticular wax. Cutin is a lipidic polymer containing C_{16} and C_{18} families of acids. The former is more abundant in growing parts, the later is present in the cuticle of slower-growing plants. These acids may be saturated, unsaturated, mono- or di-hydroxylated. In the cutin structure, a polyester structure exists where cross-linking depends on the availability of secondary hydroxyl groups. It has even been suggested that a biopolymer called "algaenan" consisting mainly of linear polyester chains cross-linked by ether bridges is present in cell wall of green microalgae.

Pyrethrins are natural or synthetic organic compounds that have potent insecticidal activity. All are formed from a cyclopropane fatty acid esterified by an allylic alcohol having a cyclopropane core. The pyrethrins are contained in all parts of several species of *Chrysanthemum*.

Waxes are largely used in cosmetics, in pharmaceutical industries, as lubricants, polishes, plasticizers and in food industries. As natural sources of waxes are expensive and limited in access, they are frequently synthesized by or chemical procedures.

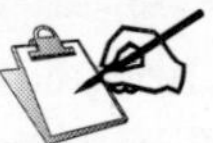

STUDY QUESTIONS

1. Explain the classification of Alkaloids.
2. Write short notes on:
   (a) Volatile oils.
   (b) Lipids.
3. Explain the methods of preparation of Volatile Oils.

■■■

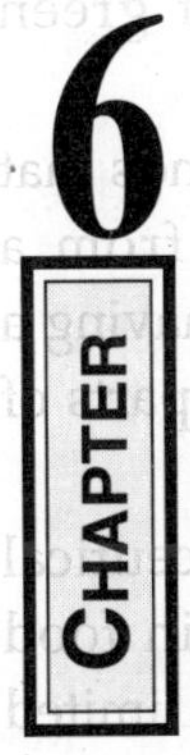

LAXATIVES

ALOES

Botanical Name	:	*Aloe Barbadensis, Aloe Indica, Aloe Vera*
Family	:	Liliaceae
Parts Used	:	Leaves, Flowers, Roots
Common Name	:	Aloe, Aloe Vera, Indian Alces, Kumari, Ghirita, Gawarpaltra, Barbados aloe, Curacao aloe, Lu hui

HABITAT

Aloes are indigenous to East and South Africa, but have been introduced into the West Indies (where they are extensively cultivated) and into tropical countries, and will even flourish in the countries bordering on the Mediterranean.

The drug Aloes consists of the liquid exuded from the transversely-cut bases of the leaves of various species of Aloes, evaporated to dryness.

DESCRIPTION

They are succulent plants belonging to the *Lily* family, with perennial, strong and fibrous roots and numerous, persistent, fleshy leaves, proceeding from the upper part of the root, narrow, tapering, thick and fleshy, usually beset at the edges with spiney teeth. Many of the species are woody and branching. In the remote districts of S.W. Africa and in Natal, Aloes have been discovered 30 to 60 feet in height, with stems as much as 10 feet in circumference.

The flowers are produced in erect, terminal spikes. There is no calyx, the corolla is tubular, divided into six narrow segments at the mouth and of a red, yellow or purplish colour. The capsules contain numerous angular seeds.

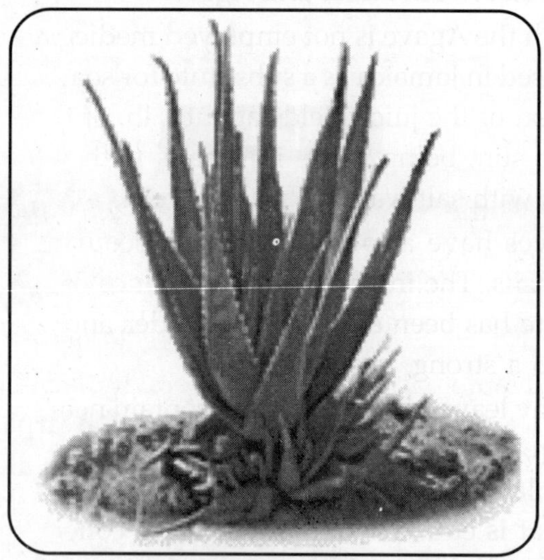

Fig. 6.1: Aloe

The true Aloe is in flower during the greater part of the year and is not to be confounded with another plant, the *Agave* or *American Aloe* (Agave Americana), which is remarkable for the long interval between its periods of flowering. This is a succulent plant, without stem, the leaves being radical, spiney, and toothed. There is a variety with variegated foliage. The flower-stalk rises to many feet in height, bearing a number of large and handsome flowers. In cold climates there is usually a very long interval between the times of its flowering, though it is a popular error to suppose that it happens only once in a hundred years for when it obtains sufficient heat and receives a culture similar to that of the pineapple, it is found to flower much more frequently.

Various species of Agave, all of which closely resemble each other, have been largely grown as ornamental plants since the first half of the sixteenth century in the South of Europe, and are completely acclimatized in Spain, Portugal and Southern Italy, but though often popularly called *Aloes* all of them are plants of the New World whereas the true Aloes are natives of the Old World. From a chemical point of view there is also no analogy at all between Aloes and Agaves.

Although the Agave is not employed medicinally, the leaves have been used in Jamaica as a substitute for soap, the expressed juice (a gallon of the juice yields about 1 lb. of the soft extract), dried in the sun, being made into balls with wood ash. This soap lathers with salt water as well as fresh.

The leaves have also been used for scouring pewter and kitchen utensils. The inner spongy substance of the leaves in a decayed state has been employed as tinder and the fibres may be spun into a strong, useful thread.

The fleshy leaves of the true Aloe contain near the epidermis or outer skin, a row of fibrovascular bundles, the cells of which are much enlarged and filled with a yellow juice which exudes when the leaf is cut. When it is desired to collect the juice, the leaves are cut off close to the stem and so placed that the juice is drained off into tubs.

This juice thus collected is concentrated either by spontaneous evaporation, or more generally by boiling until it becomes of the consistency of thick honey. On cooling, it is then poured into gourds, boxes, or other convenient receptacles, and solidifies.

Aloes require two or three years' standing before they yield their juice. In the West Indian Aloe plantations they are set out in rows like cabbages and cutting takes place in March or April, but in Africa the drug is collected from the wild plants.

CONSTITUENTS

The most important constituents of Aloes are the two Aloins, *Barbaloin* and *Isobarbaloin*, which constitute the so-called 'crystalline' Aloin, present in the drug at from 10 to 30 per cent. Other constituents are amorphous Aloin, resin and Aloe-emodin. The proportion in which the Aloins are present in the respective Aloes is not accurately known.

The manner in which the evaporation is conducted has a marked effect on the appearance of the Aloes, slow and moderate concentration tending to induce crystallization of the Aloin, thus causing the drug to appear opaque. Such Aloes is termed 'livery' or hepatic, and splinters of it exhibit minute crystals of Aloin when examined under the microscope. If, on the other hand, the evaporation is carried as far as possible, the Aloin does not crystallize and small fragments of the drug appear transparent; it is then termed 'glassy,' 'vitreous,' or 'lucid' Aloes and exhibits no crystals of Aloin under the microscope.

VARIETIES

The chief varieties of Aloes are *Curacao* or *Barbados, Socotrine* (including Zanzibar) and *Cape*. Other varieties of Aloes, such as black '*Mocha*' Aloes, occasionally find their way to the London market. Jafferabad Aloes, supposed to be the same as 'Mocha' Aloes, is of a black, pitch-like colour and a glassy, somewhat porous fracture; it is the product of *Aloe Abyssinica* and is imported to Mumbai from Arabia. It does not enter into English commerce. *Musambra Aloes* is made in India from *A. vulgaris*. *Uganda Aloes,* imported from Mossel Bay, not from Uganda, is a variety of *Cape Aloes* produced by careful evaporation. *Natal Aloes,* another South African variety, is no longer a commercial article in this country. The *A. purificata* of the United States Pharmacopoeia is prepared by adding alcohol to melted Aloes, stirring thoroughly, straining and evaporating the strained liquid. The product occurs in irregular, brittle, dull-brown or reddish pieces and is almost entirely soluble in Alcohol.

Curacoa Aloes is obtained from *A. chinensis* (Staud.) *A. vera* (Linn.) and probably other species. It was formerly produced on the island of Barbados, where it was largely cultivated, having been introduced at the beginning of the sixteenth century, and is still frequently, but improperly called *Barbados Aloes*. It is now almost entirely made on the Dutch islands of Curacoa, Aruba and Bonaire by boiling the Aloe juice down and pouring the viscid residue into empty spirit cases, in which it is allowed to solidify. Formerly gourds of various sizes were used (usually containing from 60 to 70 lb.) but Aloes in gourds is now seldom seen. It is usually opaque and varies in colour from bright yellowish or rich reddish brown to black. Sometimes it is vitreous and small fragments are then of a deep garnet-red colour and transparent. It is then known as *'Capey Barbados'* and is less valuable, but may become opaque and more valuable by keeping. Curacoa Aloes possesses the nauseous and bitter taste that is characteristic of all Aloes and a disagreeable, penetrating odour. It is almost entirely soluble in 60 per cent alcohol and contains not more than 30 per cent of substances insoluble in water and 12 per cent of moisture. It should not yield more than 3 per cent of ash.

Commercial Aloin is obtained usually from *Curacoa Aloes.* Solutions of Curacoa and other Aloes gradually undergo change, and may after a month no longer react normally, and may also lose the bitterness natural to Aloes.

Socotrine Aloes is prepared to a certain extent on the island of Socotra, but probably more largely on the African and possibly also on the Arabian mainland, from the leaves of *A. Perryi* (Baker). It is usually imported in kegs in a pasty condition and subsequent drying is necessary. It may be distinguished principally from *Curacoa Aloes* by its different odour. Much of the dry drug is characterized by the presence of small cavities in the fractured surface, but the variety of Socotrine Aloes distinguished as *Zanzibar Aloes* often very closely resembles Curacoa in appearance and is usually imported in liver-brown masses which break with a dull, waxy fracture, differing from that of Socotrine Aloes in being nearly smooth and even. When it is prepared, it is commonly poured into goat skins, which are then packed into cases.

The name 'Socotrine' Aloes is officially applied to both *Socotrine* and *Zanzibar Aloes*. Its chief constituents are *Barbaloin* (formerly called Socaloin and Zanaloin) and *B. Barbaloin*, no Isobarbaloin being present in this variety of Aloes. Resin water-soluble substances other than Aloin and Aloe-emodin are also present.

Socotrine Aloes should be of a dark, reddish-brown colour, and almost entirely soluble in alcohol. Not more than 50 per cent should be insoluble in water and it should yield not more than 3 per cent of ash. Garnet-coloured, translucent Socotrine Aloes is not now found in commerce, though fine qualities of Zanzibar Aloes are sometimes slightly translucent. Samples of the drug which are nearly black are unfit for pharmaceutical purposes. The odour of Zanzibar Aloes is strong and characteristic, and its taste nauseous and bitter.

Cape Aloes is prepared in Cape Colony from *A. ferou* (Linn.), *A. spicata* (Thumb.) *A. africana, A. platylepia* and other species of Aloe. It possesses more powerfully purgative properties than any other variety of the drug and is preferred to other varieties on the Continent, but is chiefly employed in this country for veterinary purposes only though for this purpose the Curacoa Aloes is as a rule preferred. Another form of the drug used for veterinary purposes, called *Caballine* or *Horse Aloes*, usually consists of the residue from the purification of the more valuable sorts.

Cape Aloes almost invariably occurs in the vitreous modification; it forms dark coloured masses which break with a clean glassy fracture and exhibit in their splinters a yellowish, reddish-brown or greenish tinge. Its translucent, glossy appearance and very characteristic, red-currant like odour sufficiently distinguish it from all other varieties of Aloes.

Uganda Aloes is also obtained from *A. ferox*. It occurs in bricks or fragments of hepatic, yellowish-brown colour, with a bronze gold fracture and its odour resembles that of Cape Aloes.

Cape Aloes contains 9 per cent or more of Barbaloin (formerly known as Capaloin) and *B. Barbaloin*. Only traces of Capalores combined with paracumaric acid. Cape Aloes should not contain more than 12 per cent of water; it should yield at least 45 per cent of aquoeus extract but not more than 2 per cent of ash Uganda Aloes yields about 6 per cent of Aloin, part of which is *B. Barbaloin*. The leaves of the plants from which Cape Aloes is obtained are cut off near the stem and arranged around a hole in the ground, in which a sheepskin is spread, with smooth side upwards. When a sufficient quantity of juice has drained from the leaves it is concentrated by heat in iron cauldrons (a large vessle or kettle) and subsequently poured into boxes or skins in which it solidifies on cooling. Large quantities of the drug are exported from Cape Town and Mossel Bay.

Natal Aloes. The source of this variety which is seldom imported, is not yet definitely ascertained, but it is probably prepared from one or more species of Aloe, probably including *A. ferox*. Natal Aloes is prepared with greater care than Cape Aloes the leaves being cut obliquely into slices and the juice allowed to exude or discharge in the hot sunshine, after which it is boiled down in iron pots the liquid being stirred until it becomes thick and then poured into wooden cases to solidify. Natal Aloes is much weaker than any other variety, having little purgative action on human beings, apparently because it contains no Emodin. It is no longer of commercial importance. It resembles Cape Aloes in odour and occurs in irregular pieces which are almost always opaque and have a characteristic, dull greenish-black or brown colour. It is much less soluble than Cape Aloes. It has not a glassy fracture like that of Cape Aloes and when powdered is of a greenish colour.

Both *Curacoa* and *Cape Aloes* in powder give a crimson colour with nitric acid, Socratine Aloes powder touched with nitric acid does not give a crimson colour.

MEDICINAL ACTION AND USES

The drug Aloes is one of the safest and best warm and stimulating *purgatives* to persons of sedentary habits and phlegmatic constitutions. An ordinary small dose takes from 15 to 18 hours to produce an effect. Its action is exerted mainly on the large intestine, for which reason, also it is useful as a vermifuge.

Aloe has been well known for centuries for its *healing properties*, and both oral intake and topical *dressings* have been documented to facilitate healing of any kind of skin wound, burn, or scald – even speeding recovery time after surgery. Situations to try it on include blisters, insect bites, rashes, sores, *herpes, urticaria, athlete's foot, fungus, vaginal infections, conjunctivitis, allergic reactions*, and *dry skin*.

Other topical uses include *acne, sunburn, frostbite* (it appears to prevent decreased blood flow), shingles, screening out X-ray radiation, psoriasis, preventing scarring, *rosacea, warts, wrinkles* from aging, and *eczema*.

Internally, aloe is showing real promise in the fight against *AIDS*, and the *virus* has become undetectable in some patients who used it on a regular basis, due to its immune system stimulant properties.

The National Cancer Institute has included Aloe Vera in their recommendations for increased testing because of these apparent cancer fighting properties.

Taken orally, aloe also appears to work on heartburn, arthritis and rheumatism pain and asthma, and studies have shown that it has an effect on lowering blood sugar levels in diabetics.

Other situations in which it appears to work when taken internally include congestion, intestinal worms, indigestion, stomach ulcers, colitis, hemorrhoids, liver problems such as cirrhosis and hepatitis, kidney infections, urinary tract infections, prostate problems, and as a general detoxifier.

Commercially, aloe can be found in pills, sprays, ointments, lotions, liquids, drinks, jellies, and creams, to name a few of the thousands of products available.

Aloe is safe when used in moderation, but there are a few contraindications. If you have a heart problem and use any kind of digitalis medication, consult your doctor before using any aloe product internally, as the interaction may cause irregular heartbeat. Avoid aloe preparations if you are pregnant, breast feeding, or menstruating, as it can cause uterine contractions.

RHUBARB

Botanical Name	:	*Rheum rhabarbarum*
Family	:	Polygonaceae
Part Used	:	Seeds
Common Name	:	Rhubarb, Himalayan Rubarb, Indian Rhubarb, Revat Chinni

HABITAT

Throughout the valleys in Himalayan region at altitude of 3200 m-5200 m. Rhubarb is a plant name for the many different species of *Rheum*, growing in the wild in the mountains of the Western and North-western provinces of China and in the adjoining Tibetan territory and in cultivation in much of Europe and the United States.

DESCRIPTION

Rhubarb is a perennial plant (the kind that grows from year to year) which forms large fleshy rhizomes and large leaves with long, thick (and tasty) petioles (stalks).

Rhubarb stalks are commonly found in supermarkets, fresh rhubarb is prized by gourmet cooks.

There are many species of plants called *rhubarb*. The *Rhubarb Compendium* is primarily concerned with common *garden rhubarb, Rheum cultorum.*

Rhubarb leaves grow from the ground in early spring. The leaves can grow up to a foot or more in width and length and the plant may grow to a height of several feet. The blade or green leaves of the plant are the part that is poisonous.

They contain high concentrations of oxalic acid crystals which can cause serious problems when eaten. These crystals can cause the tongue and throat to swell, preventing breathing.

The edible petioles (stalks) are up to 18 inches long, 1 to 2 inches in diameter, generally somewhat hemispherical in cross section. These petioles are cut and used in pies, jams, jellies, sauces and juice.

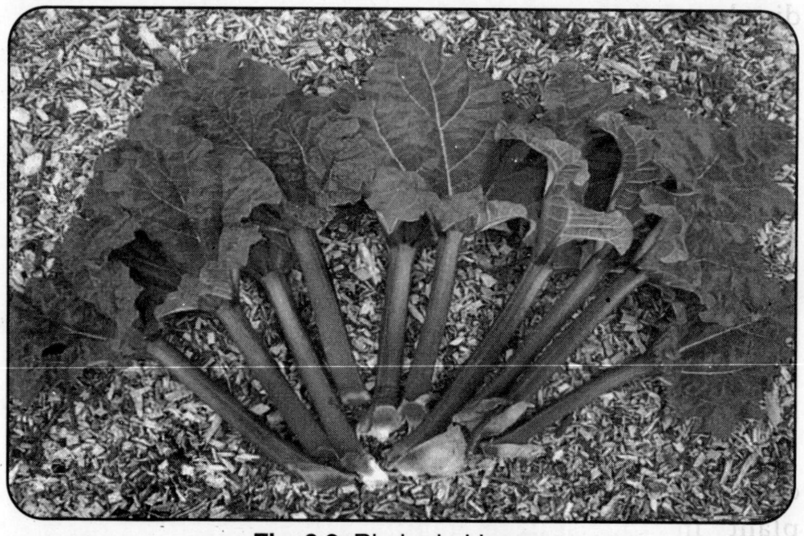

Fig. 6.2: Rhubarb rhizome

Rhubarb rhizomes and the crown persist for many years. The roots are also taken up and bedded in cellars or houses in winter, forcing growth in darkness to produce etiolated leaf-stems, which are much prized.

MEDICINAL USE

It is recognized that rhubarb not only exercises a *digestive action* but it operates directly as a conveyer of bile salts. It can therefore be classed as a *hepatic stimulant*. Rhubarb performs its first *digestive* operation in the mouth by stimulating the taste buds with its pleasantly bitter flavour which gives a sense of cleansing out the oral cavity, preparing it to taste the coming food. When it reaches the stomach its digestive effects come into full play, causing an increase of the flow of gastric juice and inducing their movement, thus favouring the processing of the contents of the stomach. Besides stimulating the secretions from the liver which convey the bile salts, it assists the intestine in regulating the absorption of fats

It is used as *purgative* and *astringent tonic*. Its stimulating effect combined with asperient properties renders it specially useful in atonic *dyspepsia*. Rhubarb is used as a laxative, antiphlogistic, and homeostatic in the treatment of constipation, diarrhea, jaundice, gastro-intestinal hemorrhage, menstrual disorders, conjunctivitis, traumatic injuries, superficial suppurative sores and ulcers. It is also applied externally for thermal burns.

CASTOR OIL

Botanical Name	:	*Ricinus communis*
Family	:	Euphorbiaceae
Parts Used	:	Seeds, Stem and Leaf
Common Name	:	Rehri, Arind

The castor oil plant, *Ricinus communis*, is a species of flowering plant in the spurge family, *Euphorbiaceae*. It belongs to a monotypic genus, *Ricinus*, and subtribe, *Ricininae*.

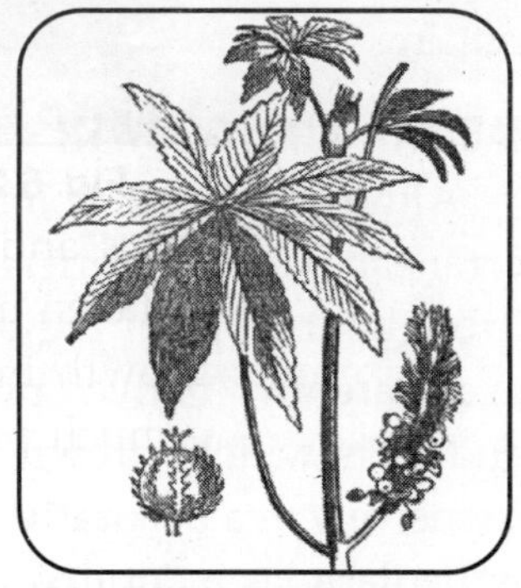
Fig. 6.3: Castor oil plant

Castor seed is the source of castor oil, which has a wide variety of uses. The seeds contain between 40% and 60% oil that is rich in triglycerides, mainly ricinolein. The seed coat contains ricin, a toxin, which is also present in lower concen-trations throughout the plant.

The toxicity of raw castor beans due to the presence of ricin is well-known. Although the lethal dose in adults is considered to be 4 to 8 seeds, reports of actual poisoning are relatively rare.

Another plant species, Fatsia japonica, looks similar to the castor oil plant and is known as the false castor oil plant.

DESCRIPTION

The glossy leaves are 15–45 centimetres (5.9–18 inch) long, long-stalked, alternate and palmate with 5–12 deep lobes with coarsely toothed segments. Their colour varies from dark green, sometimes with a reddish tinge, to dark reddish purple or bronze.

The stems and the spherical, spiny seed pods also vary in pigmentation. The pods are more showy than the flowers [the male flowers are yellowish-green with prominent creamy stamens and are carried in ovoid spikes up to 15 centimetres (5.9 inch) long; the female flowers, borne at the tips of the spikes, have prominent red stigmas].

Terminating stems are panicle-like inflorescences of green monoecious flowers, the stalked female flowers above the male flowers below, both without petals.

The fruit is a spiny, greenish capsule with large, oval, shiny, bean-like, highly poisonous seeds with variable brownish motling.

HABITAT AND GROWTH

Although castor is indigenous to the South Eastern Mediterranean Basin, Eastern Africa, and India, today it is widespread throughout tropical regions. Castor establishes itself easily as an apparently "native" plant and can often be found on wasteland. It is widely grown as a crop in Ethiopia. It is also used extensively as a decorative plant in parks and other public areas, particularly as a "dot plant" in traditional bedding schemes. It was used in Edwardian times in the parks of Toronto, Ontario, Canada. Of the red and white variety, the red is seen as an ornamental plant, the white is used medicinally. Although monotypic, the castor oil plant can vary greatly in its growth habit and appearance.

It is a fast-growing, suckering perennial shrub which can reach the size of a small tree (around 12 metres/39 feet), but it is not cold hardy. However, it grows well outside, at least in Southern England, and the leaves do not appear to suffer frost damage in sheltered spots, where it remains evergreen. In areas prone to frost it is usually shorter and grown as if it were an annual. If sown early, under glass, and kept at a temperature of around 20°C (68°F) until planted out, the castor oil plant can reach a height of 2–3 metres (6.6–9.8 ft.) in a year.

USES

The use of castor bean oil in India has been documented since 2000 B.C. in lamps and in local medicine as a laxative, purgative, and cathartic in Unani, Ayurvedic and other ethnomedical systems. Traditional Ayurvedic medicine considers castor oil the king of medicinals for curing arthritic diseases.

Castor seed and its oil have also been used in China for centuries, mainly prescribed in local medicine for internal use or use in dressings. Castor oil is also the source for undecylenic acid, a natural *fungicide*.

MEDICAL USES FOR CASTOR OIL

The most common and most frequent of the medical uses for castor oil are the way it is used for treating *constipation*. Castor oil is triglyceride of fatty acids. It contains *ricinoleic acid*. This is an unsaturated fatty acid and this unsaturated fatty acid is found in high concentration in castor oil. This makes castor oil a unique substance with great healing capabilities. Ricinoleic acid inhibits the growth of many viruses, bacteria, yeasts and molds. This makes castor oil as the best remedy for topical application in cases of *ringworm, keratoses, skin inflammation, abrasions, fungal infections*, and *acne*. For small areas of infections you can apply a bandaid that contains castor oil or soak a cloth in castor oil and wrap up the area of the infection.

The most common of the *gastrointestinal problems* that are treated with castor oil are constipation, dysentery, and inflammatory bowel disease. It is also used to treat *vaginal infections* and bladder problems. It is known that asthma is also treated with castor oil. Some other medical uses for castor oil are it relieves *arthritis* and *back pain* if the kernels of the castor seed are boiled with milk and water an taken orally. Nursing mothers used to apply castor oil to the breasts to increase *milk secretion* and relieve milk stagnation in the mammary glands. Castor oil is also applied to the *abdominal area* to relieve pains during the *menstruation cycle*.

ISPAGHULA

Botanical Name	:	*P. indica*
Family	:	Plantaginaceae
Part Used	:	Seeds
Common Name	:	Psyllium or Ispaghula and Ishabgul-ki-bhusi

Psyllium or *Ispaghula* is the common name used for several members of the plant genus Plantago whose seeds are used commercially for the production of mucilage. The genus *Plantago* contains over 200 species. *P. ovata* and *P. psyllium* are produced commercially in several European countries, the former Soviet Union, Pakistan, and India. Plantago seed, known commercially as black, French, or *Spanish psyllium*, is obtained from *P. psyllium L.*, also known as *P. arenaria*.

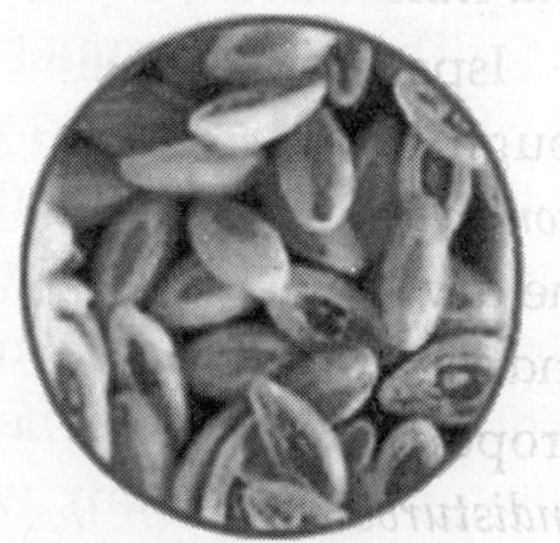

Fig. 6.4: Ispaghula seeds

Ispaghula is native to India, and has been used comprehensively in the

Indian system of medicine since prehistoric periods. It was prescribed by earliest physicians as a remedy for inflammatory and functional imbalances of the mucous membranes of the *gastro-intestinal* and *genito-urinary system.*

COMPOSITION

Ispaghula, also known as *spogel seeds,* is a nearly stemless tiny herb, covered with thick and soft bushy growth. It has extremely tapered leaves and tiny flowers in elliptical or cylindrical spikes. The upper half of its fruit opens like a lid and its seeds are boat-shaped. The seeds of this plant, also known as flea seeds, make up the drug.

The seeds contain a great amount of mucilage and a small amount of holoside planteose. The seeds also demonstrate the presence of a number of amino acids in the compounded form, viz. valine, alanine, glycine, glutamic acid, cystine, lysine, leucine and tyrosine. Valine, alanine and glutamic acid are also found in their independent forms. The Ispaghula embryo oil has been reported to be a superior source of linoleic acid.

MEDICINAL USES

Psyllium is mainly used as a *dietary fibre,* which is not absorbed by the small intestine. The purely mechanical action of psyllium mucilage absorbs excess water while stimulating normal bowel elimination. Although its main use has been as a laxative, it is more appropriately termed a true dietary fibre and as such can help reduce the syınptoms of both constipation and mild diarrhea.

Ispaghula possesses excellent properties to smoothen out tough bowel movements, and everything associated with *stomach* and *anal disorders. Ispaghula husk* (*Ishabgul-ki-bhusi*) is the dry seed-cover of the plant, received by grinding the seeds and separating the husk by winnowing. The husk has analogous properties as the seeds. It also has the *benefit of travelling undisturbed through the alimentary canal* without causing pain. The husk can be consumed dry and is easier to use compared to the whole seeds.

Due to its soothing effect on the mucous membranes, ispaghula is used in *constipation*. The seeds should be dowsed in water before use, which makes them disintegrate in the alimentary tract.

The seeds are particularly useful in acute constipation, distinguished by spasms. Ispaghula seeds are an admired cure for several kinds of acute *dysentery* and *diarrhoea*.

Ispaghula is useful in treating frequent colic in the belly, induced by *stomach ulcers*. The seeds with husk are dowsed in water or milk for a few hours. The liquid is sieved and can be taken at night.

Ispaghula seeds are one of the most efficacious remedies for *piles*. While the high mucilage content in this herb heals constipation, the rich tannin content cures swelling and ulceration in the intestinal passage up to the anus. This double action helps cure piles.

SENNA

Botanical Name	:	*Cassia angustifolia*
Family	:	Leguminosae (Fabaceae)
Parts Used	:	Dried leaflets, Pods and Stems
Common Name	:	Senna, Indian senna or Tinnevelly senna

HABITAT

Egypt, Nubia, Arabia, Sennar. The *sennas*, is a large genus of around 250 species of flowering plants in the family *Fabaceae*, subfamily *Caesalpinioideae*. Typically Senna species have yellowish flowers. They may be herbs, smallish trees or even a kind of liana, but typically are shrubs or subshrubs. Senna species make good ornamental plants and are used for landscape gardening.

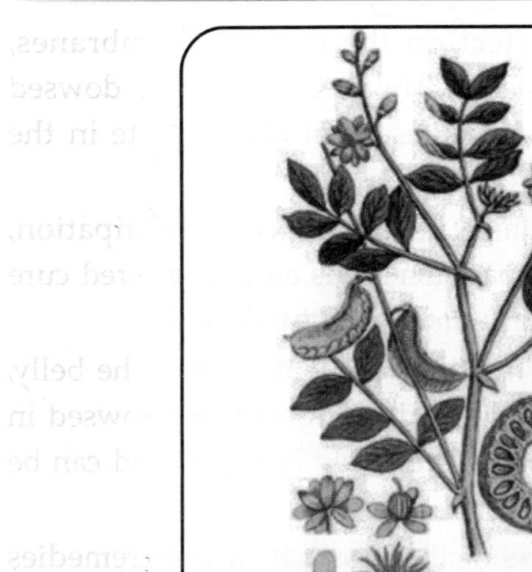

Fig. 6.5: Cassia angustifolia

Senna (*Cassia species*) can be found in the tropical and subtropical regions of the world. Most varieties are indigenous to North, Central, and South America.

DESCRIPTION

Several species of Cassia contribute to the drug of commerce, and were comprised in a single species by *Linnaeus* under the name of *Cassia Senna*. The two most widely exported and officially recognized are *C. acutifolia* and *C. angustifolia* (*Indian senna* or *Tinnevelly senna*).

C. acutifolia, yielding the finest and most valuable variety of the drug is a small shrub about 2 feet high. The stem is erect, smooth, and pale green, with long, spreading branches, bearing leaflets in four or five pairs, averaging an inch long, lanceolate or obovate, unequally oblique at the base, veins distinct on the under surface, brittle, greyish-green, of a faint, peculiar odour, and mucilaginous, sweetish taste. The form of the base, and freedom from bitterness, distinguish the Senna from the Argel leaves, which are also thicker and stiffer. The flowers are small and yellow. The pods are broadly oblong, about 2 inches long by 7/8 inch broad, and contain about six seeds.

CONSTITUENTS

Water and diluted alcohol extract the active principles of Senna. Pure alcohol only extracts them imperfectly. The leaves yield about one-third of their weight to boiling water.

The purgative constituents are closely allied to those of *Aloes* and *Rhubarb*, the activities of the drug being largely due to anthraquinone derivatives and their glucosides. It contains rhein, aloe-emedin, kaempferol, isormamnetin, both free and as glucosides together with myricyl alcohol, etc. The ash amounts to about 8 per cent, consisting chiefly of earthy and ashy carbonates.

MEDICINAL ACTION AND USES

Its action being chiefly on the lower bowel, it is especially suitable in habitual costiveness. It increases the peristaltic movements of the colon by its local action upon the intestinal wall. Its active principle must pass out of the system in the secretions unaltered, for when Senna is taken by nurses, the suckling infant becomes purged. It acts neither as a sedative nor as a refrigerant, but has a slight, stimulating influence. In addition to the nauseating taste, it is act to cause sickness, and griping pains, so that few can take it alone; but these characteristics can be overcome or removed, when it is well adapted for children, elderly persons, and delicate women. The colouring matter is absorbable, and twenty or thirty minutes after the ingestion of the drug it appears in the urine, and may be recognized by a red colour on the addition of ammonia.

The addition of cloves, ginger, cinnamon, or other aromatics are excellent correctives of the nauseous effects. A teaspoonful of cream of tartar to a teacupful of the decoction of infusion of Senna, is a mild and pleasant cathartic, well suited for women if required soon after delivery. Some practitioners add neutral laxative salts, or saccharine and aromatic substances. The purgative effect is increased by the addition of pure bitters; the decoction of guaiacum is said to answer a similar purpose. Senna is contraindicated in an inflammatory condition of the alimentary canal, hemorrhoids, prolapsus, ani, etc. The well-known 'black draught' is a combination of Senna and Gentian, with any aromatic, as cardamom or coriander seeds, or the rind of the Seville orange. The term 'black draught,' it is stated, should never be used, as mistakes have been made in reading the prescriptions, and 'black drop' or vinegar of opium has been given instead, several deaths having been caused in this way.

STUDY QUESTIONS

1. Write short notes on the following:
   (a) Aloes;
   (b) Castor oil;
   (c) Ispaghula; and
   (d) Senna.
2. Explain the medicinal action and uses of Senna and Ispaghula.

■■■

7

CHAPTER

CARDIOTONICS

DIGITALIS

Botanical Name	:	*Digitalis purpurea*
Family	:	Scrophulariaceae (Dog flower family)
Part Used	:	Leaves
Common Name	:	Foxglove

DESCRIPTION

Foxglove is a bienneial plant with soft, hairy, toothed, ovate and lance-shaped leaves in a basal rosette. The life span of the plant is 2 seasons. The first year growth remains in a basal rosette of leaves. Second year growth produces flowering stems, 3 -6 feet in height. Flower spikes have *purple* to white spotted thimble-like flowers which hang down and last about six days.

The earliest known name for this plant is the *Anglo-Saxon* "foxes glofa" (the glove of the fox). It derives its name from the flowers which resemble the fingers of a glove and possibly from a northern legend that bad fairies gave the blossoms to the fox to put on his toes, so that he might soften his tread while he hunted for prey. The *heart medication,* digitalis, was originally derived from this plant. It is now synthetically made. Today, foxglove is used mainly in *landscaping*.

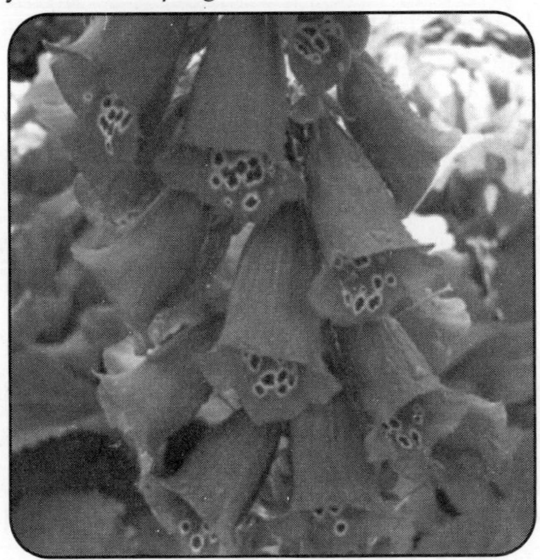

Fig. 7.1: Foxglove

CULTIVATION

The Foxglove is cultivated by a few growers in this country in order to provide a drug of uniform activity from a true type of Digitalis purpurea. It is absolutely necessary to have the true medicinal seeds to supply the drug market: crops must be obtained from carefully selected wild seed and all variations from the new type struck out.

The plant will flourish best in well drained loose soil, preferably of siliceous origin, with some slight shade. The plants growing in sunny situations possess the active qualities of the herb in a much greater degree than those shaded by trees, and it has been proved that those grown on a hot, sunny bank, protected by a wood, give the best results.

It grows best when allowed to seed itself, but if it is desired to raise it by sown seed, 2 lb. of seed to the acre are required. As the seeds are so small and light, they should be mixed with fine sand in order to ensure even distribution. They should be thinly covered with soil. The seeds are uncertain in germination, but the seedlings may be readily and safely transplanted in damp weather, and should be pricked out to 6 to 9 inches apart. Sown in spring, the plant will not blossom till the following year. Seeds must be gathered as soon as ripe. The flowers of the true medicinal type must be pure, dull pink or magenta, not pale-coloured, white or spotted externally.

It is estimated that one acre of good soil will grow at least two tons of the Foxglove foliage, producing about 1/2 ton of the dried leaves.

CONSTITUENTS

Digitalis contains four important glucosides of which three arecardiac stimulants. The most powerful is *Digitoxin,* an extremely poisonous and cumulative drug, insoluble in water, *Digitalin,* which is crystalline and also insoluble in water; *Digitalein,* amorphous, but readily soluble in water, rendering it, therefore, capable of being administered subcutaneously, in doses so minute as rarely to exceed of a grain; *Digitonin,* which is a cardiac depressant, containing none of the physiological action peculiar to Digitalis, and is identical with Saponin, the chief constituent of Senega root. Other constituents are volatile oil, fatty matter, starch, gum, sugar, etc.

The amount and character of the active constituents vary according to season and soil: 100 parts of dried leaves yield about 1.25 of Digitalin, which is generally found in a larger proportion in the wild than in the cultivated plants.

The active constituents of Digitalis are not yet sufficiently explored to render a chemical assay effective in standardizing for therapeutic activity. The different glucosides contained varying from each other in their physiological action, it is impossible to assay the leaves by determining one only of these, such as Digitoxin.

USE IN MOLECULAR BIOLOGY

Digoxigenin (DIG) is a steroid found exclusively in the flowers and leaves of the plants Digitalis purpurea and Digitalis lanata. It is used as a molecular probe to detect DNA or RNA. It can easily be attached to nucleotides by chemical modifications. DIG molecules are often linked to uridine nucleotides; DIG labeled uridine (DIG-U) can then be incorporated into RNA probes via in vitro transcription. Once hybridisation occurs in situ, RNA probes with the incorporated DIG-U can be detected with anti-DIG antibodies that are conjugated to alkaline phosphatase. To reveal the hybridised transcripts, alkaline phosphatase can be reacted with a chromogen to produce a colour precipitate.

DIGITALIS GLYCOSIDES (ADVERSE EFFECTS AND TOXICITY)

Glycosides from plants of the genus *Digitalis*. Some of these are useful as cardiotonic and anti-arrhythmia agents. Included also are semi-synthetic derivatives of the naturally occurring glycosides. The term has sometimes been used more broadly to include all *Cardiac Glycosides*, but here is restricted to those related to *Digitalis*.

Contraindications and Warnings

- *Arrhythmias*: Digitalis should not be used in patients with *ventricular tachycardia* or runs of complex ventricular premature depolarizations unless there is strong reason to believe that the arrhythmia results from a digitalis-correctable decrease in cardiac function.

- *Potassium depletion*: Digitalis arrhythmias are much more common in patients with low serum potassium (less than 3 mEq).
- *Cardioversion*: Cardioversion tends to exacerbate arrhythmias caused by digitalis. Antiarrhythmic drugs may be preferred to cardioversion if the digitalized patient is stable. However, the presence of nontoxic levels of digitalis is not a contraindication to the use of cardioversion.
- *High output failure (warning):* Congestive heart failure caused by thyrotoxicosis, beri-beri, arteriovenous shunts, and a few other conditions are associated with a higher than normal cardiac output and respond poorly to digitalis glycosides.

ARJUN TREE

Botanical Name	:	*Terminalia arjuna*
Family	:	Combretaceae
Parts Used	:	Fruits, Seeds and Bark
Common Name	:	Arjuna, Koha, Kahu, Arjan, White Marudah, White Murdh, Arjuna Myrobalan, Orjun, Yerra maddi, Sadada, Sadaru and many more.

HABITAT

Terminalia arjuna is common throughout India especially in the sub Himalayan tracts and Eastern India. They are widely grown in Bandhavgarh National Park, Pench Tiger Reserve and Kanha National Park in India. It is mainly grown on the banks of the rivers and streams.

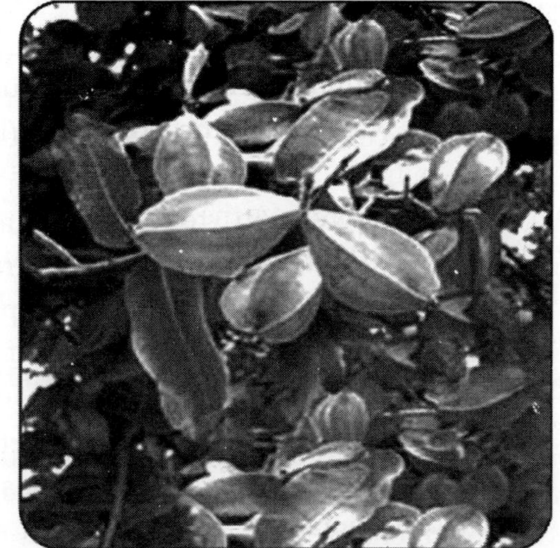

Fig. 7.2: Terminalia arjuna.

OTHER SPECIES

Terminalia chebula, T. bellrica and *T. ciliata* are the other species of Arjun tree found in India.

DESCRIPTION

Arjuna is the large size deciduous tree. The height of the Arjuna tree reaches upto 60-85 feet. It is the evergreen tree with the yellow flowers and conical leaves. It has a smooth gray bark. Fruit is 2.5-3.5 cm long, fibrous woody, glabrous with 5 hard wings, striated with numerous curved veins. It has a buttressed trunk and a vast spreading crown from which the branches drop downwards. Its leaves are dull green above and pale brown beneath. Arjuna flowers between March to June and fruits between September to November.

CULTIVATION METHODS

Its fruit is dried in the sunlight and than stored up to 6-12 months. Seeds are pretreated by soaking in the water for 48 hours before sowing in beds. 8-9 months seedlings are better to transplant in the field.

MEDICINAL USES

The Bark of the Arjuna tree contains calcium salts, magnesium salts, and glucosides has been used in traditional Ayurvedic herbalism Juice of its leaf is used to cure dysentry and earache. Arjuna helps in maintaining the cholesterol level at the normal rate, as it contains the antioxidant properties similar to the Vitamin E. It strengths the heart muscles and maintains the heart functioning properly. It also improves functioning of cardiac muscle.

Arjuna is used for the treatment of coronary artery disease, heart failure, edema, angina and hypercholesterolemia. Its bark power possesses diuretic, prostaglandin enhancing and coronary risk factor modulating properties. It is also considered as beneficial in the treatment of Asthma.

OTHER USES

Its wood is used in boat and house building as it is very hard. Its wood is also used in the making of the agricultural implements and weapons too. It is grown in the cities and towns for the purpose of shade.

CULTURAL IMPORTANCE

Arjuna is one of the sacred tree of India. It has acquired the social and religious sanctity with the passage of time. It is said that Arjuna has been born of the two sons of Kubair after saint Narada cursed him. The leaves and flowers of this tree are offered to the Lord Vishnu and Lord Ganpati on the several religious occasions. It has been used in Ayurvedic formation since ancient times.

STUDY QUESTIONS

1. Write short notes on the following:
   (a) Digitalis; and
   (b) Arjun Tree.
2. Describe the medicinal uses of bark of the Arjuna.

■■■

8

CHAPTER

Carminatives and Gastro Intestines Regulators

UMBELLIFEROUS FRUITS

CHARACTERISTIC FEATURES

1. They are usually *cremocarps* either entire or separated into its *mericarps*.
2. At the apex of fruit, there may be five small inconspicuous sepals, e.g., coriander, and in the centre are the two styles surrounded below by disc-like nectary forming the stylopod.
3. Each mericarp has 2 surfaces, a flat surface called the commissural surface and arounded one called the dorsal surface.
4. The dorsal surface shows 5 raised ridges over the vascular bundle called primary ridge between which may be found 4 ridges over the secretory canals and called secondary

ridges; primary ridges are mostly more prominent except in coriander where the secondary ridges are more conspicuous.

5. There is a minute thread lies between the 2 mericarps usually attached basally to the pedicel and apically to the stylopod, it is called carpophore.
6. Each mericarp encloses a single seed derived from anatropous ovule. The seeds shows a large oily endosperm, small apical embryo and a raphe in the middle of the commissural side.
7. Mostly, the mericarp is longitudinally traversed by 5 vascular bundles in the primary ridges and by 6 schizogenous secretory ducts called vittae, 4 on the dorsal surface and 2 on the commissural one. The vittae may be simple as in fennel, branched as in anise or almost inconspicuous as in Hemlock.
8. The *endocarp* mother cells are divided into groups of narrow parallel cells which may be parallel to each other forming parallel arrangement or variously oriented forming parquetry arrangement.
9. The endosperm cells contain aleurone grains enclosing a globoid and one or more micro- rosette crystals of calcium oxalate.

FENNEL

Botanical Name	:	*Foeniculum vulgare*
Family	:	Apiaceae (Umbellifereae)
Parts Used	:	Roots, Stalks and Leaves
Common Name	:	Saunf, Sweet fennel

HABITAT

The plant is native to the Mediterranean coasts, cultinated now in Europe, India, china and Egypt.

DESCRIPTION

Fennel seeds split into two, one sometimes remaining on the stalk. They are 4 -8 mm (1/8 - 5/16 in.) long, thin and curved, with colour varying from brown to light green (the green being superior).

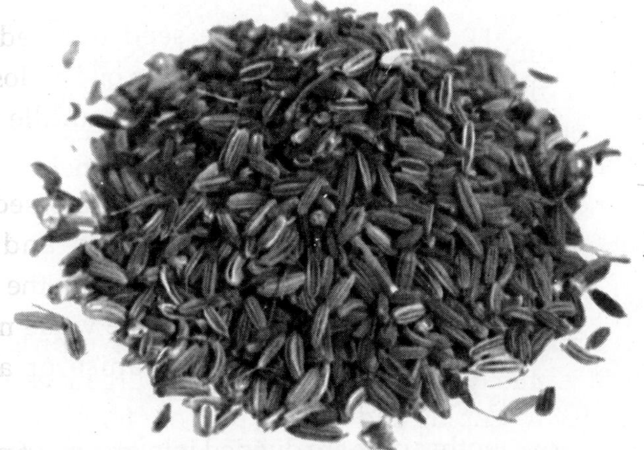

Fig. 8.1: Foeniculum vulgare

Fennel is a hardy perennial related to parsley, often cultivated as an annual, reaching heights of 1.5 - 2.5 m (5-8 ft.). It resembles dill, which it can cross-pollinate with. It should be kept at a distance from dill because the resulting seed will have a dulled flavour. The flower heads are collected before the seeds ripen and threshed out when completely dried.

Fennel is a beautiful plant. It has a thick, perennial root-stock, stout stems, 4 to 5 feet or more in height, erect and cylindrical, bright green and so smooth as to seem polished, much branched bearing leaves cut into the very finest of segments. The bright golden flowers, produced in large, flat terminal umbels, with from thirteen to twenty rays, are in bloom in July and August.

In the kitchen garden this naturally ornamental, graceful plant, generally has its stems cut down to secure a constant crop of green leaves for flavouring and garnishing, so that the plant is seldom seen in the same perfection as in the wild state. In the original wild condition, it is variable as to size, habit, shape and colour of leaf, number of rays in the flower-head or umbel, and shape of fruit, but it has been under cultivation for so long that there are now several well-marked species.

The Common Garden Fennel (*F. capillaceum* or *officinale*) is distinguished from its wild relative (*F. vulgare*) by having much stouter, taller, tubular and larger stems, and less divided leaves, but the chief distinction is that the leaf-stalks form a curved sheath around the stem, often even as far as the base of the leaf above. The flower-stalks, or pedicels, of the umbels are also sturdier, and the fruits, 1/4 to 1/2 inch long, are double the size of the wild ones.

MEDICINAL ACTION AND USES

On account of its aromatic and carminative properties, Fennel fruit is chiefly used medicinally with purgatives to allay their tendency to griping and for this purpose forms one of the ingredients of the well-known compound Liquorice Powder. Fennel water has properties similar to those of anise and dill water: mixed with sodium bicarbonate and syrup, these waters constitute the domestic 'Gripe Water', used to correct the flatulence of infants. Volatile oil of Fennel has these properties in concentration.

Fennel tea, formerly also employed as a carminative, is made by pouring half a pint of boiling water on a teaspoonful of bruised Fennel seeds.

Syrup prepared from Fennel juice was formerly given for chronic coughs.

Fennel is also largely used for cattle condiments.

CORIANDER

Botanical Name	:	*Coriandrum sativum*
Family	:	Apiaceae (Umbellifereae)
Parts Used	:	Seeds and Leaves
Common Name	:	Dhanaiya, Dhone

HABITAT

It is cultivated in Russia, Hungary, North Africa and India.

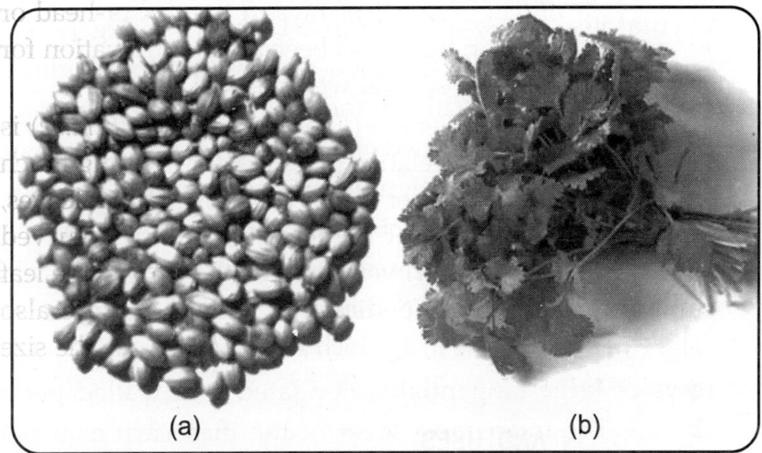

(a) (b)

Fig. 8.2: (a) and (b) Coriandrum sativum

DESCRIPTION

The drug usually consists of the whole cremocarp, which are sub-spherical, 3-5 mm in diameter, nealy glabrous, brownish-yellow or brown in colour, each is crowned by 5 small sepals and a short conical stylopod. The mericarps are usually united by their margins. The dorsal surface of each mericarp shows 5 inconspicuous wavy primary ridges and 4 more prominent straight secondary ridges. The transverse section of fully ripe mericarp shows only 2 vittae in the commissural side but no vittae in the dorsal one, an almost complete ring of sclerenchyma in the dorsal side, a large oily endosperm and a small curved apical embryo. Coriander has aromatic odour and aromatic spicy and characteristic taste.

MICROSCOPICAL CHARACTERS

I. Pericarp

(a) *Epicarp* is composed of polygonal tubular thick-walled cells and showing occasional small prismatic crystals of calcium oxalate, few anisocytic stomata and no hairs.

(b) *Mesocarp* is formed of 3 different zones, the outer zone consists of few layers of tangentially elongated parenchymatous cells usally collapsed, showing degenerated vittae as tangentially flattened cavities and longitudinally traversed by 10 vascular stands with small spiral vessels. The middle zone is formed of a broad layer of sclerenchyma consisting of strongly lignified pitted fusiform fibres in 2 sinous bands crossing each other at right angles, the outer 5 to 6 rows run longitudinally while the inner, 1 to 3 rows rung tangentially, in the secondary ridges almost all the cells runs tangentially. The inner zone is composed of 2-3 rows of large tangentially elongated thin walled parenchyma. The inner most layer of the mesocarp conists of flattened hexagonal thin-walled sclerenchyma. Mesocarp on the commissural side shows no sclerenchyma but two large elliptical yellowish brown vittae.

(c) *Endocarp* is formed of very narrow elongated thin-walled cells, arranged in variously oriented groups, i.e., parquetry arranged.

II. Seeds

The seed coat is formed of polygonal brown cells with narrow collapsed layer underneath. The endosperm is composed of thick-walled cellulosic cells containing fixed oil and aleurone grains including globoids and micro rosette crystals of calcium oxalate.

III. Carpophore

Splits, passing at the apex of each mericarp into the raphe and at the base to the pedicel.

POWDER CORIANDER

Powder coriander is light brown to brown in colour with aromatic odour and characteristic aromatic taste. It is characterised microscopically by:

1. Numerous irregular fragments of endosperm cells containing globules of fixed oils and aleurone grains containing micro-rossette crystals of calcium oxalate.
2. Fragments of endocarp cells associated with hexagonal sclerenchyma of the innermost layer of the mesocarp.
3. Fragments of characteristic irregularly curved yellowish pitted lignified fusiform fibers of the mesocarp in sinuous rows, often crossing at right angles.
4. Fragments of parenchymatous cells of the mesocarp without reticulate thickening.
5. Very few fragments showing pieces of yellowish brown vittae.
6. Hairs and starch granules are completely absent.

CONSTITUENTS

Coriander fruits of good quality yield from 0.8-1.0% of volatile oil, the chief constituent of which is the terpene alcohol linalol (65-90%). It also contains fixed oil and proteins.

USES

It is used as a flavoring agent and carminative, the powdered fruits find wide use in the Egyptian kitchen as a spice and the oil is used in perfumery.

AJOWAN

Botanical Name	:	*Trachyspermum ammi*
Family	:	Apiaceae (Umbelliferae)
Parts Used	:	Seeds
Common Name	:	Ajowan

Ajowan is a member of the *Umbelliferae* family, which has some 2,700 members including *dill, caraway* and *cumin*. It is mostly found in Indian cooking, where it is also known as bishop's weed or carom. It is particularly suited to the delicate vegetarian fare found in the state of Gujarat.

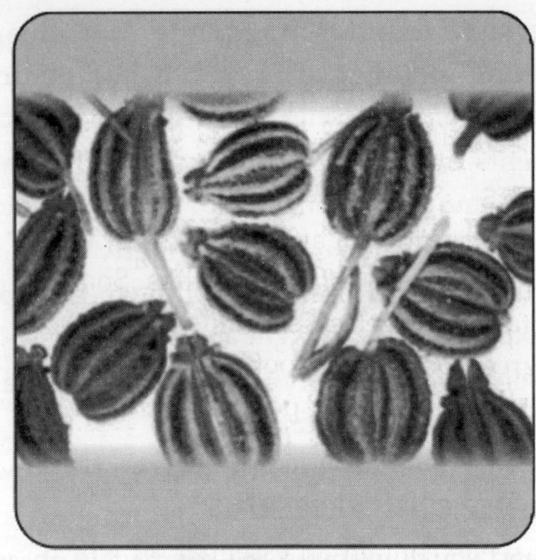

Fig. 8.3: Ajowan.

DESCRIPTION AND CULTIVATION

Ajowan is and annual herbaceous, 30-70 cm (1-2 ft) in height, bearing feathery leaves and red flowers. When the seeds are ripe, they are dried and threshed. Ajowan is native to India, but is also cultivated in Iran, Egypt Pakistan and Afghanistan.

SPICE DESCRIPTION

Ajowan seeds come from *Trachyspermum ammi*, a native plant of southern India. Ajowan seeds are used as a spice. The grayish-green seeds are striped and curved (similar to cumin or caraway seeds in appearance), often with a fine silk stalk attached. They are usually sold whole. The seeds are often chewed on their own for medicinal value, tasting bitingly hot and bitter, leaving the tongue numb for a while. Cooking ajowan when crushed, they have a strong and distinctive thyme-like fragrance.

Ajowan is usually ground in mortar and pestle, or crushed by rubbing between hands or fingertips before using. When used whole, for parathas or other breads, lightly bruise the seeds first, to release oils and increase flavour. The seeds can be stored indefinitely if kept from light in airtight containers.

FLAVOUR

A harsh thyme-like flavour with a bit of a kick, leaving a milder, pleasant aftertaste.

CULINARY USES

Ajowan has a particular affinity to starchy foods like savoury pastries and breads, especially parathas. Snacks like Bombay mix and potato balls get an extra kick from ajowan. It is also good with green beans and root vegetables. Lentil dishes and recipes using besan (chick pea flour). It is occasionally an ingredient of curry powder.

ATTRIBUTED MEDICINAL PROPERTIES

Ajowan seeds contain an essential oil which is about 50% thymol which is a strong germicide, anti-spasmodic and fungicide. Thymol is also used in toothpaste and perfumery. It is used in a steeped liquid form against diarrhea and flatulence. In India the seeds are used as a household remedy for indigestion and colic, and used in poultices to relieve asthma and arthritis. It also has aphrodisiac properties and the Ananga Ranga prescribes it for increasing a husband's enjoyment in his middle years.

CARDAMOM

Botanical Name	:	*Elettaria cardamomum*
Family	:	Zingiberaceae
Part Used	:	Seeds
Common Name	:	Chhoti elachi

Cardamom is one of the world's very ancient spices. It is native to the East originating in the forests of the western ghats in southern India, where it grows wild. Today it also grows in Sri Lanka, Guatemala, IndoChina and Tanzania. The ancient Egyptians chewed cardamom seeds as a tooth cleaner; the Greeks and Romans used it as a perfume. Vikings came upon cardamom about one thousand years ago, in Constantinople, and introduced it into Scandinavia, where it remains popular to this day.

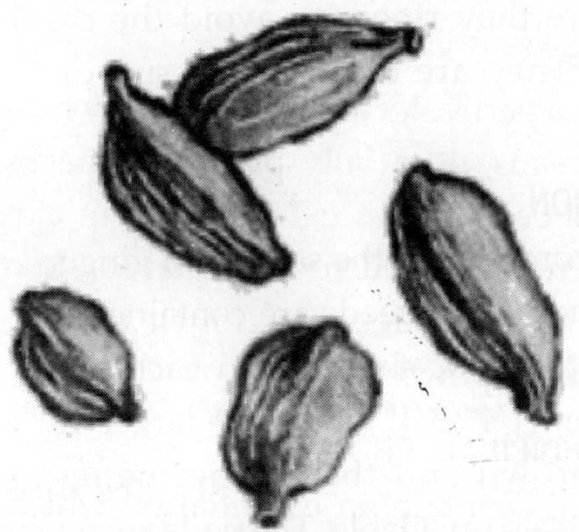

Fig. 8.4: Cardamom

Cardamom is an expensive spice, second only to saffron. It is often adulterated and there are many inferior substitutes from cardamom-related plants, such as Siam cardamom, Nepal cardamom, winged Java cardamom, and bastard cardamom. However, it is only Elettaria cardamomum which is the true cardamom. Indian cardamom is known in two main varieties: Malabar cardamom and Mysore cardamom. The Mysore variety contains higher levels of cineol and limonene and hence is more aromatic.

PLANT DESCRIPTION AND CULTIVATION

A perennial bush of the ginger family, with sheathed stems reaching 2-5 m (6-16 feet) in height. It has a large tuberous rhizome and long, dark green leaves 30-60 cm (1-2 ft) long, 5-15 cm (2-6") wide. It grows in the tropics, wild and in plantations. Trailing leafy stalks grow from the plant base at ground level. These bear the seed pods. The flowers are green with a white purple-veined tip.

Cardamoms are traditionally grown in partially cleared tropical rain forests, leaving some shade. Similarly, in plantation cultivation, forest undergrowth is cleared and trees thinned to give just enough shade and the rhizome or seeds planted at 3 m (10 ft) intervals. The plants are gathered in October-December, before they ripen, to avoid the capsules splitting during drying. They are dried in the sun or bleached with sulphur fumes.

SPICE DESCRIPTION

Cardamom comes from the seeds of a ginger-like plant. The small, brown-black sticky seeds are contained in a pod in three double rows with about six seeds in each row. The pods are between 5-20 mm (1/4"-3/4") long, the larger variety known as 'black', being brown and the smaller being green. White-bleached pods are also available. The pods are roughly triangular in cross section and oval or oblate. Their dried surface is rough and furrowed, the large 'blacks' having deep wrinkles. The texture of the pod is that of tough paper. Pods are available whole or split and the seeds are sold loose or ground. It is best to buy the whole pods as ground cardamom quickly loses flavour.

FLAVOUR

Warm and eucalyptine with camphorous and lemony undertones. Black cardamom is blunter, the eucalyptus and camphor suggestions very pronounced.

USES

The pods can be used whole or split when cooked in Indian substantial meals – such as pulses. Otherwise, the seeds can be bruised and fried before adding main ingredients to the pan, or pounded with other spices as required. Keep the pods whole until use. The pod itself is neutral in flavour and not generally used, imparting an unpleasant bitter flavour when left in dishes.

Cardamom is used mainly in the Near and Far East. Its commonest Western manifestation is in Dutch 'windmill' biscuits and Scandinavian-style cakes and pastries, and in akvavit. It features in curries, is essential in pilaus (rice dishes) and gives character to pulse dishes. Cardamom is often included in Indian sweet dishes and drinks. At least partially because of its high price, it is seen as a 'festive' spice. Other uses are; in pickles, especially pickled herring; in punches and mulled wines; occasionally with meat, poultry and shellfish. It flavours custards, and some Russian liqueurs. Cardamom is also chewed habitually (like nuts) where freely available, as in the East Indies, and in the Indian masticory, betel pan. It is a flavouring for Arab and Turkish coffee which is served with an elaborate ritual.

MEDICINAL USES

A stimulant and carminative, cardamom is not used in Western medicine for it own properties, but forms a flavouring and basis for medicinal preparations for indigestion and flatulence using other substances, entering into a synergetic relationship with them. The Arabs attributed aphrodisiac qualities to it (it features regularly in the Arabian Nights) and the ancient Indians regarded it as a cure for obesity. It has been used as a digestive since ancient times. A medicinal (perhaps aphrodisiac) cordial can be made by macerating seeds in hot water.

GINGER

Botanical Name	:	*Zingiber officinale*
Family	:	Zingiberaceae
Parts Used	:	Rhizom (Underground modified stem)
Common Name	:	Adarak, Ada, Adak

DESCRIPTION

Ginger is native to India and China. It takes its name from the Sanskrit word stringa-vera, which means "with a body like a horn", as in antlers. Ginger has been important in Chinese medicine for many centuries, and is mentioned in the writings of Confucius. It is also named in the Koran, the sacred book of the Moslems, indicating it was known in Arab countries as far back as 650 A.D. It was one of the earliest spice known in Western Europe, used since the ninth century. It became so popular in Europe that it was included in every table setting, like salt and pepper. A common article of medieval and Renaissance trade, it was one of the spices used against the plague. In English pubs and taverns in the nineteenth century, barkeepers put out small containers of ground ginger, for people to sprinkle into their beer — the origin of ginger ale. In order to 'gee up' a lazy horse, it is the time honoured practice of Sussex farmers to apply a pinch of ginger to the animal's backside.

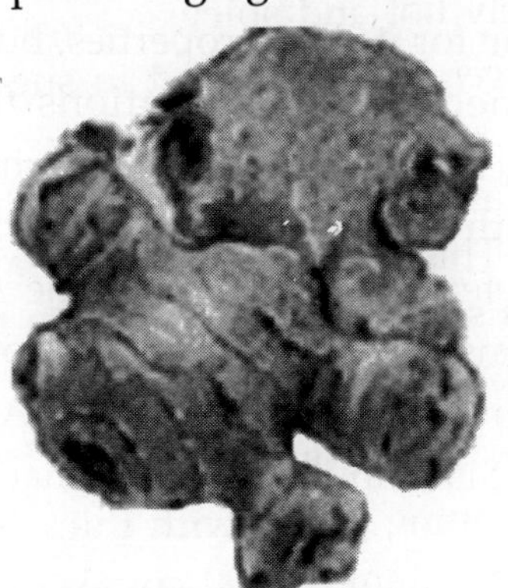

Fig. 8.5: Zingiber officinale

SPICE DESCRIPTION

Although often called "ginger root" it is actually a rhizome. It is available in various forms, the most common of which are as follows:

Whole raw roots are generally referred to as fresh ginger. A piece of the rhizome, called a 'hand'. It has a pale yellow interior and a skin varying in colour from brown to off-white. Jamaican ginger, which is pale buff, is regarded as the best variety. African and Indian ginger is darker skinned and generally inferior, with the exception of Kenya ginger. Buy fresh ginger

Whole fresh roots provide the freshest taste. The roots are collected and shipped when they are still immature, the outer skin is a light green colour. These can sometimes be found in Oriental markets.

Dried roots are sold either 'black' with the root skin left on, or 'white' with the skin peeled off. The dried root is available whole or sliced.

Powdered ginger is the buff-coloured ground spice made from dried root.

Preserved or 'stem' ginger is made from fresh young roots, peeled and sliced, then cooked in a heavy sugar syrup. The ginger pieces and syrup are canned together. They are soft and pulpy, but extremely hot and spicy.

Crystallized ginger is also cooked in sugar syrup, then air dried and rolled in sugar.

Pickled ginger has the root sliced paper-thin and pickled in a vinegar solution. This pickle is known in Japan as *gari,* which often accompanies sushi, and is served to refresh the palate between courses.

PLANT DESCRIPTION AND CULTIVATION

A perennial creeping plant, with thick tuberous rhizome, producing a an erect stem 30-100 cm (1-3 ft) tall. The lance-shaped leaves are bright green, 15-20 cm (6-8 in) long, with a prominent longitudinal rib, enclosing conical clusters of small yellow-green flowers marked with purple speckles. It is propagated from rhizome cuttings, planted on rich, well drained loam. It requires a tropical climate with both a heavy rain season and a hot dry season. Plants shoot in ten days and are harvested after nine to ten months.

PREPARATION AND STORAGE

In Asian cooking ginger is almost always used fresh, either minced, crushed or sliced. Fresh ginger can be kept for several weeks in the salad drawer of the refrigerator. Dried ginger should be 'bruised' by beating it to open the fibers, then infused in the cooking or making ginger beer and removed when the flavour is sufficient. Store dried and powdered ginger in airtight containers.

USES

Fresh ginger is essential to Asian and oriental cookery. It is used in pickles, chutneys and curry pastes and the ground dried root is a constituent of many curry powders. Tender young ginger can be sliced and eaten as a salad. Sometimes the roots will produce green sprouts which can be finely chopped and added to a green salad. In the West, dried ginger is mainly used in cakes and biscuits, especially ginger snaps and gingerbread. Ginger is also used in puddings, jams, preserves and in some drinks like ginger beer, ginger wine and tea. Pickled ginger is a delicious accompaniment to satays and a colourful garnish to many Chinese dishes. Preserved ginger is eaten as a confection, chopped up for cakes and puddings, and is sometimes used as an ice cream ingredient.

MEDICINAL USES

Ginger is most commonly known for its effectiveness as a digestive aid. By increasing the production of digestive fluids and saliva, Ginger helps relieve indigestion, gas pains, diarrhea and stomach cramping. The primary known constituents of Ginger Root include gingerols, zingibain, bisabolenel, oleoresins, starch, essential oil (zingiberene, zingiberole, camphene, cineol, borneol), mucilage, and protein. Ginger root is also used to treat nausea related to both motion sickness and morning sickness. Ginger has been found to be even more effective than Dramamine® in curbing motion sickness, without causing drowsiness. Ginger's anti-inflammatory properties help relieve pain and reduce inflammation associated with arthritis, rheumatism and muscle spasms. Ginger's therapeutic properties effectively stimulate circulation of the blood, removing toxins from the body, cleansing the bowels and kidneys, and nourishing the skin. Other uses for Ginger Root include the treatment of asthma, bronchitis and other respiratory problems by loosening and expelling phlegm from the lungs. Ginger Root may also be used to help break fevers by warming the body and increasing perspiration.

BLACK PEPPER

Botanical Name	:	*Piper nigrum*
Family	:	Piperaceae
Parts Used	:	Fruit
Common Names	:	Black pepper, White pepper, Green pepper, Peppercorn, pepper, Kali mirch

A pinch of black pepper is added to almost every type of recipe imaginable. Once used as currency and presented to the gods as a sacred offering, it is fortunate that this most popular of spices is available throughout the year.

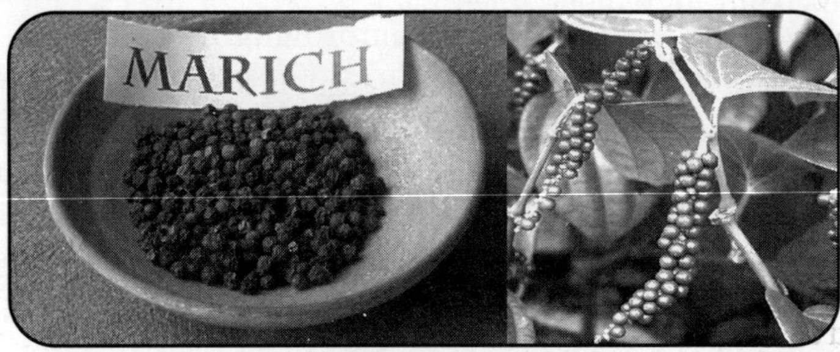

Fig. 8.6: Piper nigrum

Black pepper comes from the pepper plant, a smooth woody vine that can grow up to 33 feet in hot and humid tropical climates. They begin to bear small white clustered flowers after 3 to 4 years and develop into berries known as *peppercorns*.

DESCRIPTION

Black pepper comes from the berries of the pepper plant. Black pepper, green pepper and white peppercorns are actually the same fruit (*Piper nigrum*); the difference in their color is a reflection of varying stages of development and processing methods.

Black peppercorns are made by picking the pepper berries when they are half ripe and just about to turn red. They are then left to dry which causes them to shrivel and become dark in color. Alternatively, green peppercorns are picked while still unripe and green in color, while white peppercorns are picked when very ripe and subsequently soaked in brine to remove their dark outer shell leaving just the white pepper seed.

Pink peppercorns are actually from a completely different plant species (Schinus molle) that is related to ragweed.

Black pepper is the most pungent and flavorful of all types of peppers and it is available as whole or cracked peppercorns or ground into powder.

IMPROVE DIGESTION AND PROMOTE INTESTINAL HEALTH

Black pepper (*Piper nigrum*)stimulates the taste buds in such a way that an alert is sent to to the stomach to increase hydrochloric acid secretion, thereby improving digestion. Hydrochloric acid is necessary for the digestion of proteins and other food components in the stomach. When the body's production of hydrochloric acid is insufficient, food may sit in the stomach for an extended period of time, leading to heartburn or indigestion, or it may pass into the intestines, where it can be used as a food source for unfriendly gut bacteria, whose activities produce gas, irritation, and/or diarrhoea or constipation.

Black pepper has long been recognized as a carminitive, (a substance that helps prevent the formation of intestinal gas), a property likely due to its beneficial effect of stimulating hydrochloric acid production. In addition, black pepper has diaphoretic (promotes sweating), and diuretic (promotes urination) properties.

Good for the Stomach

Black pepper is used traditionally to treat stomach acid and prevent the formation of intestinal gas. It is sometimes made into preparations with other substances including cow's urine.

TRADITIONAL MEDICINE

In Ayurveda the fruits are valued for a range of properties including its hot, light and anti-flatulent effects. In Ayurvedic medicine black pepper has been used to aid digestion, improve the appetite, treat coughs, colds, breathing and heart problems, colic, diabetes, anaemia and piles. Stomach ailments such as dyspepsia, flatulence, constipation and diarrhoea are all treated with black pepper, which may be mixed with other substances such as castor oil, cow's urine or ghee.

Black pepper has been prepared in the form of pills as a remedy for *cholera* and *syphilis*, sometimes combined with other substances. It has also been used in tooth powder for toothache and an infusion of black pepper has been described as a remedy for sore throat and hoarseness. Alternatively black pepper could be chewed to reduce *throat inflammation*.

External Application

Externally it has been applied in paste form to boils and *to treat hair loss* and some *skin diseases*. Oil of pepper is reputed to alleviate itching. A mixture of *sesame oil* and powdered black pepper is described as an application for areas affected by *paralysis*. A mixture of black pepper and honey is regarded as a remedy for *night blindness*. In comatose patients black pepper has been given by inhalation. It is also believed to be useful in *hepatitis, urinary* and *reproductive disorders*. In Ayurveda and Siddha medicine, a paste is made using *white pepper* is applied to treat some *eye diseases*.

ASAFOETIDA

Botanical Name	:	*Ferula asafoetida*
Family	:	Apiaceae
Parts Used	:	Resin extracted from rhizome and thickened root
Common Name	:	Hing and Hingra

DESCRIPTION

Asafoetida, the gum resin prized as a condiment in India and Iran, is obtained chiefly from plant Ferula asafoetida. The Latin name 'ferula' means "carrier" or "vehicle". 'Asa' is a latinized form of Farsi *asa* "resin", and Latin *foetidus* means "smelling, fetid".

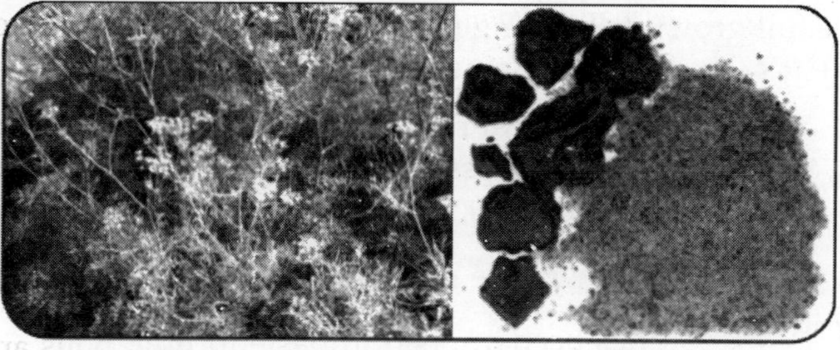

Fig. 8.7: Asafoetide (Ferula asafoetida)

A related species (*F. vulgaris*), native to the Mediterranean, is mentioned in the Greek mythology as the plant that helped Prometheus to carry the stolen fire from the Sun to the Earth earth and hence has great significance in the Greek mythology. All central Asia from Iran to Afghanistan has the use of Ferula as important spice in food and as an essential ingredient for home remedies. Although the smell of fresh asafoetida does not seem to qualify as a valuable food enhancement, but after frying (and in small dosage) the taste becomes pleasant.

Asafoetida or asafoetida (Devil's Dung) is dried latex (oleo-gum-resin) exuded from the living rhizome, rootstock or taproot of an umbelliferous plant of varied species. Being a unique blend of finest ingredients, Indian asafoetida from Kashmir enjoys an exalted position in the international market.

Commercially, Indian asafoetida comes in three forms on the basis of quality :

1. Tears.
2. Mass.
3. Paste.

Another forms names two varieties on the basis of place of origin, flavour and colour:

1. Hing
2. Hingra.

AROMA AND FLAVOUR

The whole plant is used as a fresh vegetable, the inner portion of the full-grown stem being regarded as a delicacy. The horrible smell of fresh asafoetida does not seem to qualify as a valuable food enhancement, but after frying (and in small dosage), the resin, the taste becomes rather pleasant, even for Western taste buds. The so-called "powdered asafoetida" is the resin mixed with rice fiour and therefore much less strong in taste, but more easy in application.

MEDICINAL PROPERTIES

Antispasmodic, Aromatic, Carminative, Digestive, Expectorant, Laxative, Sedative, Nervine, Analgesic, Anthel-mintic, Aphrodisiac, Antiseptic.

MED!CINAL AND OTHER USE

Asafoetida is an interesting alternative to onion and garlic, even for Western dishes. In ancient Rome, asafoetida was stored in jars together with pine nuts, which were alone used to flavour delicate dishes. Another method is dissolving asafoetida in hot oil and adding the oil drop by drop to the food.

If used with sufficient moderation, asafoetida enhances mushroom and vegetable dishes, but can also be used to give fried or barbecued meat a unique flavour. Asafoetida is a useful antidote for flatulence. There are claims for it being used to cure bronchitis and even hysteria.

Gum resin of the plant is used as spice and as medicine. It is well known for its effects on the digestive system. It is observed that asafoetida do not have a marked effect on the gas producing bacteria in the intestine. However, it alters the proportion of the hydrogen to carbon dioxide formed by these organisms. Thus, it acts as an ideal option to leave the flatulence.

Its' other uses indicated in chronic Bronchitis, Colic, Dyspepsia, Hysteria, Tympanitis, infantile convulsions, and whooping cough. It is used as a stimulant to the brain and nervous and gastric systems. Its paste is useful on the itching surface of the skin. it calms skin eruptions. Taken internally it cools the body and mind, while helping to improve the concentration.

Tagara (*Valeriana Wallichii*) has long been used as a sedative and anti-spasmodic. Being a natural tranquillizer, it is particularly useful in the treatment of hysteria and epilepsy.

It also stimulates regular flow of menstrual cycle, as well as cleanliness of the uterus after labour (Childbirth). It is employed in preparation of large number of Ayurvedic formulation

Asafoetida is a popular spice in Europe since the Roman times and a much-preferred spice of the Middle Ages. All over Persia and India, people who do not prefer to eat onion and garlic make asafoetida an essential ingredient of their cuisine and hence it is used as an alternative or substitute for onion and garlic in almost all vegetable dishes.

A pea-sized amount is considered to be large or sufficient to add the asafoetida flavor to a large pot of food whereas powdered asafoetida is less intense and can be without frying. The aroma of this spice is less when used in powdered form but the resin has a non-perishable fragrance. The resin is strongly scented and must be fried shortly in hot oil.

The reason being that the resin dissolves in the hot fat and gets better dispersed in the food and the high temperature changes the taste to a more pleasant impression. If used with sufficient moderation, asafoetida enhances mushroom and vegetable dishes but can also be used to give fried or barbecued meat a unique flavor.

NUTMEG

Botanical Name	:	*Myristica fragrans*
Family	:	Myristicaceae
Part Used	:	Seed
Common Name	:	Jaiphal, Nutmug

DESCRIPTION

Nutmeg or *Myristica fragrans* is an evergreen tree indigenous to the Banda Islands in the Moluccas of Indonesia, or Spice Islands. The nutmeg tree is important for two spices derived from the fruit, nutmeg and mace.

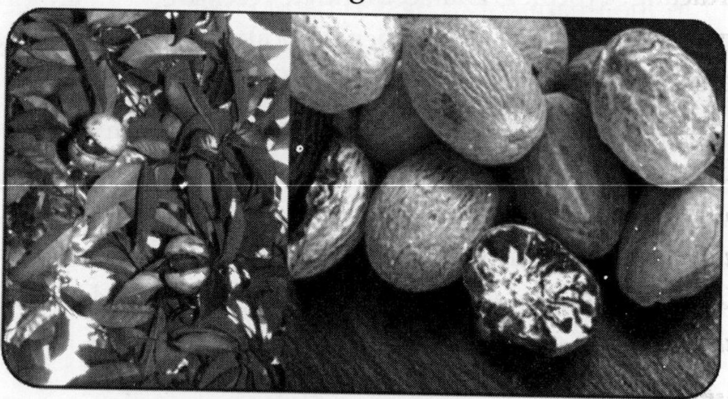

Fig. 8.8: Nutmeg

Nutmeg is the actual seed of the tree, roughly egg-shaped and about 20 to 30 mm (0.8 to 1 inch) long and 15 to 18 mm (0.6 to 0.7 inch) wide, and weighing between 5 and 10 g (0.2 and 0.4 oz) dried, while mace is the dried "lacy" reddish covering or arillus of the seed. This is the only tropical fruit that is the source of two different spices.

Several other commercial products are also produced from the trees, including essential oils, extracted oleoresins, and nutmeg butter.The outer surface of the nutmeg bruises easily.

The *pericarp* (fruit/pod) is used in Grenada to make a jam called *'Morne Delice'*. In Indonesia, the fruit is also made into jam, called selei *buah pala,* or sliced finely, cooked and crystallised to make a fragrant candy called *manisan pala* ('nutmeg sweets').

CULINARY USES

Nutmeg and mace have similar taste qualities, nutmeg having a slightly sweeter and mace a more delicate flavour. Mace is often preferred in light dishes for the bright orange, saffron-like hue it imparts. Nutmeg is a tasty addition to cheese sauces and is best grated fresh. Nutmeg is a traditional ingredient in mulled cider, mulled wine, and eggnog.

In Penang cuisine, nutmeg is made into pickles and these pickles are even shredded as toppings on the uniquely Penang Ais Kacang. Nutmeg is also blended (creating a fresh, green, tangy taste and white colour juice) or boiled (resulting in a much sweeter and brown juice) to make Iced Nutmeg juice or as it is called in Penang Hokkien, 'Lau Hau Peng'.

In Indian cuisine, nutmeg is used in many sweet as well as savoury dishes (predominantly in Mughlai cuisine). It is known as *Jaiphal* in most parts of India and as *Jatipatri* and *Jathi* seed in Kerala. It may also be used in small quantities in *garam masala*. Ground nutmeg is also smoked in India.

NUTMEG SEEDS

The essential oil is obtained by the steam distillation of ground nutmeg and is used heavily in the perfumery and pharmaceutical industries. The oil is colourless or light yellow, and smells and tastes of nutmeg. It contains numerous components of interest to the oleochemical industry, and is used as a natural food flavouring in baked goods, syrups, beverages, and sweets. It replaces ground nutmeg as it leaves no particles in the food. The essential oil is also used in the cosmetic and pharmaceutical industries, for instance, in toothpaste, and as a major ingredient in some cough syrups. In traditional medicine nutmeg and nutmeg oil were used for illnesses related to the nervous and digestive systems.

NUTMEG BUTTER

Nutmeg butter is obtained from the nut by expression. It is semi-solid, reddish brown in colour, and tastes and smells of nutmeg. Approximately 75% (by weight) of nutmeg butter is trimyristin, which can be turned into myristic acid, a 14-carbon fatty acid which can be used as a replacement for cocoa butter, can be mixed with other fats like cottonseed oil or palm oil, and has applications as an industrial lubricant.

PSYCHOACTIVITY AND TOXICITY OF NUTMEG

In low doses, nutmeg produces no noticeable physiological or neurological response. Large doses can be dangerous (potentially inducing convulsions, palpitations, nausea, eventual dehydration, and generalized body pain). In large amounts it is reputed to be a strong deliriant. Users may feel a sensation of blood rushing to the head, or a strong euphoria and dissociation. Nutmeg contains myristicin, a weak monoamine oxidase inhibitor.

Nutmeg contains no amphetamine derivatives nor are any formed in the body from the main chemical components of nutmeg. Use of nutmeg as a recreational drug is unpopular due to its unpleasant taste and its possible negative side effects, including dizziness, flushes, dry mouth, accelerated heartbeat, temporary constipation, difficulty in urination, nausea, and panic. In addition, experiences usually last well over 24 hours making recreational use rather impractical.

A risk in any large-quantity ingestion of nutmeg is the onset of 'nutmeg poisoning', an acute psychiatric disorder marked by thought disorder, a sense of impending doom/death, and agitation. Some cases have resulted in hospitalization.

Nutmeg was once considered an abortifacient, but may be safe for culinary use during pregnancy. However, it inhibits prostaglandin production and contains hallucinogens that may affect the fetus if consumed in large quantities.

CLOVES

Botanical Name	:	*Eugenia caryophyllus* or *Syzygium aromaticum*
Family	:	Myrtaceae
Parts Used	:	Dried and unexpanded flower bud
Common Name	:	Laung, Labanga

HABITAT

It is cultivated in Brazil, West Indies, Mauritius, Madagascar, India, Sri Lanka, Zanzibar and Pemba. The Chinese wrote of cloves as early as 400 B.C. and there is a record from 200 B.C. of courtiers keeping cloves in their mouths to avoid offending the emperor while addressing him. Arab traders delivered cloves to the Romans.

DESCRIPTION AND CULTIVATION

A conical tropical evergreen myrtaceous tree reaching heights of up to 14 m (45 ft.). The bark is gray, the leaves are a shiny dark green, elliptical in shape and very fragrant. Small crimson flowers grow in triple clusters at the ends of branches. The fruit is a purple drupe, about 2.5 cm (1") long. Cloves grow in the tropics and best near the sea. Rainfall must be at least sixty inches per year and a dry season is needed for harvesting and curing. The clove clusters are picked by hand before the buds open and dried on palm mats.

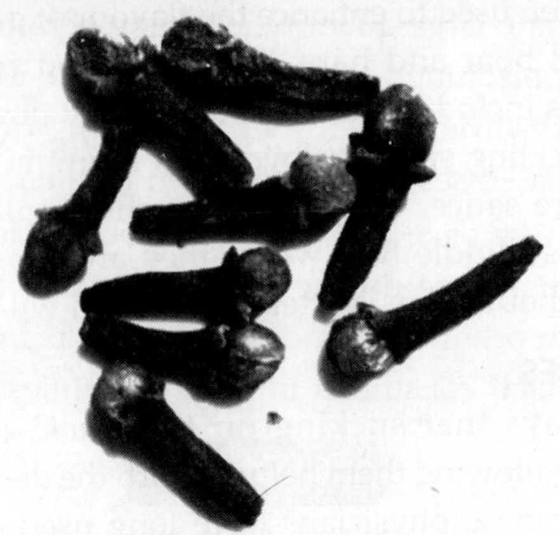

Fig. 8.9: Eugenia caryophyllus

SPICE DESCRIPTION

Cloves are the immature unopened flower buds of a tropical tree. When fresh, they are pink, dried, they turn to a rust-brown colour. Measuring 12-16 mm (1/2"-5/8") long, they resemble small nails, with a tapered stem. The large end of the clove is the four-pointed flower bud.

FLAVOUR

Sweetly pungent, astringent and strongly aromatic.

PREPARATION AND STORAGE

Cloves are best bought whole. As a powder flavour quickly deteriorates. Being extremely hard, it is difficult to grind cloves with a mortar and pestle so an electric grinder such as a coffee grinder is recommended. Store in an airtight container out of direct light.

CULINARY USES

Cloves can easily overpower a dish, particularly when ground, so only a few need be used. Whole cloves are often used to "stud" hams and pork, pushing the tapered end into the meat like a nail. A studded onion is frequently used to impart an elusive character to courts-bouillons, stocks and soups.

Cloves are often used to enhance the flavour of game, especially venison, wild boar and hare. They are used in a number of spice mixtures including ras el hanout, curry powders, mulling spices and pickling spices. Cloves also figure in the flavour of Worcestershire sauce. They enjoy much popularity in North Africa and the Middle East where they are generally used for meat dishes, though rice is often aromatized with a few cloves.

MEDICINAL USES

Folklore says that sucking on *two whole cloves* without chewing or swallowing them helps to curb the desire for alcohol. Traditional Chinese physicians have long used cloves to treat *indigestion, diarrhea, hernia,* and *ringworm,* as well as *athlete's foot* and other *fungal infections.* India's traditional Ayurvedic healers have used Cloves since ancient times to treat *respiratory* and *digestive ailments.* The medieval German herbalists used cloves as part of *anti-gout mixture.* Early American Eclectic physicians used cloves to treat digestive complaints, and they added it to bitter herbal medicines to make them more palatable. They were also the first to extract clove oil from the herbal buds, which they used on the *gums to relieve toothache.* A few drops of the oil in water will stop *vomiting,* and an infusion will relieve *nausea.* Essential oil of clove is effective against strep, staph and *pneumomocci bacterias.* Contemporary herbalists recommend vloves for digestive complaints and its oil for toothache. The primary chemical constituents include eugenol, caryophyllene, and tannins.

Cloves are said to have a positive effect on *stomach ulcers, vomiting, flatulence,* and *to stimulate the digestive system.* It has powerful local antiseptic and mild anesthetic actions. Japanese researchers have discovered that like many spices, clove contains antioxidants. Antioxidants help prevent the cell damage that scientists believe eventually causes cancer.

On the other hand, in laboratory tests, the chemical eugenol, has been found to be a weak tumor promoter, making clove one of many healing herbs with both pro- and anti-cancer effects. At this point, scientists aren't sure which way the balance tilts. Until they are, anyone with a history of cancer should not use medicinal amounts of clove.

For otherwise healthy non-pregnant, non-nursing adults, powdered clove is considered nontoxic.

Additionally, dentists have used clove oil as an oral anesthetic. They also used it to disinfect root canals.

Clove oil still is an active ingredient in several mouthwash products and a number of over-the-counter toothache pain-relief preparations.

Cloves kill intestinal parasites and exhibits broad anti-microbial properties against fungi and bacteria, thus supporting its traditional use as a treatment for diarrhea, intestinal worms, and other digestive ailments.

Like many culinary spices, *Cloves* helps relax the smooth muscle lining of the digestive tract. And finally, eating cloves is said to be aphrodisiac.

HEALTH BENEFITS OF CLOVE OIL

Clove oil is often used for a number of medicinal reasons, one of which is for the relief of certain aches and pains. Since it has analgesic properties, it is useful for exactly this purpose.

Clove oil has also been used as a remedy for problems with respiration. Asthma and bronchitis are two of the respiratory problems that are being treated naturally with the use of clove oil.

The ingredient that is used in the making of clove oil is not the clove itself but the flower of the red clove plant. Some people believe that clove oil is simply any kind of edible oil that has cloves in them but this is not the case. Clove oil is the oil that is extracted from the clove plant's flower.

·Other ailments that use clove oil for treatment include muscle pains, strains and sprains and other painful ailments like *toothaches*, *rheumatism*, and *arthritis*.

Clove oil is well known for its analgesic properties and has been widely used because of this. Clove oil has more to it than just killing pain.

OTHER BENEFITS

- Clove oil has anti-inflammatory properties that make it ideal for use on such aches and pains like toothaches and sprains since these often have swelling associated with the pain.
- Not only is clove oil good for toothaches and other pains in the mouth, it is also a good mouth antiseptic and mouthwash that can kill germs that cause bad breath.
- Clove oil has been seen to offer a person better blood circulation, which in turn gives him the much needed boost in the immune system. This makes a person less prone to illnesses.
- Diabetic patients have been known to use clove oil to help in controlling the sugar levels in blood.
- Clove oil is also widely used for treating skin problems.

CINNAMON

Botanical Name	:	*Cinnamomum cassia*
Family	:	Lauraceae
Parts Used	:	The dried bark
Common Name	:	Dal chhini

Although available throughout the year, the fragrant, sweet and warm taste of cinnamon is a perfect spice to use during the winter months.

Cinnamon has a long history both as a spice and as a medicine. It is the brown bark of the cinnamon tree, which is available in its dried tubular form known as a quill or as ground powder. The two varieties of cinnamon, *Chinese* and *Ceylon*, have similar flavor, however, the cinnamon from Ceylon is slightly sweeter, more refined and more difficult to find in local markets.

DESCRIPTION

Cinnamon is the brown bark of the cinnamon tree, which when dried, rolls into a tubular form known as a quill. Cinnamon is available in either its whole quill form (cinnamon sticks) or as ground powder.

While there are approximately one hundred varieties of *Cinnamonum verum* (the scientific name for cinnamon), *Cinnamonum zeylanicum* (Ceylon cinnamon) and *Cinna-momun aromaticum* (Chinese cinnamon) are the leading varieties consumed. (Ceylon cinnamon is also referred to as "true cinnamon", while the Chinese variety is known as "cassia". While both are relatively similar in characteristics and both feature a fragrant, sweet and warm taste, the flavor of the Sri Lanka variety is more refined and subtle. Sri Lanka cinnamon is more rare in North America than the cassia, the less expensive variety, which is the most popular in the United States.

HEALTH BENEFITS

Cinnamon's unique *healing abilities* come from three basic types of components in the essential oils found in its bark. These oils contain active components called *cinnamaldehyde, cinnamyl acetate,* and *cinnamyl alcohol,* plus a wide range of other volatile substances.

Anti-Clotting Actions

Cinnamaldehyde (also called cinnamic aldehyde) has been well-researched for its effects on blood platelets. Platelets are constituents of blood that are meant to clump together under emergency circumstances (like physical injury) as a way to stop bleeding, but under normal circumstances, they can make blood flow inadequate if they clump together too much. The cinnaldehyde in cinnamon helps prevent unwanted clumping of blood platelets. (The way it accomplishes this health-protective act is by inhibiting the release of an inflammatory fatty acid called arachidonic acid from platelet membranes and reducing the formation of an inflammatory messaging molecule called *thromboxane*). Cinnamon's ability to lower the release of arachidonic acid from cell membranes also puts it in the category of an "anti-inflammatory" food that can be helpful in lessening inflammation.

Anti-Microbial Activity

Cinnamon's essential oils also qualify it as an "anti-microbial" food, and cinnamon has been studied for its ability to help stop the growth of bacteria as well as fungi, including the commonly problematic yeast Candida. In laboratory tests, growth of yeasts that were resistant to the commonly used anti-fungal medication fluconazole was often (though not always) stopped by cinnamon extracts.

Blood Sugar Control

Cinnamon slows the rate at which the stomach empties after meals, reducing the rise in blood sugar after eating. Researchers measured how quickly the stomach emptied after 14 healthy subjects ate 300 grams (1.2 cups) of rice pudding alone or seasoned with 6 grams (1.2 teaspoons) of cinnamon. Adding cinnamon to the rice pudding lowered the gastric emptying rate from 37% to 34.5% and significantly lessened the rise in blood sugar levels after eating.

Cinnamon may also significantly help people with *type 2 diabetes* improve their ability to respond to insulin, thus normalizing their blood sugar levels.

Studies to confirm cinnamon's beneficial actions in humans are currently underway with the most recent report coming from researchers from the *US Agricultural Research Service*, who have shown that *less than half a teaspoon per day of cinnamon reduces blood sugar levels in persons with type 2 diabetes.*

In humans with type 2 diabetes, consuming as little as 1 gram of cinnamon per day was found to reduce blood sugar, triglycerides, LDL (bad) cholesterol, and total cholesterol, in a study published in the December 2003 issue of *Diabetes Care.*

Cinnamon is so powerful an *antioxidant* that, when compared to six other antioxidant spices (anise, ginger, licorice, mint, nutmeg and vanilla) and the chemical food preservatives (BHA (butylated hydroxyanisole), BHT (butylated hydroxytoluene), and propyl gallate), cinnamon prevented oxidation more effectively than all the other spices (except mint) and the chemical antioxidants.

Specifically, cinnamon improved participants' scores on tasks related to attentional processes, virtual recognition memory, working memory, and visual-motor speed while working on a computer-based program.

Calcium and Fiber Improve Colon Health and Protect Against Heart Disease

In addition to its unique essential oils, cinnamon is an excellent source of the trace mineral manganese and a very good source of dietary fiber, iron and calcium. The combination of calcium and fiber in cinnamon is important and can be helpful for the prevention of several different conditions. Both calcium and fiber can bind to bile salts and help remove them from the body. By removing bile, fiber helps to prevent the damage that certain bile salts can cause to colon cells, thereby reducing the risk of colon cancer. In addition, when bile is removed by fiber, the body must breakdown cholesterol in order to make new bile. This process can help to lower high cholesterol levels, which can be helpful in preventing atherosclerosis and heart disease. For sufferers of irritable bowel syndrome, the fiber in cinnamon may also provide relief from constipation or diarrhea.

A Traditional Warming Remedy

In addition to the active components in its essential oils and its nutrient composition, cinnamon has also been valued in energy-based medical systems, such as *Traditional Chinese Medicine*, for its warming qualities. In these traditions, cinnamon has been used to provide relief when faced with the onset of a cold or flu, especially when mixed in a tea with some fresh ginger.

STUDY QUESTIONS

1. Write short notes on the following:
   (a) Ajowan;
   (b) Cardamom;
   (c) Cloves; and
   (d) Cinnamon.
2. How can calcium and fiber improve colon health and protect against heart disease?
3. Explain the medicinal uses of the follwing:
   (a) Ferula Asafoetida;
   (b) Piper nigrum; and
   (c) Foeniculum vulgare.

■■■

9 CHAPTER

ASTRINGENTS

CATECHU, BLACK

Botanical Name	:	*Catechu nigrum, Acacia catechu*
Family	:	Leguminosae
Parts Used	:	Bark
Common Name	:	Katha

HABITAT

Acacia catechu found in Burma and India. Pale Catechu is an extract made from the leaves and young shoots of Uncaria Gambier (Roxb.), a member of the order *Rubiaceae*, not an Acacia. It occurs in commerce in dark or pale-brown cubes with a dull, powdery fracture, or sometimes in lozenge form. Black Catechu occurs in black, shining pieces or cakes. Both substances are sold under the name of *Catechu*.

DESCRIPTION

Cutch occurs in nearly black masses, the outer portions of which are hard and brittle, but the interior often still soft. It breaks easily, the fractured surface having a dull gloss, and containing a number of small cavities. It yields a dull brown powder and has no odour, but an astringent and subsequently sweetish taste. When macerated with cold water it forms a brown magma, which exhibits under the microscope numerous minute crystals similar to those found in gambier. Boiling water dissolves it almost entirely but on cooling deposits a crystalline sediment.

CONSTITUENTS

Cutch closely resembles gambier in chemical composition. It contains as principal constituents catechutannic acid and acacatechin, but the former is usually present in much larger quantity than the latter. Acacatechin differs from the catechin of gambier in its formula, $C_{15}H_{14}O_6$, $3H_{10}$, and melting point. The drug contains in addition catechu-red and small quantities of quercetin, but is free from the fluorescent substance that is present in gambier. Although the two drugs, gambier and cutch, as usually found on the market have little resemblance to one another, this is due solely to the manner of preparation, the syrupy liquor being in the case of gambier allowed to crystallise. This method is sometimes pursued in India with Cutch, and the resulting drug, 'katha', then closely resembles gambier, but can always be distinguished from it by the absence of the fluorescent substance.

SOURCE

Cutch is an extract prepared from the heartwood of *Acacia Catechu, Willdenow* (*Leguminosoe*), a tree of medium size common in India and Burma. It yields a valued timber, and also an astringent bark that is used for tanning.

This drug must be carefully distinguished from the foregoing (gambier), which is official under the name of catechu. The two substances are quite distinct, and that obtained from

Acacia Catechu is to be regarded as true catechu. To avoid confusion it would be well to adhere to the terms 'gambier' and 'cutch' for the two drugs, thus avoiding the use of the term 'catechu', which has been applied to both.

To obtain the drug the tree is felled, the bark and sapwood stripped from the trunk, the dark red heartwood cut into chips and boiled in water in earthen pots. The decoction is then strained and boiled down in iron pots with continual stirring until it attains the consistency of syrup. When sufficiently cool to handle, the extract is spread upon leaves arranged within a wooden frame or mould and left for the night. In the morning the cutch is dry, and forms brick-like masses weighing about 20 kilograms, which are broken up for the market.

MEDICINAL ACTION AND USES

Both the dark and the pale Catechu are employed in medicine, the former is more astringent, the latter, being sweeter, is less disagreeable. It depends almost entirely for its virtues upon the tannic acid it contains and is hence employed as an astringent to overcome relaxation of mucous membranes in general.

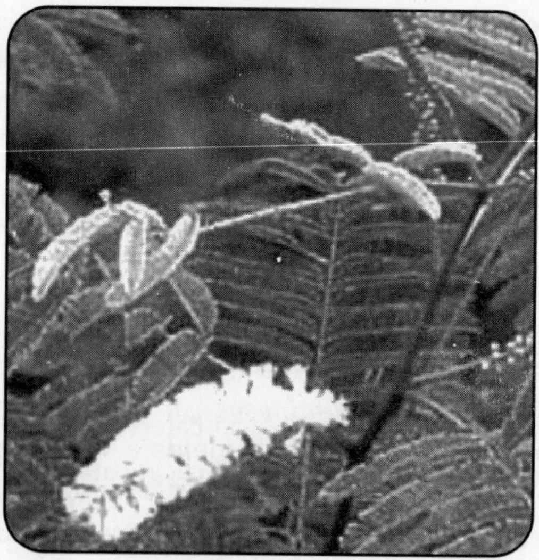

Fig. 9.1: Acacia catechu

An infusion can be employed to stop nosebleeding, and is also employed as an injection for uterine haemorrhage, leucorrhoea and gonorrhoea.

Externally, it is applied in the form of powder, to boils, ulcers and cutaneous eruptions, and also used for the same purposes mixed with other ingredients, in an ointment.

A small piece, held in the mouth and allowed slowly to dissolve, is an excellent remedy in relaxation of the uvula and simple pharyngitis.

In powder, applied to spongy gums, it often proves of use and has been recommended as a dentifrice with powdered charcoal, myrrh, etc.

The pharmaceutical preparations are: Powdered Catechu, dose 5 to 15 grains; Compound Powder of Catechu, B.P., dose 10 to 40 grains; Tincture of Catechu, B.P., dose 1/2 to 1 drachm; Comp. Tincture, U.S.P., dose 1 drachm. Catechu Lozenges are also official preparations in both the British and United States Pharmacopoeias.

Like *Acacia arabica*, the wood-extract of this species has, however, a larger field in the tanning industry than in medicine. The Pale Catechu (Gambier Catechu) is largely used in the arts, for dyeing purposes, yielding a colour known as 'Cutch Brown'.

Cutch is subject to the most extensive adulteration, though this exists chiefly in the tanning grades. The chief adulterants are Than (an extract obtained by boiling the bark of Buceras oliverii), dried blood, ashes, sand, clay and starch, and their detection is provided for in the official tests.

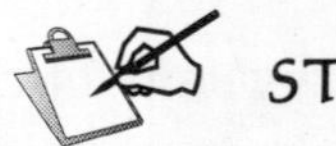

STUDY QUESTIONS

1. Write a detailed note on Acacia catechu.
2. Explain the medicinal uses of Acacia catechu.

■■■

10

CHAPTER

Drugs Acting on Nervous System

HYOSCYAMUS

Botanical Name	:	*Hyoscyamus niger*
Family	:	Solanaceae
Parts Used	:	Fresh leaves, Flowering tops and Branches and Seeds.
Common Name	:	Henbane

DESCRIPTION

H. niger is susceptible of considerable diversity of character, causing varieties which have by some been considered as distinct species. Thus, the plant is sometimes annual, the stem almost unbranched, smaller and less downy than in the biennial form, the leaves shorter and less hairy and the flowers often yellow, without any purple markings. The annual plant also flowers in July or August, the biennial in May and June.

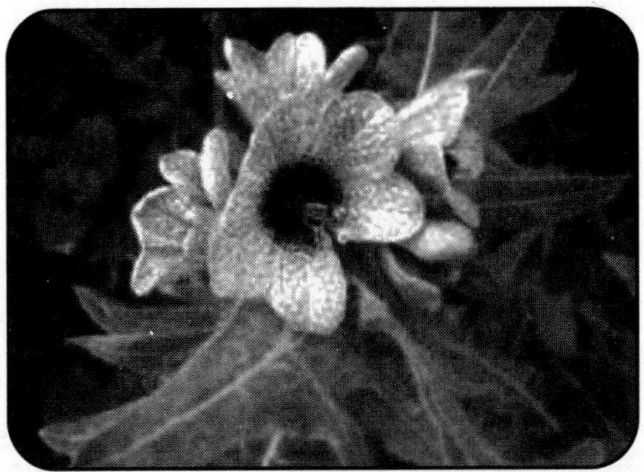

Fig. 10.1: Hyoscyamus niger

The annual and biennial form spring indifferently from the same crop of seed, the former growing during summer to a height of from 1 to 2 feet, and flowering and perfecting seed, the latter producing the first season only a tuft of radical leaves, which disappear in winter, leaving underground a thick, fleshy root, from the crown of which arises in spring a branched, flowering stem, usually much taller and more vigorous than the flowering stems of the annual plants. The annual form is apparently produced by the weaker and later developed seeds formed in the fruit at the ends of the shoots; it is considered to be less active than the typical species and differs in being of dwarfed growth and having rather paler flowers. The British drug of commerce consists of dense flowering shoots only, and of larger size.

Both varieties are used in medicine, but the biennial form is the one considered official. The leaves of this biennial plant spread out flat on all sides from the crown of the root like a rosette; they are oblong and egg-shaped, with acute points, stalked and more or less sharply toothed, often more than a foot in length, of a greyish-green colour and covered with sticky hairs. These leaves perish at the appearance of winter.

The flowering *stem* pushes up from the root-crown in the following spring, ultimately reaching from 3 to 4 feet in height, and as it grows, becoming branched and furnished with alternate, oblong, unequally lobed, stalkless leaves, which are stem-clasping and vary considerably in size, but seldom exceed 9 or 10 inches in length. These leaves are pale green in colour, with a broad conspicuous mid-rib, and are furnished on both sides (but particularly on the veins on the under surface) with soft, glandular hairs, which secrete a resinous substance that causes the fresh leaves to feel unpleasantly clammy and sticky. Similar hairs occur on the sub-cylindrical branches.

The *flowers* are shortly stalked, the lower ones growing in the fork of the branches, the upper ones stalkless, crowded together in onesided, leafy spikes, which are rolled back at the top before flowering, the hairy, leafy, coarsely-toothed bracts becoming smaller upwards. The flowers have a hairy, pitchershaped calyx, which remains round the fruit and is strongly veined, with five stiff, broad, almost prickly lobes. The corollas are obliquely funnel-shaped, upwards of an inch across, of a dingy yellow or buff, marked with a close network of lurid purple veins. A variety sometimes occurs in which the corolla is not marked with these purple veins. The seed-capsule opens transversely by a convex lid and contains numerous small seeds. The whole plant has a powerful, oppressive, nauseous odour.

CULTIVATION

Henbane is in such demand for medicinal purposes that it is necessary to cultivate it, the wild plants not yielding a sufficient supply. Henbane will grow on most soils, in sandy spots near the sea, on chalky slopes, and in cultivation flourishing in a good loam.

In some maritime localities it can be grown without any trouble. It requires a light, moderately rich and well-drained soil for successful growth and an open, sunny situation, but does not want much attention beyond keeping the ground free from weeds.

The seed should be sown in the open early in May or as soon as the ground is warm, as thinly as possible, in rows 2 to $2^1/_2$ feet apart, the seedlings thinned out to 2 feet apart in the rows, as they do not stand transplanting well. Only the larger seedlings should be reserved, especially those of a bluish tint. The soil where the crop is to be, must have been well manured, and must be kept moist until the seeds have germinated, and also during May and June of the first year. It is also recommended to sow seeds of biennial Henbane at their natural ripening time, August, in porous soil.

The ground must never be water-logged, especially in the first winter; it runs to stalk in a wet season. Drought and late frosts stunt the growth and cause it to blossom too early, and if the climatic conditions are unsuitable, especially in a dry spring and summer, the biennial Henbane will flower in its first year, while the growth is quite low, but wellmanured soil may prevent this.

CARE MUST BE TAKEN IN SELECTING THE SEED

Commercial Henbane seed is often kiln-dried and useless for sowing. In order to more readily ensure germination, it is advisable to soak the seeds in water for twenty-four hours before planting: the unfertile seeds will then float on the top of the water and may thus be distinguished. Ripe seed should be grey, and yellowish or brown seeds should be rejected, as they are immature.

Henbane seed being very small and light should be well mixed with fine dry soil as it is sown. As seedlings often die off, a reserve should be kept in a box or bed to fill gaps, even though they do not always transplant success fully.

If it is desired to raise a crop of the annualvariety the plants, being smaller and not branching so freely, may be grown at a distance of 18 inches apart each way, but the annual is very little cultivated in this country.

If any annuals come up among the biennials sown, the flowers should be cut off until the leaves get larger and the stem branches.

There is usually some difficulty in growing Henbane owing to its destruction by insects: sometimes the whole of the foliage is destroyed by the larvae of a leaf-mining fly, Pegomyia

Hyoscyami, and the crop is rendered worthless in a week. And when the large autumnal leaves of the first-year plants of the biennial variety decay, the large terminal bud is often destroyed by one of the various species of macro-lepidopterous caterpillars which hide themselves in the ground. The crown or bud should be covered as soon as the leaves have rotted away with soil mixed with soot or naphthaline, to prevent the depredations of these and other insects.

Floods may also rot the plants in winter, if grown on level ground. Potato pests are fond of the prickly leaves and will leave a potato patch to feed on the Henbane plant.

If mildew develops on the foliage in summer, dust the plants with powdered sulphur or spray with 1/2 oz. (ouznce) of liver of sulphur in 2 gallons of water.

When it is desired to preserve seed for propagation, it is well to cut off the top flowering shoots at an early stage of flowering (these may be dried and sold as flowering tops), and allow only about six seed-capsules to ripen. This will ensure strong seed to the capsules left, and this seed will probably produce biennial Henbane, weaker seeds being apt to produce the less robust and less valuable annual Henbane.

Seeds sown as soon as ripe in August may germinate in autumn, and thus constitute a biennial by growing on all through the winter and flowering the next summer.

Although the cultivation of Henbane in sandy ground near the sea, especially on the rich soil of estuaries, would probably pay well, it is hardly a profitable plant to grow in small gardens, more especially as the yield of dried leaf is very small. It is estimated that about 15 cwt. of dry herb are obtained from an acre of ground.

CONSTITUENTS

The chief constituent of Henbane leaves is the alkaloid Hyoscyamine, together with smaller quantities of Atropine and Hyoscine, also known as *Scopolamine*.

The proportion of alkaloid in the British Pharmacopoeia dried drug varies from 0.045 to 0.14 per cent. Higher yields are exceptional. The amount of Hyoscyamine is many times greater than that of Hyoscine.

Other constituents of Henbane are a glucosidal bitter principle called hyoscytricin, choline, mucilage, albumin, calcium oxalate and potassium nitrate. On incineration, the leaves yield about 12 per cent of ash. By destructive distillation, the leaves yield a very poisonous empyreumatic oil.

The chief constituent of the seeds is about 0.5 to 0.6 per cent of alkaloid, consisting of Hyoscyamine, with a small proportion of Hyoscine. The seeds also contain about 20 per cent of fixed oil.

MEDICINAL ACTION AND USES

Antispasmodic, hypnotic, mild diuretic. The leaves have long been employed as a narcoticmedicine. It is similar in action to belladonna and stramonium, though milder in its effects.

The drug combines the therapeutic actions of its two alkaloids, *Hyoscyamine* and *Hyoscine*. Because of the presence of the former, it tends to check secretion and to relax spasms of the involuntary muscles, while through the narcotic effects of its hyoscine it lessens pain and exercises a slight somnifacient action.

Its most important use is in relief of painful *spasmodic* affections of the unstriped muscles, as in lead *colic* and irritable bladder. It will also relieve pain in *cystitis*.

It is much employed to allay *nervous irritation*, in various forms of hysteria or irritable cough, the tincture or juice prepared from the bruised, fresh leaves and tops being given in mixtures as an antispasmodic in asthma.

Combined with silver nitrate, it is especially useful in the treatment of *gastric ulcer*.

It is used to relieve the griping caused by drastic *purgatives*, and is a common ingredient of aperient pills, especially those containing aloes and colocynth.

In small repeated doses Henbane has been found to have a tranquillizing effect upon persons affected by severe nervous irritability, producing a tendency to sleep, not followed by the disorder of the digestive organs and headache, which too frequently result from the administration of repeated doses of opium, to which Henbane is often preferred when an anodyne or sedative is required.

A watery solution of the extract applied to the eye has a similar effect to that of atropine, in dilating the pupil and thus preparing the eye for an operation, or assisting the cure of its internal inflammation. This dilution leaves no injurious effect afterwards.

ATROPA BELLADONNA

Botanical Name	:	*Atropa belladonna*
Family	:	Solanaceae
Parts Used	:	Leaf and Roots
Common Name	:	Dhatura

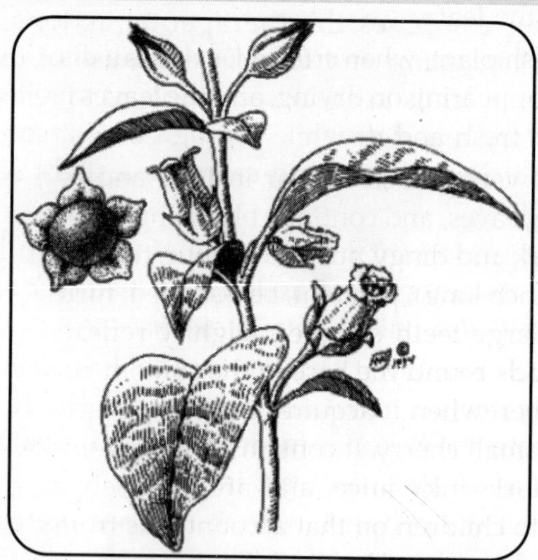

Fig. 10.2: Atropa belladonna

DESCRIPTION

The root is thick, fleshy and whitish, about 6 inches long, or more, and branching. It is perennial. The purplishcoloured stem is annual and herbaceous. It is stout, 2 to 4 feet high, undivided at the base, but dividing a little above the ground into three branches freely. More rarely two or four branches, each of which again branches freely.

The leaves are dull, darkish green in colour and of unequal size, 3 to 10 inches long, the lower leaves solitary, the upper ones in pairs alternately from opposite sides of the stem, one leaf of each pair much larger than the other, oval in shape, acute at the apex, entire and attenuated into short petioles.

First-year plants grow only about $1^1/_2$ feet in height. Their leaves are often larger than in full-grown plants and grow on the stem immediately above the ground. Older plants attain a height of 3 to 5 feet, occasionally even 6 feet, the leaves growing about 1 to 2 feet from the ground.

The whole plant is glabrous, or nearly so, though soft, downy hairs may occur on the young stems and the leaves when quite young. The veins of the leaves are prominent on the under surface, especially the midrib, which is depressed on the upper surface of the leaf.

The fresh plant, when crushed, exhales a disagreeable odour, almost disappearing on drying, and the leaves have a bitter taste, when both fresh and dry.

The flowers, which appear in June and July, singly, in the axils of the leaves, and continue blooming until early September, are of a dark and dingy purplish colour, tinged with green, large (about an inch long), pendent, bell-shaped, furrowed, the corolla with five large teeth or lobes, slightly reflexed. The five-cleft calyx spreads round the base of the smooth berry, which ripens in September, when it acquires a shining black colour and is in size like a small cherry. It contains several seeds. The berries are full of a dark, inky juice, and are intensely sweet, and their attraction to children on that account, has from their poisonous properties, been attended with fatal results.

CULTIVATION

Belladonna herb and root are sold by analysis, the value depending upon the percentage of alkaloid contained. A wide variation occurs in the amount of alkaloid present. It is important, therefore, to grow the crop under such conditions of soil and temperature as are likely to develop the highest percentage of the active principle.

It has been found, on the contrary, that artificial aids, such as the judicious selection of manure, the cleansing and preparation of the soil, destruction of weeds, etc., in accordance with the latest scientific practice, have improved the plants in every respect, not only in bulk, but even in percentage weight of alkaloidal contents.

CONSTITUENTS

The medicinal properties of Belladonna depend on the presence of *Hyoscyamine* and *Atropine*. The root is the basis of the principal preparations of Belladonna.

The total alkaloid present in the root varies between 0.4 and 0.6 per cent, but as much as 1 per cent has been found, consisting of Hyoscyamine and its isomer Atropine, 0.1 to 0.6 per cent; Belladonnine and occasionally, Atropamine. Starch and Atrosin, a red colouring principle, are also present in the root.

Scopolamine (hyoscine) is also found in traces, as is a fluorescent principle similar to that found in horse-chestnut bark and widely distributed through the natural order *Solanaceae*. The greater portion of the alkaloidal matter consists of Hyoscyamine, and it is possible that any Atropine found is produced during extraction.

The amount of alkaloids present in the leaves varies somewhat in wild or cultivated plants, and according to the methods of drying and storing adopted, as well as on the conditions of growth, soil, weather, etc.

The proportion of the total alkaloid present in the dried leaves varies from 0.3 to 0.7 per cent. The greater proportion consists of Hyoscyamine, the Atropine being produced during extraction, as in the root. Belladonnine and Apoatropine may also be formed during extraction from the drug. The leaves contain also a trace of Scopolamine, Atrosin and starch.

A standardized liquid extract is prepared, from which the official plaster, alcoholic extract, liniment, suppository, tincture and ointment are made. The green extract is prepared from the fresh leaves.

MEDICINAL ACTION AND USES

Narcotic, diuretic, sedative, antispasmodic, mydriatic. Belladonna is a most valuable plant in the treatment of *eye diseases,* Atropine, obtained during extraction, being its most important constituent on account of its power of dilating the pupil.

The various preparations of Belladonna have many uses. Locally applied, it lessens irritability and pain, and is used as a lotion, plaster or liniment in cases of *neuralgia, gout, rheumatism* and *sciatica*. As a drug, it specially affects the brain and the bladder. It is used to check excessive secretions and to allay inflammation and to check the sweating of phthisis and other exhausting diseases.

It is a powerful *antispasmodic* in *intestinal colic* and *spasmodic asthma*. Occasionally the leaves are employed as an ingredient of cigarettes for relieving the latter. It is well borne by children, and is given in large doses in *whooping cough* and false croup.

For its action on the circulation, it is given in the collapse of *pneumonia, typhoid fever* and other *acute diseases*. It increases the rate of the heart by some 20 to 40 beats per minute, without diminishing its force. It is of value in acute *sore throat,* and relieves local *inflammation* and *congestion*. A mixture of Belladonna plaster, Salicylic acid and Lead plaster is recommended as an application for *corns* and *bunions*.

ACONITE

Botanical Name	:	*Aconitum napellus*
Family	:	Ranunculaceae (Buttercup family)
Parts Used	:	Leaves, Stem, Flowering tops and Roots
Common Name	:	Monkshood, Wolfsbane

HABITAT

Lower mountain slopes of North portion of Eastern Hemisphere. From Himalayas through Europe to Great Britain. Aconite is now found wild in a few parts of England, mainly in the western counties and also in South Wales, but can hardly be considered truly indigenous. It was very early introduced into England, being mentioned in all the English vocabularies of plants from the tenth century downwards, and in Early English medical recipes.

DESCRIPTION

The plant is a hardy perennial, with a fleshy, spindle-shaped root, palecoloured when young, but subsequently acquiring a dark brown skin.

The *stem* is about 3 feet high, with dark green, glossy leaves, deeply divided in palmate manner and flowers in erect clusters of a dark blue colour.

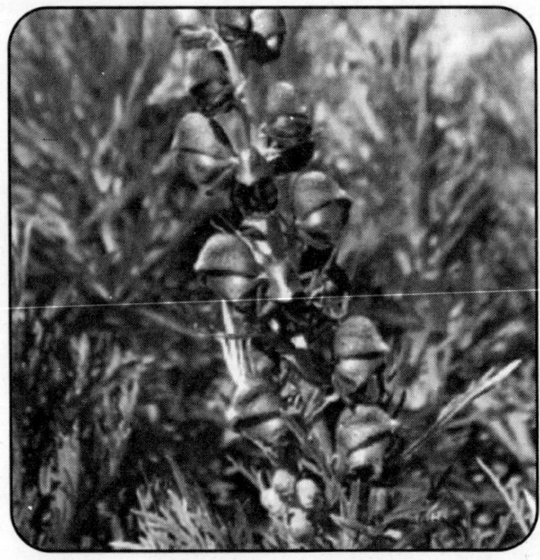

Fig. 10.3: Aconite

The *shape* of the flower is specially designed to attract and utilize bee visitors, especially the humble bee.

The *sepals* are purple-purple being specially attractive to bees and are fancifully shaped, one of them being in the form of a hood.

The *petals* are only represented by the two very curious nectaries within the hood, somewhat in the form of a hammer; the stamens are numerous and lie depressed in a bunch at the mouth of the flower. They are pendulous at first, but rise in succession and place their anthers forward in such a way that a bee visiting the flower for nectar is dusted with the pollen, which he then carries to the next flower he visits and thereby fertilizes the undeveloped fruits, which are in a tuft in the centre of the stamens, each carpel containing a single seed.

CULTIVATION

The chief collecting centres for foreign Aconite root have been the Swiss Alps, Salzburg, North Tyrol and Vorarlberg. Much was also formerly collected in Germany. Supplies from Spain and Japan are imported, so that the demand for English Aconite is somewhat restricted. The official Aconite is directed by the British Pharmacopceia to be derived only from plants cultivated in England, and a certain amount of home-grown Aconite has been regularly produced by the principal drug-farms, though good crops are grown with some difficulty in England, and cultivation of Aconite has not paid very well in recent years.

Aconite prefers a soil slightly retentive of moisture, such as a moist loam, and flourishes best in shade. It would probably grow luxuriantly in a moist, open wood, and would yield returns with little further trouble than weeding, digging up and drying.

In preparing beds for growing Aconite, the soil should be well dug and pulverized by early winter frosts - the digging in of rotten leaves or stable manure is advantageous.

It can be raised from seed, sown 1/2 inch deep in a cold frame in March, or in a warm position outside in April, but great care must be exercised that the right kind is obtained, as there are many varieties of Aconite—about twenty-four have been distinguished — and they have not all the same active medicinal properties. It takes two or three years to flower from seed.

Propagation is usually by division of roots in the autumn. The underground portion of the plants are dug up after the stem has died down, and the smaller of the 'daughter' roots that have developed at the side of the old roots are selected for replanting in December or January to form new stock, the young roots being planted about a foot apart each way. The young shoots appear above ground in February. Although the plants are perennial, each distinct root lasts only one year, the plant being continued by 'daughter' roots.

This official Aconite is also the species generally cultivated in gardens, though nearly all the species are worth growing as ornamental garden flowers, the best perhaps being *A. napellus*, both white and blue, *A. paniculatum*, *A. japonicum* and *A. autumnale*. All grow well in shade and under trees. Gerard grew four species in his garden: *A. lyocotonum*, *A. variegatum*, *A. napellus* and *A. pyrenaicum*.

PARTS USED

The leaves, stem, flowering tops and root. The leaves and flowering tops are of less importance, they are employed for preparing extract of Aconitum, and for this purpose are cut when the flowers are just breaking into blossom and the leaves are in their best condition, which is in June.

The roots should be collected in the autumn, after the stem dies down, but before the bud that is to produce the next year's stem has begun to develop. As this bud grows and forms a flowering stem, in the spring, some of the lateral buds develop into short shoots, each of which produces a long, slender, descending root, crowned with a bud.

These roots rapidly thicken, filled with reserve material produced by the parent plant, the root of which dies as the 'daughter' roots increase in size. Towards the autumn, the parent plant dies down and the daughter roots which have then reached their maximum development are now full of starch. If allowed to remain in the soil, the buds that crown the daughter roots begin to grow, in the late winter, and this growth exhausts the strength of the root, and the proportion of both starch and alkaloid it contains is lessened.

On account of the extremely poisonous properties of the root, it is considered desirable that the root should be grown and collected under the same conditions, so that uniformity in the drug is maintained.

The British Pharmacopceia specifies, therefore, that the roots should be collected in the autumn from plants cultivated in Britain and should consist of the dried, full-grown 'daughter' roots—much of the Aconite root that used to come in large quantities from Germany was the exhausted parent root of the wild-flowering plants.

When the roots are dug up, they are sorted over, the smallest laid aside for replanting and the plumper ones reserved for drying. They are first well washed in cold water and trimmed of all rootlets, and then dried, either entire, or longitudinally sliced to hasten drying.

Drying may at first be done in the open air, spread thinly, the roots not touching. Or they may be spread on clean floors or on shelves in a warm place for about ten days, turning frequently. When somewhat shrunken, they must be finished more quickly by artificial heat in a drying room or shed near a stove or gas fire, care being taken that the heated air can escape at the top of the room. Drying in an even temperature will probably take about a fortnight or more. It is not complete till the roots are dry to the core and brittle, snapping when bent.

Dried Aconite root at its upper extremity, when crowned with an undeveloped bud, enclosed by scaly leaves, is about 3/4 inch in diameter, tapering quickly downwards. It is dark brown in colour and marked with the scars of rootlets. The surface is usually longitudinally wrinkled, especially if it has been dried entire. The root breaks with a short fracture and should be whitish and starchy within. A transverse section shows a thick bark, separated from the inner portion by a well-marked darker line, which often assumes a stellate appearance. Aconite root as found in commerce is, however, often yellowish or brownish internally with the stellate markings not clearly shown, probably from having been collected too early. It should be lifted in the autumn of the second year.

Aconite root is liable to attack by insects, and after being well dried should be kept in securely closed vessels.

MEDICINAL ACTION AND USES

Anodyne, diuretic and diaphoretic. The value of Aconite as a medicine has been more fully realized in modern times, and it now rank as one of our most useful drugs. It is much used in homoeopathy.

Both tincture and liniment of Aconite are in general use, and Aconite is also used in ointment and sometimes given as hypodermic injection. Preparations of Aconitc are employed for outward application locally to the skin to diminish the pain of *neuralgia, lumbago* and *rheumatism.*

The official tincture taken internelly diminishes the rate and force of the pulse in the early stages of fevers and slight local inflammations, such as *feverish cold, larnyngitis,* first stages of *pneumonia* and *erysipelas*; it relieves the pain of neuralgia, pleurisy and aneurism.

In *cardiac failure* or to prevent same it has been used with success, in acute tonsilitis children have been well treated by a dose of 1 to 2 minims for a child 5 to 10 years old; the dose for adults is 2 to 5 minims, three times a day.

ASHWAGANDHA

Botanical Name	:	*Withania somnifera*
Family	:	Solanaceae
Parts Used	:	Seeds
Common Name	:	Ashwagandha

DESCRIPTION

Seed—Sow early spring in a greenhouse. There is usually a high germination rate within 2 weeks. Prick out the seedlings into individual pots once they are large enough to handle and plant them out after the last expected frost. The seeds are used to curdle plant milks in order to make vegetarian cheeses.

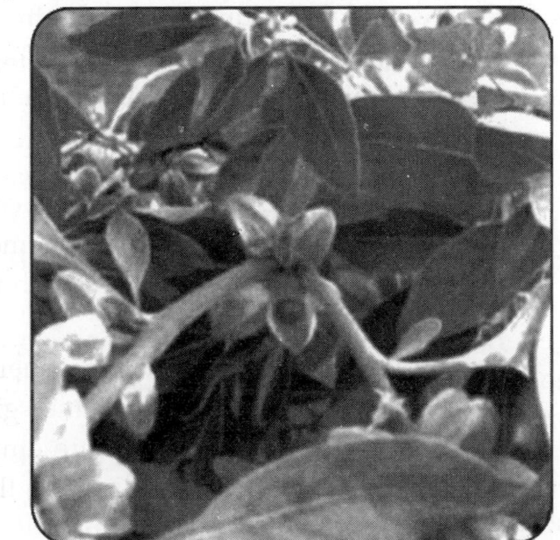

Fig. 10.4: Withania somnifera

CULTIVATION

A fairly easily grown plant, it requires a warm sheltered position in full sun and a well-drained moderately fertile soil. Prefers a dry stony soil. This species is not hardy in temperate climates but it can be grown as an annual, flowering and fruiting in its first year from seed.

Ashwagandha is a beautiful delicate plant native to India, Pakistan, and Sri Lanka. Defined by deep green leaves, branched limbs, and topped by seeded yellow flowers. Ashwagandha is a stunning in appearance and of vital importance in Ayurveda or Indian medicine. *Withania somnifera* has a long history, about 4000 years, as a holistic herb used to treat a variety of ailments.

The shoots of the Ashwagandha shrub are used in food and in India seeds of the Ashwagandha are used to thicken milk. African tribes also use *Withania somnifera* to treat fevers, and other inflammations.

Ashwagandha is usually crushed and used in a traditional Ayurvedic formula called *shilajit*.

The active ingredients in Ashwagandha are *alkaloids* and *withanoloids*. It the *withanoloids* within Ashwagandha that give it all it's medicinal qualities. Withanoloids consist of steroidal molecules which act to fight inflammation. Aswagandha is often compared to Asian ginseng which contain molecules like withanoloids called *ginsenosides*. For this reason Aswagandha is occasionally called *Indian ginseng*.

Therefore, both *ginseng* and *Ashwagandha stimulate* the *immune system*, stop inflammation, *increase memory*, and helps maintain general healthy and wellness. It is also known to increase the production of *bone marrow, semen*, and inhibit's the *aging process*.

MEDICINAL USES

Ashwagandha is one of the most widespread *tranquillisers* used in India.

It acts mainly on the *reproductive* and *nervous systems*, having a rejuvenative effect on the body, and is used to improve vitality and aid recovery after chronic illness.

Internally, it is used to tone the uterus after a miscarriage and also in treating post-partum difficulties.

It is also used to treat *nervous exhaustion, debility, insomnia*, wasting diseases, *failure to thrive* in *children, impotence, infertility, multiple sclerosis* etc. Externally it has been applied as a poultice to boils, swellings and other painful parts

Ashwagandha possesses *anti-inflammatory, antitumor, antistress, antioxidant, immunomodulatory, hemopoietic*, and *rejuvenating properties*. It also appears to exert a positive influence on the endocrine, *cardiopulmonary*, and *central nervous systems*. Some researchers suggest ashwagandha exhibits a variety of *therapeutic effects* with limited side effects or toxicity. It's naturally occurring *steroidal content* is much higher than that of hydrocortisone which is a common treatment in cancer cases.

Note—When taking Ashawagandha, like any medicine to be careful. Overuse and abuse of a herbal medication can be equally as dangerous and deadly as with any traditional medicine.

EPHEDRA

Botanical Name	:	*Ephedra sinica*
Family	:	Ephedraceae
Parts Used	:	Herb and Roots
Common Name	:	Chinese ephedra, Ma Huang

Ephedra, from the plant *Ephedra sinica,* has been used as an herbal remedy in traditional Chinese medicine for 5,000 years for the treatment of asthma and hay fever, as well as for the common cold. Known in Chinese as *ma huang*. Ephedra is a stimulant which constricts blood vessels and increases blood pressure and heart rate. Several additional species belonging to the genus Ephedra have traditionally been used for a variety of medicinal purposes, and are a possible candidate for the Soma plant of Indo-Iranian religion.

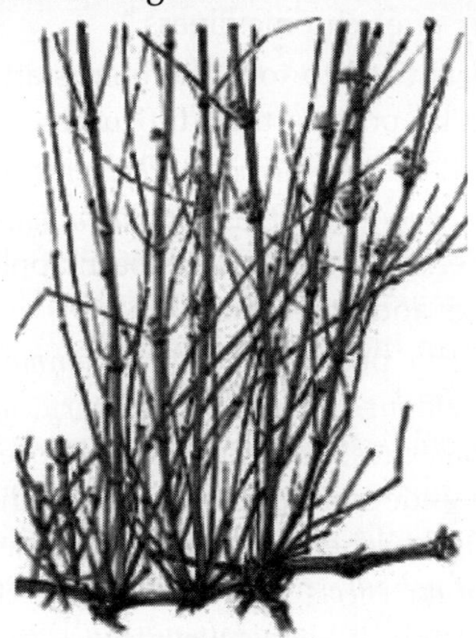

Fig. 10.5: Ephedra

Ephedra—containing dietary supplements have been linked to a high rate of serious side effects and a number of deaths, leading to concern from the U.S. Food and Drug Administration (FDA), the National Center for Complementary and Alternative Medicine, and the medical community.

Some species in the Ephedra genus have no alkaloid content and are therefore essentially inert; however, the most commonly used species, *E. sinica,* has a total alkaloid content of 1–3% by dry weight.

CONSTITUTES

Ephedrine constitutes 40–90% of the alkaloid content, with the remainder consisting of pseudoephedrine and the demethylated forms of each compound.

PHARMACOLOGY

The alkaloids ephedrine and pseudoephedrine are the active constituents of the plant. Pseudoephedrine is used in over-the-counter decongestants. Derivatives of ephedrine are used to treat low blood pressure, but alternatives with reduced cardiovascular risk have replaced it for treating *asthma*.

MEDICINAL USES

Ephedra is both a *stimulant* and a *thermogenic*; its biological effects are due to its ephedrine and pseudoephedrine content. These compounds stimulate the brain, increase heart rate, constrict blood vessels (increasing blood pressure), and expand bronchial tubes (making breathing easier). Their thermogenic properties cause an increase in metabolism, evidenced by an increase in body heat.

Ephedra is widely used by *athletes,* despite a lack of evidence that it enhances athletic performance. Ephedra may also be used as a precursor in the illicit manufacture of metha-mphetamine.

Side effects of ephedra may include— severe skin reactions, hypertension, irritability, nervousness, dizziness, trembling, headache, insomnia, profuse perspiration, dehydration, itchy scalp and skin, vomiting, hyperthermia, irregular heartbeat, seizures, heart attack, stroke, or death.

OPIUM POPPY

Botanical Name	:	*Papaver sominiferum*
Family	:	Papaveraceae
Parts Used	:	Capsule and Seed
Common Name	:	Afim

DESCRIPTION

Annual or biennial herb, 50–150 cm tall, glabrous or glaucous, sometimes with a few spreading bristles; stems slightly branched, erect leaves large, numerous, ovate to oblong, serrate to dentate-serrate, clasping at base, glaucous, the lower ones pinnatifid; flowers on long peduncles with nodding buds that expand into erect flowers; petals 4–8, white to purplish, in varieties also pink, violet, bluish, or red, 5–7 cm long; sepals glabrous, 1.5–2 cm long; fruit a capsule, ovoid to globose, glabrous, 4–6 cm long, 3.5–4 cm in diameter, with 8–12 rayed sessile stigmas; seeds oily, white, dark gray to black, or bluish.

Opium poppy has been cultivated for several thousand years and many cultivars have resulted, differing in flower color, opium production, color of seeds, oil content of seeds, and cultural requirements. Many variants are named, the best known are the "White Poppy" and the "Black Poppy" ("Blue Poppy"), named for color of seed. "White Poppy" has white to silvery-gray flowers, white seeds, and the capsule is somewhat flattened both at top and bottom. "Black Poppy" usually has violet flowers, seeds a slate color, and the capsule is smaller and and more globular. Many new hybrids being produced and classified according to seed yield, morphine content, and oil content.

DISTRIBUTION

Native and cultivated in Mediterranean region east to Iran; now cultivated in many tropical, subtropical, and warm temperate countries. Presently known to be cultivated for the opium in India, Iran, Turkey, Yugoslavia, Macedonia, Bulgaria, China, Manchuria, and Asia, and in other parts of Europe and India for the seeds. Cultivated in Japan and Australia for medicinal purposes.

CULTIVATION

Propagated from seed. Seeds germinate best at 15°C and are less sensitive to temperature than most poppy species. Seed sown in shallow furrows, at rate of 4–6 kg/ha. In some areas poppy seed, mixed with sand, is often broadcast over tilled fields in early autumn at rate of about 0.5 kg/ha, as in Asia Minor. Then fields are weeded in the spring when the poppy has grown to about 15 cm tall, and plants are thinned then to stand about 60 cm apart. They flower in April and May and the capsules are ripe in June to July. Optimum yields are obtained when plants are spaced 10 cm between plants and rows 32 cm apart, thus allowing space for mechanical cultivation. Yields of seeds are slightly higher when plants are spaced 30 cm apart than when 40 cm apart. Thinning and spacing do not affect the oil content of the seeds. Fertile soil is essential for good growth and land should be fertilized accordingly.

USES

Opium is the air-dried milky exudation obtained from excised unripe fruits. It is extensively smoked as an intoxicant. Commercial products are called *Turkey Opium, Indian Opium, Persian Opium, Chinese Opium,* and *Egyptian Opium,* and they differ in appearance and quality.

Opium is largely used for manufacture of morphine, codeine, narcotine, laudenine, papaverine, and many other alkaloids. It is also the source of the toxic and extremely habitforming narcotic heroin or dimorphine, prohibited in some countries. Seeds contain no opium and are used extensively in baking and sprinkling on rolls and bread. Seeds are a good source of energy.

They are also the source of a drying-oil, used for manufacture of paints, varnishes, and soaps, and in foods and salad dressing.

Oil cake is a good fodder for cattle. Seeds used for preparation of emulsions (white-seeded varieties preferred); the bluish-black varieties are generally used for baking. Stems used for straw. Lecithin has been extracted from poppy seed meal. Seedlings are eaten as a potherb in Iran. As the peony flowered poppy, the opium poppy is widely grown as an ornamental, even here in the U.S., where it is illegal to grow.

FOLK MEDICINE

Regarded as analgesic, anodyne, antitussive, aphrodisiac, astringent, bactericidal, calmative, carminative, demulcent, emollient, expectorant, hemostat, hypotensive, hypnotic, narcotic, nervine, sedative, sudorific, tonic, poppy has been used in folk remedies for asthma, bladder, bruises, cancer, catarrh, cold, colic, conjunctivitis, cough, diarrhea, dysentery, dysmenorrhea, enteritis, enterorrhagia, fever, flux, headache, hemicrania, hypertension, hypochondria, hysteria, inflammation, insomnia, leucorrhea, malaria, mania, melancholy, nausea, neuralgia, otitis, pertussis, prolapse, rectitis, rheumatism, snakebite, spasm, spermatorrhea, sprain, stomachache, swelling, toothache, tumor, ulcers, and warts.

Hartwell mentions opium as a remedy for such cancerous conditions as cancer of the skin, stomach, tongue, uterus, carcinoma of the breast, polyps of the ear, nose, and vagina; scleroses of the liver, spleen, and uterus; and tumors of the abdomen, bladder, eyes, fauces, liver, spleen, and uvula. The plant, boiled in oil, is said to aid indurations and tumors of the liver. The tincture of the plant is said to help cancerous ulcers. Smoking the plant is said to cure cancer of the tongue. The capsule decoction and an injection of the seed decoction are said to help uterine cancer.

Egyptians claim to become more cheerful, talkative, and industrious following the eating of opium. When falling asleep, they have visions of "orchards and pleasure gardens embellished with many trees, herbs, and various flowers." Lebanese use their opium wisely; to quiet excitable people, to relieve toothache, headache, incurable pain, and for boils, coughs, dysentery, and itches.

In *Ayurvedic medicine,* the seeds are considered aphrodisiac, constipating, and tonic; the fruit antitussive, binding, cooling, deliriant, excitant, and intoxicant, yet anaphrodisiac if freely indulged; the plant is considered aphrodisiac, astringent, fattening, stimulant, tonic, and good for the complexion.

In *Unani medicine,* the fruit is suggested as well for anemia, chest pains, dysentery, fever, but is correctly deemed hypnotic, narcotic, and perhaps harmful to the brain. The plant provides a narcotic that induces sleep; a sleep so heavy that the person becomes insensible.

Its compounds are used in medicine as analgesic, anodyne, antipasmodic, hypnotic, narcotic, sedative, and as respiratory depressants and to relieve severe pain.

CANNABIS SATIVA

Botanical Name	:	*Cannabis sativa*
Family	:	Cannabinaceae
Parts Used	:	Leaf, Flowering shoot and Inflorescence
Common Name	:	Ganja, Bhang, Charas

HABITAT

In Britain, and formerly elsewhere, only 'Hemp' grown in India was recognized as official, but the heavy tax has resulted in the admission by the United States of any active *Cannabis sativa,* whether grown in the States or in Africa, Turkey, Turkestan, Asia Minor, Italy, or Spain.

DESCRIPTION

The plant is an annual, the erect stems growing from 3 to 10 feet or more high, very slightly branched, having greyish-green hairs. The leaves are palmate, with five to seven leaflets (three on the upper leaves), numerous, on long thin petioles with acute stipules at the base, linear-lanceolate, tapering at both ends, the margins sharply serrate, smooth and dark green on the upper surface, lighter and downy on the under one. The small flowers are unisexual, the male having five almost separate, downy, pale yellowish segments, and the female a single, hairy, glandular, five-veined leaf enclosing the ovary in a sheath. The ovary is smooth, one-celled, with one hanging ovule and two long, hairy thread-like stigmas extending beyond the flower for more than its own length. The fruit is small, smooth, light brownish-grey in colour, and completely filled by the seed.

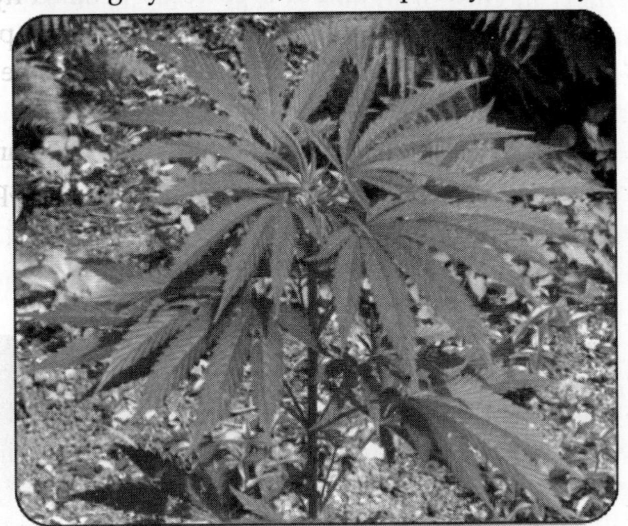

Fig. 10.6: Cannabis sativa

It is imported in parcels of small masses, with flowers, smaller leaves and a few ripe fruits pressed together by sticky, resinous matter. It is rough, brittle, dull-green in colour and almost tasteless, with a peculiar, slightly narcotic odour. It should be freed from resin by macerating in spirit and then soaking in water. The leaves are said to be picked off to form *bhang*, and the little shoots which follow these are used as above, and called *ganja*.

Ganja is smoked like tobacco. *Bhang*, sidhee, or subjee is the dried, larger leaves, broken or mixed with a few fruits. It is pounded with water to make a drink, and is the chief ingredient of the sweetmeat majun. *Churrus* or charas is the resin which exudes spontaneously from the leaves, tops and stems.

In *Nepal* the plant is squeezed between the palms of the hands, and in *Baluchistan* the resin is separated by rubbing the dried plant carefully between carpets. This is the hashish, haschisch, or hashash of the Arabians, the word 'assassin' being said to be derived from it, owing to the wild, fanatical courage given by its use.

Flat cakes called *hashish* by the Russians are a preparation made from Hemp in Central Asia, and also called *nasha.*

In Thibet momea or mimea is said to be made with *Hemp* and human fat.

Hemp Fibre is best produced by the plants in cooler latitudes, the best being obtained from Italy, but much from Russia. About one and a half million hundredweight are imported annually for cordage, sacking, and sail-cloths.

A varnish is made from the pressed seeds.

Two or three green twigs collected in spring and placed in beds will drive bedbugs from the room.

CONSTITUENTS

Cannabinone or *Hemp* resin is soluble in alcohol and ether. Cannabinol is separated from it. It is fawn-coloured, in thin layers, and burns with a clear, white flame, leaving no ash. This is the active principle. There is a small amount of ambercoloured volatile oil, one of the linseed-oil group. It has been resolved into a colourless liquid called cannabene, and a solid hydride of this.

It is said that a *volatile alkaloid* has been found in the tops, resembling nicotine. It also contains alcoholic extract, ash, and the alkaloid Choline.

MEDICINAL ACTION AND USES

The principal use of Hemp in medicine is for easing pain and inducing sleep, and for a soothing influence in *nervous disorders*. It does not cause constipation nor affect the appetite like opium. It is useful in *neuralgia, gout, rheumatism, delirium tremens, insanity, infantile convulsions, insomnia,* etc.

The tincture helps parturition, and is used in senile catarrh, gonorrhoea, menorrhagia, chronic cystitis and all painful urinary affections. An infusion of the seed is useful in after pains and prolapsus uteri. The resin may be combined with ointments, oils or chloroform in inflammatory and neuralgic complaints.

The drug deteriorates rapidly and hence is very variable, so that it is best given in ascending quantities to produce its effect. The deterioration is due to the oxidation of cannabinol and it should be kept in hermetically-sealed containers.

The action is almost entirely on the higher nerve centres. It can produce an exhilarating intoxication, with hallucinations, and is widely used in Eastern countries as an intoxicant, hence its names 'leaf of delusion,' 'increaser of pleasure,' 'cementer of friendship,' etc. The nature of its effect depends much on the nationality and temperament of the individual. It is regarded as dangerous to sleep in a field of hemp owing to the aroma of the plants.

NUX VOMICA

Botanical Name	:	*Strychnos Nux-vomica*
Family	:	Loganiaceae
Parts Used	:	Dried ripe seeds
Common Name	:	Poison nut, Quaker buttons

HABITAT

India, in the Malay Archipelago.

DESCRIPTION

A medium-sized tree with a short, crooked, thick trunk, the wood is white hard, close grained, durable and the root very bitter.

Branches irregular, covered with a smooth ash-coloured bark; young shoots deep green, shiny; leaves opposite, short stalked, oval, shiny, smooth on both sides, about 4 inches long and 3 broad; flowers small, greeny-white, funnel shape, in small terminal cymes, blooming in the cold season and having a disagreeable smell.

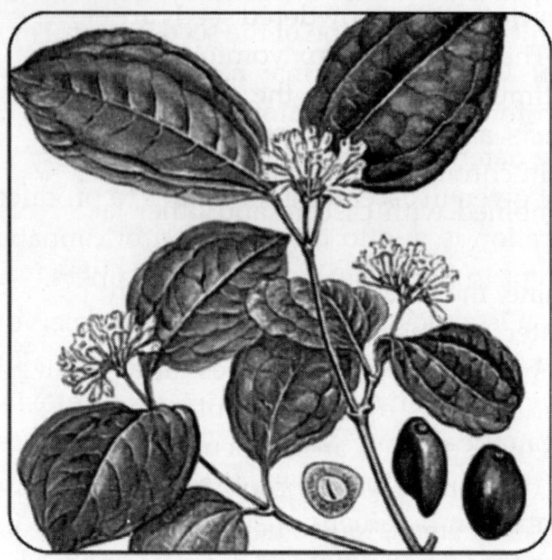

Fig. 10.7: Strychnos Nux-vomica

Fruit about the size of a large apple with a smooth hard rind or shell which when ripe is a lovely orange colour, filled with a soft white jelly-like pulp containing five seeds covered with a soft woolly-like substance, white and horny internally. The seeds are removed when ripe, cleansed, dried and sorted; they are exported from Cochin, Madras (Chennai) and other Indian ports. The seeds have the shape of flattened disks densely covered with closely appressed satiny hairs, radiating from the centre of the flattened sides and giving to the seeds a characteristic sheen; they are very hard, with a dark grey horny endosperm in which the small embryo is embedded; no odour but a very bitter taste.

CONSTITUENTS

Nux Vomica contains the alkaloids, Strychnine and Brucine, also traces of strychnicine, and a glucoside Loganin, about 3 per cent fatty matter, caffeotannic acid and a trace of copper. The pulp of the fruit contains about 5 per cent of loganin together with the alkaloid strychnicine.

MEDICINAL ACTION AND USES

The propertiesof Nux vomica are substantially those of the alkaloid Strychnine. The powdered seeds are employed in atonic dyspepsia. The tincture of Nux vomica is often used in mixtures – for its stimulant action on the gastro-intestinal tract. In the mouth it acts as a bitter, increasing appetite; it stimulates peristalsis, in chronic constipation due to atony of the bowel it is often combined with cascara and other laxatives with good effects.

Strychnine, the chief alkaloid constituent of the seeds, also acts as a bitter, increasing the flow of gastric juice; it is rapidly absorbed as it reaches the intestines, after which it exerts its characteristic effects upon the central nervous system, the movements of respiration are deepened and quickened and the heart slowed through excitation of the vagal centre.

The senses of smell, touch, hearing and vision are rendered more acute, it improves the pulse and raises blood pressure and is of great value as a tonic to the circulatory system in cardiac failure. Strychnine is excreted very slowly and its action is cumulative in any but small doses; it is much used as a gastric tonic in dyspepsia.

The most direct symptom caused by strychnine is violent convulsions due to a simultaneous stimulation of the motor or sensory ganglia of the spinal cord; during the convulsion there is great rise in blood pressure; in some types of chronic lead poisoning it is of great value. In cases of surgical shock and cardiac failure large doses are given up to 1/10 grain by hypodermic injection; also used as an antidote in poisoning by chloral or chloroform. Brucine closely resembles strychnine in its action, but is slightly less poisonous, it paralyses the peripheral motor nerves. It is said that the convulsive action characteristic of strychnine is absent in brucine almost entirely. It is used in pruritis and as a local anodyne in inflammations of the external ear.

The world's best *hang-over remedy*. It use anytime that too much rich food and/or alcohol upsets our digestion resulting in nausea, gas, diarrhoea or constipation.

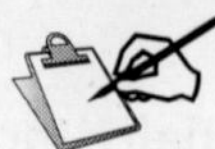

STUDY QUESTIONS

1. Write short notes on the following:
   (a) Atropa belladonna;
   (b) Ashwagandha;
   (c) Opium poppy; and
   (d) Cannabis sativa.
2. Explain the medicinal uses of Ashwagandha.

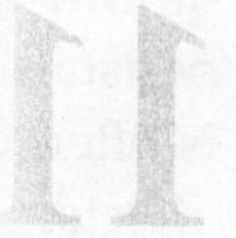

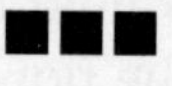

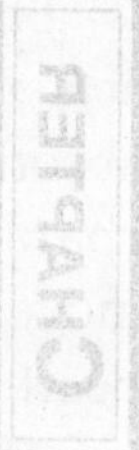

11

CHAPTER

ANTIHYPERTENSIVES

RAUWOLFIA SERPENTINA

Botanical Name	:	*Rauwolfia serpentina*
Family	:	Apocynaceae
Parts Used	:	Roots
Common Names	:	Indian Snakeroot, Rauwolfia, Serpentwood, Sarpagandha

DISTRIBUTION

In India, Rauwolfia serpentina is widely distributed in the sub-Himalayan tract from Punjab eastwards to Nepal, Sikkim, Bhutan and Assam; lower hills of Gangetic plains; Eastern and Western Ghats; parts of Central India and in the Andamans. Extensive collection of the species from the wild has led to its becoming endangered.

Rauwolfia serpentina; a famous *tranquilizer* and *antipsychotic* herb of India for the treatment of paranoia and schizophrenia, as well as a substance that controls hypertension. Rauwolfia serpentina being pronounced as the "Wonder Drug of India" in 1949, when the British Heart Journal reported the plant to be "clinically effective in treating high blood pressure". Rauwolfia has been long used in India for treating mental illness known as the "Insanity herb" and snake bites known as the "snakeroot".

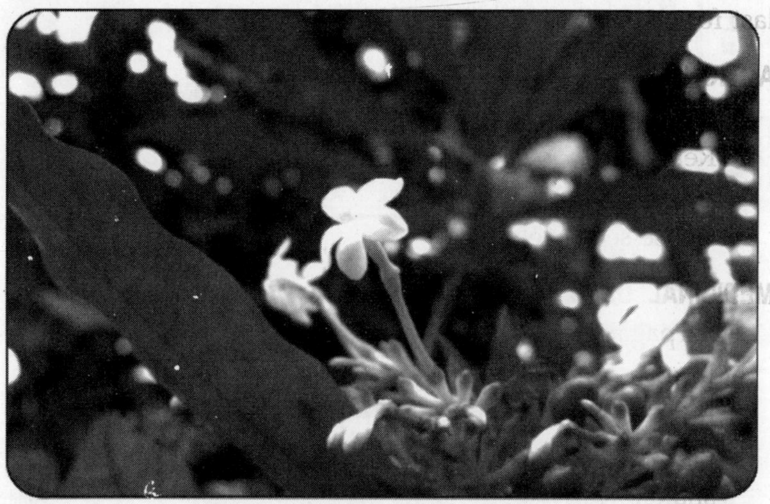

Fig. 11.1: Rauwolfia serpentina

PLANT DESCRIPTION

Rauwolfia serpentina in India, is an erect, evergreen shrub, merely 15 to 45 cm high. Its leaves are large, in whorls of three dark green above and pale green below. The flowers are white, pinkish or red, occurring in whorls. Its fruit are tiny, oval, fleshy which turn a shiny purple-black when ripe. It is the roots of the plant that are mainly used for medicinal purposes.

CHEMICAL CONSTITUENTS

The key active ingredients are reserpine, rescinnamine, deserpidine and rauhimbine. Other alkaloids are reserpinine, ajmaline, isoajmaline, rauwolfinine. More than 50 kinds of alkaloids can be extracted from Rauwolfia serpentina roots.

PHARMACOKINETICS

Rauwolfia serpentina is absorbed rapidly from the GI tract following oral administration, but the hypotensive effects usually are not observed for 2-3 weeks. The drug distributes throughout the body tissues and is completely metabolized in the liver to inactive derivatives. Metabolites of the drug are excreted gradually in the urine and feces; antihypertensive effects can last for weeks following discontinuance of therapy.

ACTIONS

- Reduces cardiac output.
- Relaxes capacitance vessels and reduces total peripheral resistance.
- Cause sedative effect.

MEDICINAL USES

- Sarpagandha acts on mild to moderate hypertension.
- In case of insomnia sarpagandha is used with precaution.
- It is used as a tranquilizer in psychiatric disorder.
- Sarpagandha has extensive use as an antidote for snakebites.
- The root is believed to stimulate uterine contraction, recommended for use in child-birth.
- It is used in treatment of intestinal disorders, particularly diarrhoea and dysentery, cholera, colic and fever. It is also an antihelmintic.
- The juice of the leaves has been used as a remedy for opacity of the cornea.

STUDY QUESTIONS

1. Write a detailed note on Rauwolfia serpentina.
2. Explain the medicinal uses of Rauwolfia serpentina.

12 CHAPTER

ANTITUSSIVES

VASAKA

Botanical Name	:	*Adhathoda vasica*
Family	:	Acanthaceae
Parts Used	:	Leaves, Whole plant
Common Names	:	Vasaka, Adulsa, Malabar Nut

DESCRIPTION

Vasaka, also called *adhatoda*, adalodakam malabar nut, consists of dried, as well as fresh, leaves of the plant Justicia adhatoda, belonging to family Acanthaceae. The plant has been recommended by Ayurvedic physicians for the management of various types of *respiratory disorders*.

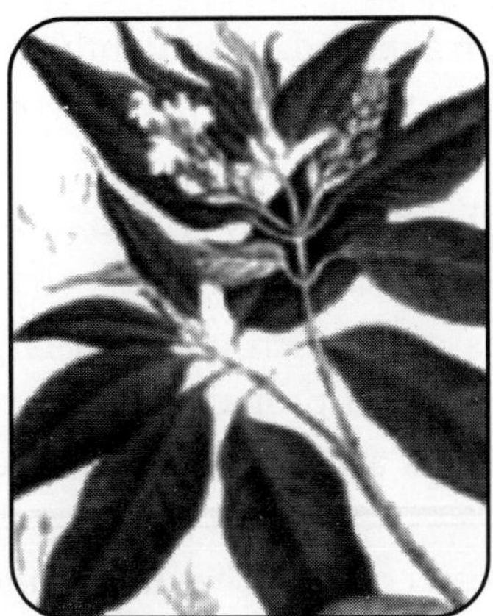

Fig. 12.1: Vasaka

ORIGIN

The plant is distributed all over the plains of India and in lower Himalayan ranges, ascending to a height of 1,500 m. The leaves of this plant was not eaten by goats as it is bitter (Hence the name Adu (Goat)—Thoda (not touch). This herb is very widely found and it was common to have a brew made with these leaves boiled in water with black pepper corns added. The benefits were captured in the western system of medicine and the extracts are used in expectorants.

CHEMICAL COMPOSITION/KEY ACTIVE CONSTITUENTS

A bioactive pyrroloquinazoline alkaloid, vaccine about 1.3%, includes other alkaloids viz., vasicol, adhatonine, vsicinone, vasicinol, vasiciolone, aliphatic hydroketones viz., hydroxy-hexateracont-l-en-15 one and 37 hydroxy hentetracontam-19-one.

PHARMACOLOGY

The bronchodilatory and expectorant properties of the leaves are attributed to vasicine. The Drug possesses abortifacient activity and significant antimicrobial activity against gingival inflammation and pyorrhoea.

Vasaka is used in ayurveda abundantly for different diseases, this is the only herb which can pacify both pitta and kapha doshas.

The details of this herb in Ayurveda is as follows—

Sanskrit Name: *Vasa Vasaka*

- *Vasika*—Means one which covers a large area, here area coverage stands for a protective cover on the body.
- *Singhasya*—Means a plant having flowers like the mouth of the lion.
- *Vajidanta*—Means a plant having white flowers like the teeth of a horse.
- *Vrusha*–Means one that showers the honey, i.e., having a lot of nectar Aatrushaka

It is used as *antimicrobial, antitussive, anticancer,* useful in infinite atopical *dermatitis, bronchodilatory, expectorant.*

DOSAGE

1-2 gm of the drug is prescribed as an expectorant either in the form of liquid extract (1-2 ml) or syrup (2-4 ml).

TOLU BALSAM

Botanical Name	:	*Myroxylon toluifera balsamum*
Family	:	Fabaceae
Parts Used	:	Oleo resin (Balsam - brittle)
Common Name	:	Tolu Balsam

DESCRIPTION

An evergreen tree growing to about 40 ft. (12 m) It's often planted as a wind-break or shade tree. All parts of the tree are aromatic. The balsam is discharged from V-shaped cuts in the bark and is collected.

CULINARY USES

Resin is used in chewing gum, ice cream, candy, soft drinks, bakery products, etc.

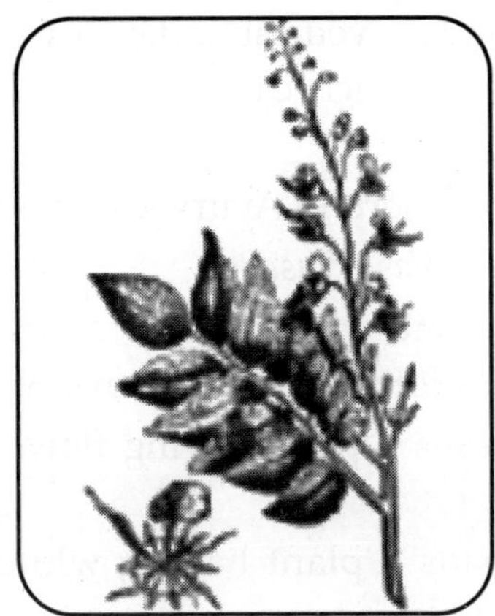

Fig. 12.2: Tolu balsam

MEDICINAL USES

Treats lung congestion, coughs and colds. Was used to treat headaches, gout and stomach problems. Can cause allergic reactions.

Tolu balsam is a balsamic type of a natural oleoresin. Its content of essential oil is so low that the product could justly be called a balsamic resin or a Balsam. Balsam Tolu is formed after injuries in the trunk of Myroxylon Balsamum tree, native of the jungles of northern South America, particularly in Colombia and Venezuela.

TULSI OR HOLY BASIL

Botanical Name	:	*Occimum sanctum*
Family	:	Labiatae
Parts Used	:	Leaves, Seeds
Common Name	:	Tulsi, Holy basil

HABITAT AND CULTIVATION

It is grown and found almost all over the world. In India the plant of Tulsi is cultivated in almost every house and is also worshipped. Usually the plant is 1-2 ft high with fragrant small oval shaped leaves, flat seeds red in colour, flowers blossoming on inflorescence (manjari).

White Tulsi and *Black Tulsi* are most commonly found although there are also *Vanatulsi, Rama-tulsi* & *Kappori Tulsi* and *Black Tulsi* is the best as regards its properties.

DESCRIPTION

The colloquial name in India for *holi basil* is *tulsi* and its botanical name is *ocimum sanctum.* Holi basil is a herb with multiple branching of stems and a typical aromatic smell.

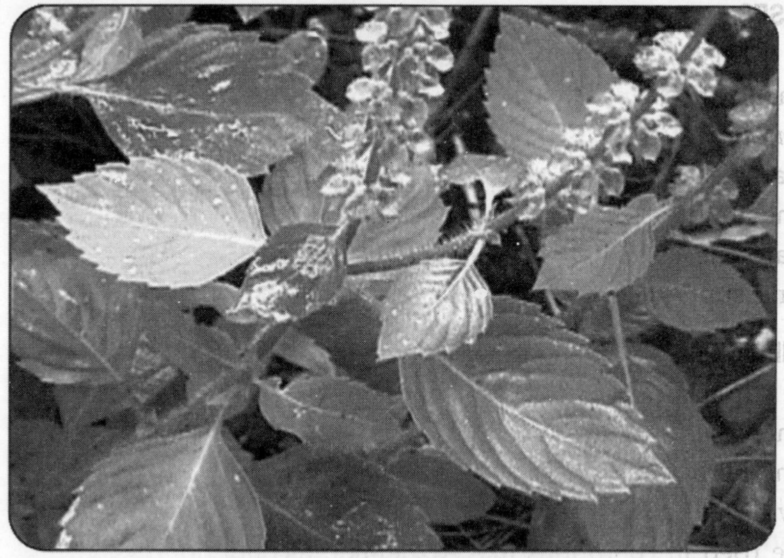

Fig. 12.1: Occimum sanctum

Leaves are hairy, green, smooth and pungent in taste. The small compact clusters of flowers are arranged on branches which are called mangiri. These bear *fruits* and seeds which are brownish in color and have typical odor. Leaves and manjiri are edible part of the plant and have medicinal value.

This medicinal herb is known to Indians from vedic period. (Vedas = songs of life written by Indian sages) Hindu religion has given special honor to Holy basil in their life and the plant itself is treated as god at some places. The leaves are included in many religious performances. They are included in tirth (holy liquid) and prasad (Holy food) of pooja (worshiping god) and the custom is followed by generations after generations.

Tulsi has *antioxidant* properties, and helps boost the body's ability to fight off damaging free radicals, which have been linked to disease and aging. It is an adaptogen that helps the body fight the effects of ongoing stress and also balances the mind, nerves and emotions. It is known to maintain the health of the throat chest and lungs. In fact, it helps protect the entire respiratory tract.

USES

Tulsi maintains the health of the throat chest and lungs. In fact, it helps protect the entire respiratory tract. It is an *anti-inflammatory*. Tulsi helps protect the physiology from garavisha—environmental toxins and pollution. It helps purify the atmosphere. Tulsi is also a skin rasayana. With vitamin C, carotene, calcium and phosphorus, Tulsi helps skin stay healthy and supple. It also helps maintain the digestive agni (fire).

MEDICINAL USES

It acts as an *appetizer* and helps digestion. Holy basil has many *medicinal properties*. The leaves are included in most of the herbal nervo-tonics. A fresh juice/decoction of holy basil with few other herbs is taken for *improving memory*. Herb can be tried in conditions like Alzheimer, alcohol brain syndrome which are modern diseases and until now there are no perfect remedies for these disorders.

Holy Basil is of two types. According to some experts there are many other types of basil namely *white* and *black*. Both have the same qualities. Basil is hot, bitter, increases the digestive fire, beneficial for the heart, spicy, increases the bile and cures leprosy, burning sensation in the urine, blood impurities, pain due to stones, kapha and vata.

Holy Basil is mainly used for curing *cold* and *kapha*. *Black basil* also known as *shyama tulsi* is used along with black pepper to remove kapha from the lungs. It is effective in curing fever. The dry basil leaves powder is used for curing kapha. The oil cooked with bails paste is useful in ear pain and nose problem. Along with lemon it is used for curing eczema and ringworm. The seeds are useful for increasing the potency in men. The leaves, seeds, flowers, skin, stem and roots are useful for curing all diseases of the body. The atmosphere is absolutely clean and pure where basil plant is grown and the lightning does not strike that place. It protects from smallpox and malaria as well.

Regular use of this medicine cures cough, cold, chronic or new catarrh, nausea, cold by birth, respiratory problem, pain in the eyes and head, low or high blood pressure, ear disease, acidity, constipation, gas, weakness of the kidneys, stones, deficiency of vitamin A or C and the diseases caused thereby, skin diseases, fever.

Basil is the best medicine for *jaundice*. Take ten basil leaves with 10gm of radish juice and consume 10 gm with jaggery regularly for one month thrice daily to cure jaundice.

Eat three to five basil leaves everyday. Put five basil leaves in drinking water before half an hour. This cures *piles*. Grind the basil leaves and apply the lep on the haemorrhoids. And half a piece of camphor in this paste and avoid hot and spicy food items. Restrict sour food items totally for complete relief.

Basil leaves cure the *stomachache*. Consuming one spoon each of basil and ginger juice cures cramps and stomachache.

Heat the basil and ginger juice and take one spoon for two days at an interval of three hours to cure stomach worms, they are evacuated with stools.

Make a powder out of flower of basil, skin of neem, small pipal and black pepper and take three gm of this powder on empty stomach to cure *acidity*. This cures the disease within 4-5 days.

Basil cures *seminal problems,* take 50gm each of basil seeds and sugar candy and take 2.5 gm of this powder with milk every morning. If the basil seeds are not available then basil roots can be taken with sugar candy. The basil roots are also beneficial for strengthening and thickening the sperm and bring back the masculinity.

STUDY QUESTIONS

1. Write a short note on Occimum sanctum.
2. What are the medicinal uses of Tulsi?

■■■

13

CHAPTER

ANTIRHEUMATICS

GUGGUL

Botanical Name	:	*Commiphora Mukul*
Family	:	Burseraceae
Parts Used	:	Whole Plant
Common Names	:	Commiphora, Mukul, Guggul, Balsamodendrom Mukul, Indian Bdellium Tree, Moql, Moqle-arzagi

HABITAT

Rocky tracks of Western India and Eastern Himalayas.

DESCRIPTION

Guggul is the yellowish resin (or gum) that is produced by the *mukul Commiphora* mukul tree, a small, thorny plant that grows throughout northern India. Guggul is also referred as guggul gum, guggal, gugglesterone, guggul, gugulu and gum gugal.

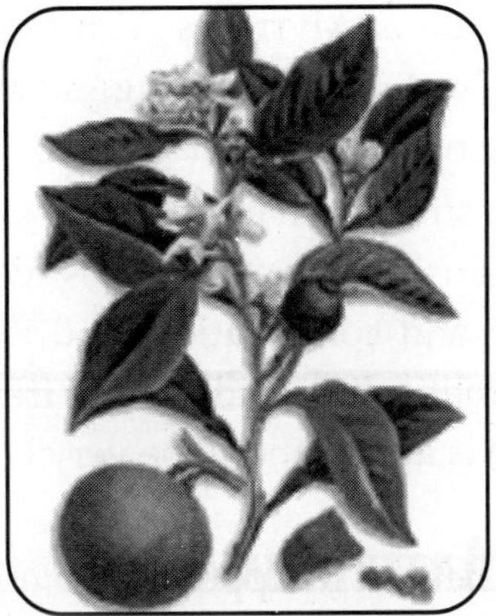

Fig. 13.1: Guggul

Analysis of guggul gum shows the active ingredients are plant sterones or "guggulsterones". In addition, the data supports the idea that the two compounds, Z and E-guggulsterones, work with the body to significantly lower serum triglycerides and cholesterol as well as LDL and VLDL cholesterols (the 'bad' cholesterols) as it raises levels of HDL cholesterol (the 'good' cholesterol). Since guggul is also an antioxidant, guggulsterones also keep LDL cholesterol from oxidizing, which protects against atherosclerosis. Guggul has also been shown to reduce the stickiness of platelets—another effect that lowers the risk of coronary artery disease.

MEDICINAL USE

Guggul plays a major role in the *traditional herbal medicine* of India. It is often combined with other herbs and used in the treatment of arthritis, skin diseases, pains in the nervous system, obesity, digestive problems, infections in the mouth, and menstrual problems.

The mukul myrrh tree is closely related to the Commiphora Mukul tree (or common myrrh). Myrrh was one of the first medicines with hieroglyphic notation of use during ancient

Egyptian times depicting its many uses. With such a close relation, many scientists believe that Guggul may have many of the same properties as Myrrh as even their ancient status is similar. In the Sushruta Samhita, guggul was also suggested for fat loss and the relief of *arthritis*.

It also works to strengthen our *digestive system*, it even helps in the easy secretions of digestive juices, works as appetizer, avoids indigestion and constipation, and is also beneficial in hemorrhoids and colitis. It provides relief from *hyperacidity* and belching. This herb is also found to be very beneficial in various liver problems.

Guggul is also helpful in upper *respiratory tract infection*. Its expectorant action helps in the suppression of the kapha dosha, which is the main cause of wet cough. Benefits are also seen in asthmatic conditions.

It works as a *diuretic* for the patients suffering from renal calculi by means of crushing the calculus therefore relieving and treating the renal stones.

COLCHICUM

Botanical Name	:	*Colchicum autumnale*
Family	:	Liliaceae
Parts Used	:	Root, seeds
Common Name	:	Saffron, Meadow

HABITAT

Grows wild in meadows, especially on limestone.

DESCRIPTION

It has lanceolate leaves, dark green, glabrous, often a foot long. Flowers light purple or white, like crocus but for their six stamens; the ovaries remain underground until the spring after flowering, when they are borne up by the elongating peduncles and ripen. It flowers in September and October. The leaves and fruit are poisonous to cattle.

The root is called a *corm,* from which in autumn the light-purplish mottled flowers arise.

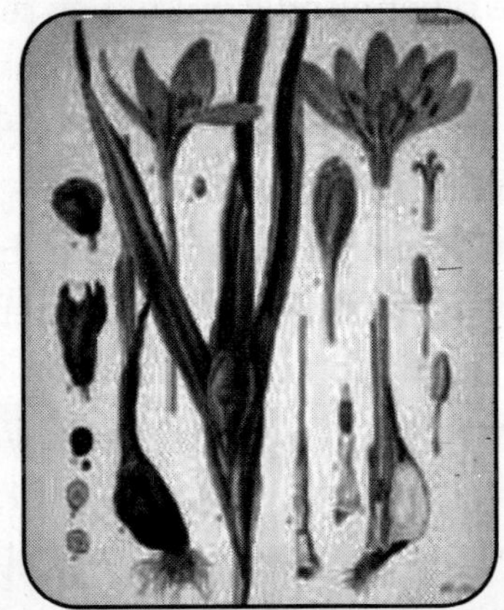

Fig. 13.2: Colchicum autumnale

CULTIVATION

Requires light, sandy loam, enriched with decayed manure or leafmould. Plant the bulbs 3 inches deep and 3 inches apart in July or August, in moist beds or rockeries, shrubbery, borders or lawns near shade of trees. The foliage dies down in June and July, and does not reappear until after the plant has flowered. It may also be propagated by seeds sown 1/8 inch deep in a bed of fine soil outdoors in August or September, or in pans or boxes of similar soil in cold frame at the same time, transplanting seedlings 3 inches apart when two years old; or by division of bulbs in August. Seedling bulbs do not flower till four or five years old.

MEDICINAL ACTION AND USES

The Colchicum is valued for its medicinal properties. The parts used are the root and seeds, these being anti-rheumatic, cathartic, and emetic. Its reputation rests largely upon its value in acute gouty and rheumatic complaints. It is mostly used in connexion with some alkaline diuretic; also in pill form. Overdoses cause violent purging, etc.

The active principle is said to be an alkaline substance of a very poisonous nature called *Colchinine*. It is acrid, sedative, and acts upon all the secreting organs, particularly the bowels and kidneys. It is apt to cause undue depression, and in large doses acts as an irritant poison. Dr. Lindley relates the case of a woman who was poisoned by the sprouts of Colchicum, which had been thrown away in Covent Garden Market and which she mistook for onions.

The Hermodactyls of the Arabians, formerly celebrated for soothing pains in the joints, are said to be this plant.

The corm or root is usually sold in transverse slices, notched on one side and somewhat reniform in outline, white and starchy internally, about 1/8 inch thick, and varying from 3/4 to 1 inch in diameter. Taste sweetish, then bitter and acrid. Odour radish-like in fresh root, but lost in drying.

STUDY QUESTIONS

1. Write short notes on the following:
   (a) Guggul; and
   (b) Colchicum autumnale.
2. Explain the medicinal action of guggul and Colchicum autumnale.

■■■

14 CHAPTER

ANTITUMOUR AGENTS

VINCA ROSEA

Botanical Name	:	*Vinca rosea*
Family	:	Apocynaceae
Parts Used	:	Leaves, Roots.
Common Name	:	Periwinkle, Madagascar Periwinkle, Sadabahar.

HABITAT

Grows throughout India and found as an escape in waste places and sandy tracts.

DESCRIPTION

Catharanthus roseus (Madagascar periwinkle) is a species of Catharanthus native and endemic to Madagascar. In the wild, it is an endangered plant; the main cause of decline is habitat destruction by slash and burn agriculture. It is also however widely cultivated and is naturalised in subtropical and tropical areas of the world.

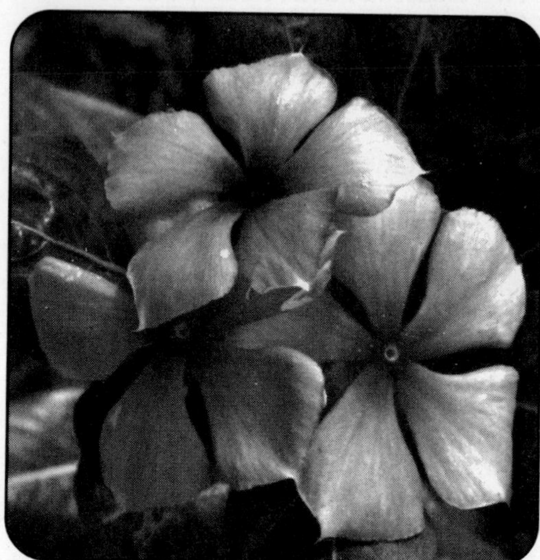

Fig. 14.1: Vinca rosea

It is an evergreen subshrub or herbaceous plant growing to 1 m tall. The leaves are oval to oblong, 2.5–9 cm long and 1–3.5 cm broad, glossy green, hairless, with a pale midrib and a short petiole 1–1.8 cm long; they are arranged in opposite pairs. The flowers are white to dark pink with a darker red centre, with a basal tube 2.5-3 cm long and a corolla 2–5 cm diameter with five petal-like lobes. The fruit is a pair of follicles 2–4 cm long and 3 mm broad.

MEDICINAL USE

The species has long been cultivated for herbal medicine and as an ornamental plant. In traditional Chinese medicine, extracts from it have been used to treat numerous diseases, including *diabetes*, *malaria*, and *Hodgkin's disease*. The substances vinblastine and vincristine extracted from the plant are used in the treatment of *leukemia*.

Taken as a daily supplement, it improves the blood supply to the brain, increases oxygen and glucose for the brain to use, helps prevent abnormal coagulation of blood, and it *raises brain levels of the neurotransmitter serotonin.*

There are two classes of active compounds in Vinca: *alkaloids* and *tannins.*

The major alkaloid is known as *vincamine.*

A closely related semi-synthetic derivative of vincamine widely used as medicine is known as *ethyl-apovincaminate* or *vinpocetine*. It has *vasodilating, blood thinning, and memory-enhancing actions*. It has been shown in double-blind studies to help alleviate a type of dementia known as *vascular dementia,* in which the arteries supplying blood to the brain develop atherosclerotic plaques.

Extracts of Vinca have significant anticancer activity against numerous cell types.

The greatest activity is seen against multi-drug resistant tumor types which suggest that there are compounds in Vinca rosea that are synergistic or additive with anti-neoplastic elements by inhibiting resistance to them.

STUDY QUESTIONS

1. Write a detailed note Vinca rosea.
2. Explain the medicinal uses of Vinca rosea.

■■■

15 CHAPTER

ANTILEPROTICS

CHAULMOOGRA

Botanical Name	:	*Hydnocarpus laurifolia, H. kurzii, Taraktogenos kurzii*
Family	:	Flacourtiaceae
Parts Used	:	The oil from the seeds
Common Name	:	Chaulmoogra

HABITAT AND CULTIVATION

Chaulmoogra is native to the tropical areas of Malaysia and the Indian subcontinent.

DESCRIPTION

Seeds are ovoid, irregular and angular, 1 to $1^1/_4$ inches long, 1 inch wide, skin smooth, grey, brittle; kernel oily and dark brown. A fatty oil is obtained by expression, known officially as *Gynocardia* oil in Britain, as *OleumChaulmoograe* in the U.S.A.

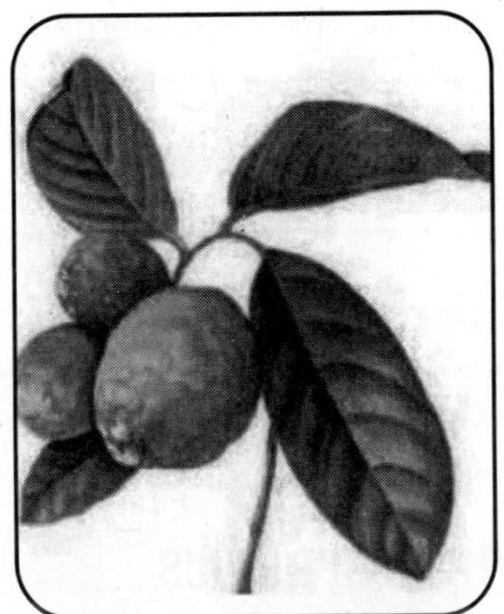

Fig. 15.1: Chaulmoogra

CONSTITUENTS

The oil contains chaulmoogric acid and palmitic acid, and the fatty oil has been found to yield glycerol, a very small quantity of phytosterol and a mixture of fatty acids. The chaulmoogra tree bears brown, velvety, round fruit and irregular grayish seeds that are angled with blunt ends. Chaulmoogra oil can also come from *Tarak-togenos kurzii*, an allied species.

MEDICINAL ACTION AND USES

Chaulmoogra Oil is pressed from the seeds of the Chaulmoogra tree. The antimicrobial properties of this oil is used to treat *eczema, psoriasis, arthritis, sprains, bruises* and *skin inflammations*. This oil is an effective treatment for *leprosy*. This oil can be well utilized in creams, lotions, balms, ointments, lip balms, massage oils and wound care balms. It is also used in veterinary practice. Dose of oil, 5 or 10 to 60 minims.

Some of the commercial oil on the market probably comes from the allied species *Hydnocarpus*.

Chaulmoogra contains strongly antibacterial chemicals, two of which, *hydnocarpic* and *chaulmoogric acids*, are responsible for destroying the bacterium, Mycobacterium leprae, that causes leprosy.

In Indian medicine, the oil has also been used to treat intestinal worms and skin diseases.

In many places today, the ingredients of chaulmoogra oil, modified by chemists, are still used to cure early cases of leprosy-advanced cases do not yield to the treatment, but they have generally been replaced by synthesized sulfones.

STUDY QUESTIONS

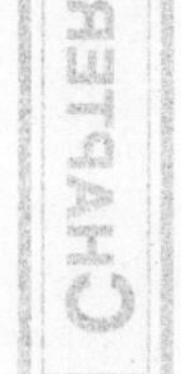

1. Write a detailed note on Chaulmoogra.
2. Explain the medicinal uses of Chaulmoogra.

■■■

16

CHAPTER

ANTIDIABETICS

PTEROCARPUS MARSUPIUM

Botanical Name	: *Pterocarpus marsupium*
Family	: Fabaceae
Parts Used	: Heart Wood, Leaves, Flowers
Common Name	: Indian Kino Tree, Malabar Kino Tree, Kino

HABITAT

Found commonly in hilly regions throughout the Deccan Peninsula, and extending to Gujarat, Madhya Pradesh, Uttar Pradesh, Bihar and Orissa.

DESCRIPTION

A moderate-sized to large deciduous tree. The bark is grey, rough, longitudinally fissured and scaly. The older trees exude a blood red gum-resin. The leaves are imparipinnate: the leaflets are oblong; the flowers occur in large panicles, they are yellowish and fragrant; the pods are orbicular, flat, winged.

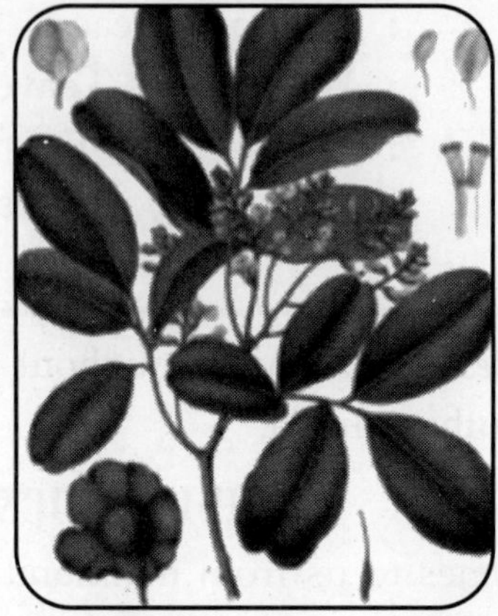

Fig. 16.1: Pterocarpus Marsupium

INDICATIONS

An aqueous infusion of the wood is said to be of use in diabetes. Tests on mice and rabbits with alcohol and aqueous extracts of the heartwood are said to have shown hypoglycemic action, probably by hindering the absorption of glucose in the intestine.

MEDICINAL USES

The heartwood is astringent, bitter acrid, anti inflammatory, anthelmintic and anodyne. An aqueous infusion of the wood is used in *diabetes*. It has been found to reduced the glucose absorption from the gastrointestinal tract and improve insulin and pro-insulin levels. It is effective in beta cell regeneration and has also been found to have a *hypocholesteremic effect*. It turns the water blue as soon as it comes in contact with the water. It is good for *elephantiasis, leucoderma, diarrhoea, dysentery, rectalgia, cough* and *greyness of hair*. The bark is used as an *astringent* and in *toothache*.

The bruised leaves are considered useful as an external application for boils, sores and *skin diseases*.

GYMNEMA SYLVESTRE

Botanical Name	:	*Gymnema sylvestre*
Family	:	Asclepiadaceae
Parts Used	:	Whole plant, Leaves and Roots
Common Names	:	Gurmarbooti, Gurmar, periploca of the woods, meshasring.

DISTRIBUTION

Gymnema sylvestre is found throughout the tropical forests of central and southern India.

DESCRIPTION

Gymnema comes to us from mainland India and several parts of Africa and has a deep history rooted in Ayurvedic medicine. Currently it is one of the major botanicals being administered for those suffering from *diabetes*, in boosting insulin levels and controlling healthy blood sugar levels.

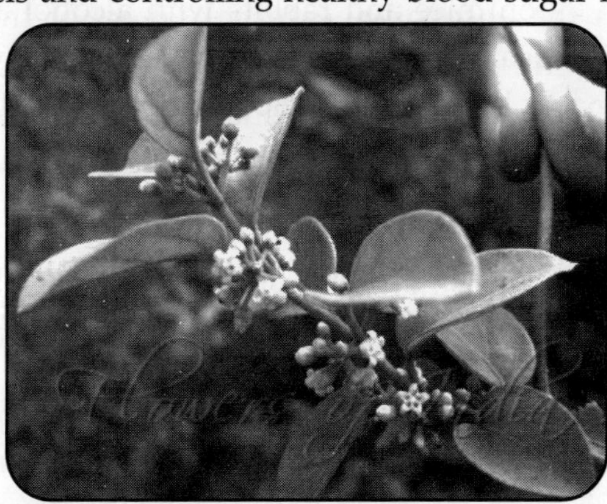

Fig. 16.2: Gymnema sylvestre

Gymnema sylvestre is a woody climbing plant that grows in the tropical forests of central and southern India. The leaves lamina is ovate, elliptic or ovate-lanceolate, with both surfaces pubescent. The flowers are small bell-shaped yellow color. The leaves of gurmar are used medicinally, for its unique property to directly mask the tongue's ability to taste sweet foods; at the same time suppresses glucose absorption from the intestine. This is the reason it is known in Hindi as *gurmar,* actually means *diabetes killer* or *"destroyer of sugar"*.

Historically, gymnema sylvestre has been used to treat conditions ranging from malaria to snake bites. Sushruta, the classic book on Ayurveda, describes G. *sylvestre,* as a destroyer of "Madhumeha" (glycosuria) and other urinary disorders.

PHARMACOLOGY

The hypoglycemic extract of Gymnema sylvestris brings about blood glucose homeostasis, which in turn prevents increased glycosylation of proteins thus reversing the onset of changes leading to micro and macroangiopathy. Control of Diabetes mellitus and the associated complications are mediated through the revival or regeneration of the insulin, producing beta-cells in the islets of langerhans. The glucose-like molecules in Gurmar known as the gymnemic acid fills the receptor locations in the absorptive external layers of the intestine, thereby preventing the intestine from absorbing the sugar molecules. Due to the change in the absorption level of sugar, there is a consequent change in the blood sugar level.

MEDICINAL USES

Gymnema is anti-diabetic, astringent, stomachic, tonic and refrigerant. In Ayurveda the plant has been described as an anti-diabetic, antiperiodic, stomachic and diuretic.

- This is one of the main herbs used for healing diabetes mellitus.
- It removes sugar from pancrease, restores pancreatic function.
- Gymnema stimulate the circulatory system, increases urine secretion.
- It is also useful for the treatment of swollen glands, cough, and fever.

STUDY QUESTIONS

1. Write short notes on the following:
   (a) Pterocarpus marsupium; and
   (b) Gymnema sylvestris.
2. Describe the medicinal uses of Gymnema sylvestris.

■■■

17 CHAPTER

DIURETICS

SMALL GOKHRU

Botanical Name	:	*Tribulus terrestris*
Family	:	Zygophyllaceae
Parts Used	:	Whole plant, Seeds and Root
Common Name	:	Gokshur, Puncture vine, Chhota gokhru, Land caltrop

HABITAT

The trailing plant is common in sandy soil throughout India and Ceylon (Sri Lanka).

DESCRIPTION

An annual herb with diffused or prostrates stems. The branches are flexuous covered with silky thread like hairs. The leaves are pari-pinnate having 6 to 7 pairs of leaflets that are narrow-elliptic with round base and apex. The yellow flowers are borne solitary and axillary. The fruit is weapon-wheel shaped containing five parts. Each part has two long sharp rigid spines, several shorter spines and surface covered with many hairs.

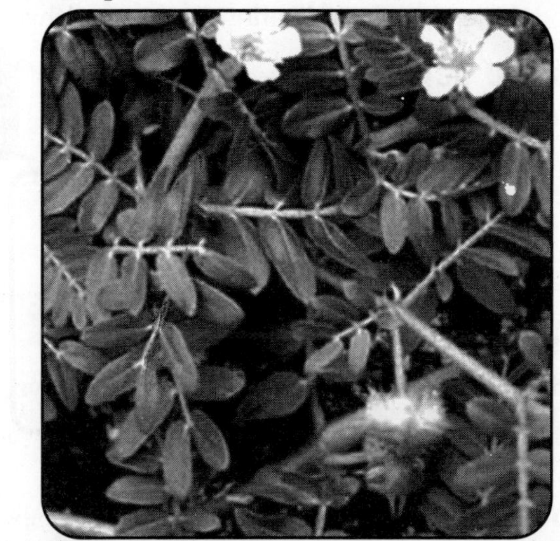

Fig. 17.1: Tribulus terrestris

The name "Gokshura" signifies "cow hoof" from its resemblance of the cocci when adhering together in pairs. It is also called "Ikshugandha" for its aroma which resembles the sugarcane. The entire plant but especially the fruit and roots are used in Ayurvedic formulations for urinary disorders, calculus formation, impotence and other urinary tract infection.

Tribulus is a prostrate, annual herb grows upto 90 cm in length with paripinnate leaves. The flowers are small, yellowish, and solitary. The fruits of tribulus are typically five angled and spinous. Tribulus is cooling, sweet and strengthening. It is common throughout India and found to be growing as weed along roadside and waste places.

PHARMACOLOGICAL ACTION

The roots and fruits are sweet, cooling, emollient (softening and soothing), appetizer, alternate, laxative, cardiotonic, styptic, lithontriptic and tonic. They are useful in strangury, dysuria, vitiated conditions of vat and pitta, renal and vesical calculi, anorexia, dyspepsia, helminthiasis, cough, asthama. The seeds are astringent, strengthening and are useful in epistaxis, hemorrhages and ulcerative stomatitis. The ash of the whole plant is good for external application in rheumarthritis.

PROPERTIES AND ACTION

Rasa—madhur

Guna—guru, snigdh

Virya—shit

Vipaka—madhura

Karma—vatanashak, vrsya, brmhana, mutral

MEDICINAL USES

- **Digestive system:** It is used in diarrhea and dysentery.
- **Reproductive system:** It is used to promote lactation.
- **Skin:** It is used in psoriasis and eczema
- **Genito-urinary system:** The diuretic properties of plant are due to large amount of nitrates and essential oils present in seeds. Plant and dried spiny fruit is used for spermatorrhea, phosphateuria, dysuria, gonorrhea, gleet, chronic cystitis, calculous affections, incontinence of urine and impotency. It is used in inflammation of urinary passage

Tribulus Terrestris has the action of *dilating coronary artery* and improving coronary circulation, and thus has better effects on improving ECG of myocardial ischemia. If taken for a long time, it has no adverse reaction on blood system and hepatic and renal functions. Neither does it have side effects. It is one of the ideal medicines to treat angina pectoris.

Tribulus Terrestris is used in impotency as a *testosterone enhancer*. Studies show that it works very well when stacked with DHEA and androstenedione Instead of being a testosterone precursor, it leads to the production of the *luteinizing hormone* (LH). When LH levels are increased, the natural production of testosterone also increases. LH is a hormone that also deals with sex drive. Laboratory animal studies found that Tribulus Terrestris *increased sperm* count as well as motility levels after taking it for 30 days.

BURRA GOOKERO

Botanical Name	:	*Pedalium murex*
Family	:	Pedaliaceae
Parts Used	:	Seeds
Common Name	:	Bada gokshur, til kul

HABITAT

It is found throughout India.

DESCRIPTION

Fruits taste mucilaginous, odourless. It is a creeper that is about 2 to 3 feet long having branches spread all over, leaves are in pairs of 5 to 8 and is of irregular shape. Flowers are small and yellow coloured.

Fruits are round brown, two-celled with four narrow, long seeds. and possess 5 to 12 compartments and each compartment contains a seed. The seeds contain aromatic oil. Roots are 4 to 5 inch long, brown in color and bear a sweet aroma. The plant flowers in early winters followed by fruiting.

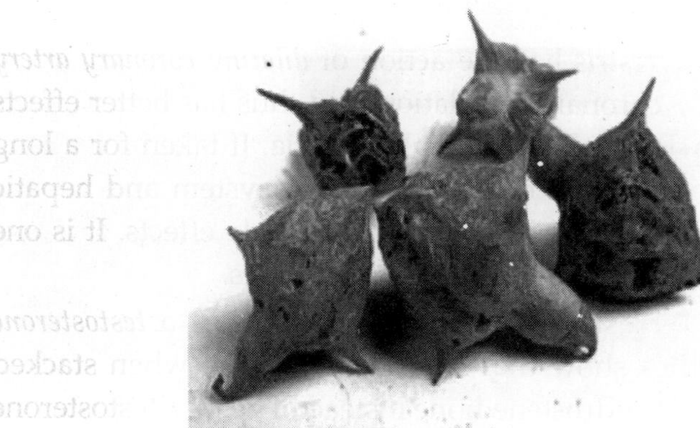

Fig. 17.2: Pedalium murex

PHARMACOLOGY

It is *vata* and *pitta* suppressant. It helps in suppressing pain and inflammation due to its sweet taste. It also provides strength to the body due to presence of slimy properties and sweet taste. It also has a good effect on the respiratory and digestive system. It is a good aphrodisiac agent. It is a diuretic agent

According to ayurveda it contains:

Gunna (properties) – guru (heavy), snigdh (slimy)

Rasa (taste) – madhur (sweet)

Virya (potency) – sheet (cold)

MEDICINAL USES

Diuretic, demulcent, aphrodisiac. It is used for *impotence* in males, nocturnal emissions, gonorrhoea, gleet and incontinence of urine.

USES

Paste: It is applied on the head incase of nervine weakness. It also relives from the pain and inflammation when applied on the affected part.

Powder: It helps in regularizing the digestive activities. It also regulates the circulatory system and strengthens the heart muscles. It helps in cleaning the respiratory tract. It provides strength to the uterus. It is also helpful in increasing the strength of the body.

PUNARNAVA

Botanical Name	:	*Boerhavia diffusa*
Family	:	Nyctaginaceae
Parts Used	:	Whole herb and Root
Common Name	:	Hog-weed, Beshakapore, Punarnava

HABITAT

It is found throughout India, especially during the rainy season.

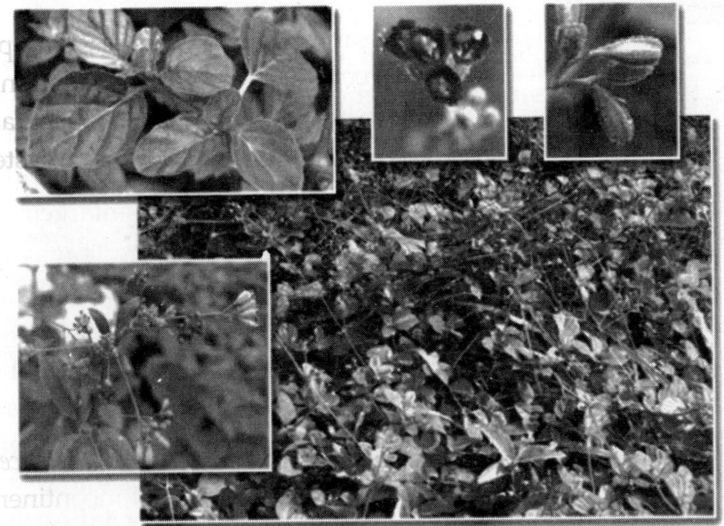

Fig. 17.3: Boerhavia diffusa

BIO ENERGETICS

Rasa (Taste)—Madhura (Sweet); Tikta (Bitter); Kashaya (Astringent)

Guna (Characteristics)—Laghu (Light); Ruksha (Rough)

Veerya (Potency)—Ushna (Warm)

Vipaka (Post digestion effect)—Madhura (Sweet)

TRADITIONAL AYURVEDIC USES

The root of this plant is a powerful Rasayana (*longevity enhancer*). It is good for the kidneys, especially the nephron cells which are damaged by long-term hyperglycemia (diabetes). And it pacifies two of the main laws of physiology (*Vata* and *Kapha*).

Punarnava enhances the quality of 6 of the 7 categories of bodily tissues, including nutrient plasma (Rasa Dhatu), blood (Rakta Dhatu), muscle (Mamsa Dhatu), fat (Meda Dhatu), bone marrow and nerves (Majja Dhatu), and reproductive fluids (Shukra Dhatu).

MEDICINAL USES

According to *Ayurveda* Boerhavia is bitter, anaemia, cooling, heart diseases, astringent to bowels, useful in biliousness (disorder of the liver or gallbladder), blood impurities, leucorrhoea, asthma, alternatives etc. The leaves are useful in dyspepsia, tumours, abdominal pains, and spleen enlargement.

According to *Unani* system of medicine, the leaves are appetizers, alexiteric, useful in opthalmia and in joint pains. Seeds are tonic expectorant, carminative, useful in lumbago, scabies. The seeds are considered as promising blood purifier. Roots are used to treat gonorrhea, all internal inflammation and edema. Roots stimulate the emptying of the gall bladder, as a diuretic, for all types of liver disorders (including jaundice and hepatitis), gall bladder pain and stones, urinary tract disorders, renal disorders, kidney stones, cystitis, and nephritis.

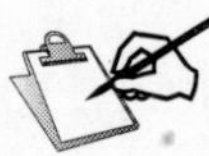

STUDY QUESTIONS

1. Write short notes on the following:
   (a) Small Gokhru;
   (b) Burra Gookero; and
   (c) Punarnava.
2. Explain the medicinal uses of small Gokhru and Punarnava.

■■■

18

CHAPTER

ANTIDYSENTRICS

IPECACUANHA

Botanical Name	:	*Psychotria ipecacuanha*
Family	:	Rubiaceae
Parts Used	:	Root
Common Name	:	Ipecac

HABITAT

The root used in medicine under this name is that of a small, shrubby plant about a foot high, belonging to the order Rubiaceae, which is found in most parts of Brazil, growing in clumps or patches, in moist, shady woods.

DESCRIPTION

Ipecacuanha (*Psychotria ipecacuanha*) of family *Rubiaceae* is a flowering plant, the root of which is most commonly used to make syrup of ipecac, a powerful *emetic.* The plant has a slender stem which grows partly underground and is often procumbent at the base, the lower portion being knotted. Fibrous rootlets are given off from the knots, and some of them develop an abnormally thick bark, in which much starch is deposited. The thickened rootlets alone are collected and dried for medicinal use, since the active constituents of the drug are found chiefly in the bark. Ipecacuanha roots are collected, chiefly by the Indians, during the months of January and February, when the plant is in flower and are prepared by separation from the stem, cleaning and hanging in bundles to dry in the sun.

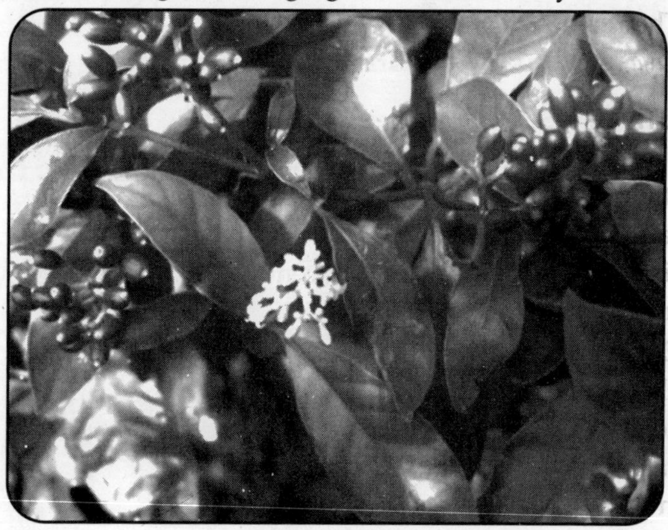

Fig. 18.1: Psychotria ipecacuanha

SUBSTITUTES

In addition to the Cartagena Ipecacuanha, various other roots have been offered as substitutes, but all differ considerably. East Indian Ipecacuanha, from Cryptocarpus spiralis, exhibits a typically monocotyledous structure in transverse section, scattered bundles running the pith, and a white starchy bark. The name poaya is applied in Brazil to emetic roots of several genera belonging to the natural orders Rubiaceae, Violaceae and Polygalaceae, and hence several roots have from time to time been sent over to England as Ipecacuanha, but none of them possess the ringed or annulated appearance of the true drug. Of these, the root of Ionidium Ipecacuanha, Richardsonia scabra and *P. emetica* are those which have most frequently been exported from Brazil or Colombia.

White Ipecacuanha, from *I. ipecacuanha* is greyish-white, or yellowish in colour and is also free from starch. This likewise was for long believed to be the plant which produces the genuine drug. It is a member of the order Violaceae. The root is almost insipid and inodorous and is used in Brazil as an emetic, though it has been considered doubtful whether it possesses any well-defined properties.

The roots of several species of Borreria, as *B. ferruginia* and *B. poaya*, are also used in Brazil as substitutes for Ipecacuanha.

CONSTITUENTS

The chief constituents of Ipecacuanha root are the alkaloids Emetine, Cephaelin and Psychotrine, of which the bark may contain from 1.5 to 2 per cent, of which about 72 per cent consists of Emetine and 26 per cent of Cephaelin, while only 2 per cent consists of Psychotrine.

Emetine, to which Ipecacuanha owes its properties and which, with the exception of traces, occurs only in the cortical portion of the root, is an amorphous white powder, but it forms crystalline salts. It has a bitter taste, no odour and turns yellow when exposed to air and light.

Other constituents are a crystalline saponin-like glucoside, an amorphous, bitter glucoside, which is a modification of tannin, and is known as Ipecacuanhic acid, choline, resin, pectin, starch, sugar, calcium oxalate, odorous, fatty matter and a disagreeable-smelling volatile oil.

Cartagena Ipecacuanha contains 2 to 3 per cent more alkaloidal matter than the Brazilian drug, but a smaller proportion of Emetine, Cephaelin being the alkaloid present in largest quantities.

East Indian Ipecacuanha and White Ipecacuanha contain minute quantities of emetic principles, which differ from the alkaloids of true Ipecacuanha, but the Undulated and Striated Ipecacuanha contain Emetine.

MEDICINAL USES

In large doses, Ipecacuanha root is emetic; in smaller doses, diaphoretic and expectorant, and in still smaller, stimulating to the stomach, intestines and liver, exciting appetite and facilitating digestion.

The dose of the powdered root is 1/4 to 2 grains when an expectorant action is desired (it is frequently used in the treatment of bronchitis and laryngitis, combined with other drugs, aiding in the expulsion of the morbid product), and from 15 to 30 grains when given as an emetic, which is one of its most valuable functions.

When applied to the skin, Ipecacuanha powder acts as a powerful irritant, even to the extent of causing pustulations.

When inhaled, it causes sneezing and a mild inflammation of the nasal mucous membrane.

Toxic doses cause gastro-enteritis, cardiac failure, dilation of the blood-vessels, severe bronchitis and pulmonary inflammation.

This plant is used by the negroes as an emetic and the root is purgative; the juice of the plant, made into a syrup, is said to be a powerful anthelmintic, and as such is given to children in the West Indies.

STUDY QUESTIONS

1. Write a detailed note Psychotria ipecacuanha.
2. Discuss the medicinal uses of Psychotria ipecacuanha

■■■

19

CHAPTER

Antiseptic and Disinfectants

BENZOIN

Botanical Name	:	*Styrax benzoin*
Family	:	Styraceae
Parts Used	:	Resin
Common Name	:	Gum benzoin, Gun benjamin, Siam benzoin, Sumatra benzoin.

HABITAT

Siam, Sumatra and Java.

DESCRIPTION

Benzoin is a balsamic resin. Normally the trees do not produce it or any substance analogous to it, but the infliction of a wound sufficiently severe to injure the cambium results in the formation of numerous oleoresin ducts in which the secretion is produced, it is, therefore, a pathological product.

The trunk of the tree is hacked with an axe, and after a time the liquid Benzoin either accumulates beneath the bark or exudes from the incisions. When it has sufficiently hardened it is collected and exported, either in the form of loose pieces (tears) or in masses packed in oblong boxes or in tins; several varieties are known, but Siam and Sumatra Benzoins are the most important. The incisions are made when the tree is seven years old, and in Sumatra each tree yields about 3 lb. annually for ten or twelve years. The first three years collections give the finest Benzoin; after that the runnings are known as the 'belly,' and finally the tree is cut down and the resin scraped out, this being termed the 'foot.' Siam Benzoin externally is reddish yellow, internally milky white, has an agreeable odour, recalling vanilla, contains benzoic acid but not cinnamic acid. Sumatra Benzoin is always in blocks of a dull reddish or greyish-brown colour. Fine qualities have a strong storax-like odour, quite distinct from the vanilla odour of the Siamese variety. Sumatra Benzoin contains cinnamic acid.

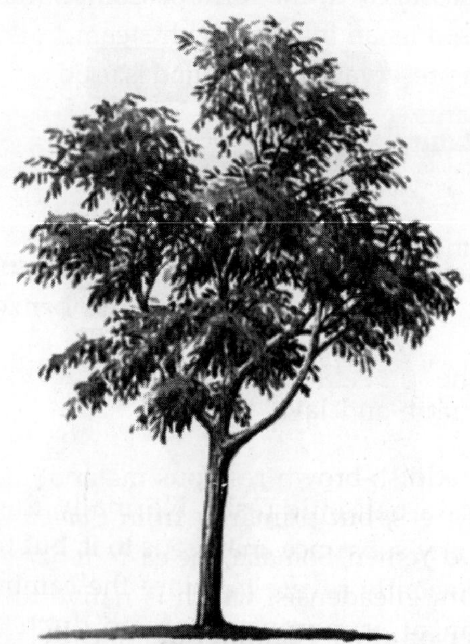

Fig. 19.1: Styrax benzoin

CONSTITUENTS

The chief constituent of Siam Benzoin is benzoic acid (up to 38 per cent), partly free and partly combined with benzoresinol and siaresinotannol; it also contains vanillin and an oily aromatic liquid. When quite pure it should be entirely soluble in alcohol and yield only traces of ash. Sumatra benzoin contains 18 per cent or more of benzoic acid and about 20 per cent of cinnamic acid the latter partly free and partly combined with benzoresinol and sumarisinotannol; it also contains 1 per cent of vanillin, styrol, styracin, phenyl-prophyl cinnamate and benzaldehyde, all of which combine to produce its characteristic odour.

MEDICINAL ACTION AND USES

It is used externally in the form of a tincture, diluted with water as a mild stimulant and antiseptic in irritable conditions of the skin. It acts as a carminative when taken internally is rapidly absorbed, and mildly expectorant diuretic and antiseptic to the urinary passages. In the form of Compound Tincture of Benzoin, it is used as an inhalant with steam in laryngitis and bronchitis. It is a preservative of fats, and is used for that purpose in Adips Benzoatus.

MYRRH

Botanical Name	:	*Commiphora myrrha*
Family	:	Burseraceae
Parts Used	:	Oleo-gum-resin from the stem
Common Name	:	Myrrh

DESCRIPTION

Myrrh is a reddish-brown resinous material, the dried sap of a number of trees, but primarily from *Commiphora myrrha,* which is native to Yemen, Somalia, the eastern parts of Ethiopia, and Commiphora gileadensis, which is native to Jordan. The sap of a number of other Commiphora and Balsamodendron species is also known as *myrrh,* including that from *Commiphora erythraea* (sometimes called East Indian myrrh), *Commiphora opobalsamum* and *Balsamodendron kua*. The name "myrrh" is also applied to the potherb Myrrhis odorata otherwise known as "Cicely" or "Sweet Cicely".

High quality myrrh can be identified through the darkness and clarity of the resin. However, the best method of judging the resin's quality is by feeling the stickiness of freshly broken fragments directly to determine the fragrant-oil content of the myrrh resin. The scent of raw myrrh resin and its essential oil is sharp, pleasant, somewhat bitter and can be roughly described as being "stereotypically resinous". When burned, it produces a smoke that is heavy, bitter and somewhat phenolic in scent, which may be tinged with a slight vanillic sweetness. Unlike most other resins, myrrh expands and "blooms" when burned instead of melting or liquefying.

Commiphora myrrha tree, one of the primary trees from which myrrh is harvested.

The scent can also be used in mixtures of incense, to provide an earthy element to the overall smell, and as an additive to wine, a practice alluded to by ancient authorities such as *Fabius Dorsennus*. It is also used in various perfumes, toothpastes, lotions, and other modern toiletries.

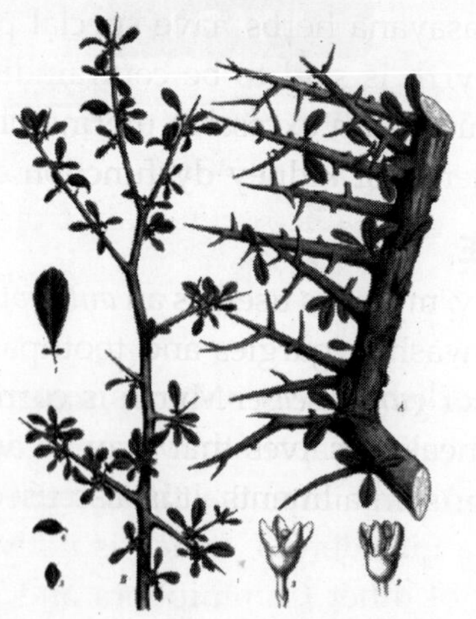

Fig. 19.2: Myrrh

TRADITIONAL MEDICINE

In Chinese medicine, myrrh is classified as bitter, spicy, neutral in temperature and affecting the *heart, liver,* and *spleen* meridians. Its uses are similar to those of frankincense, with which it is often combined in decoctions, liniments and incense. Myrrh also has been used in the treatment of *amenorrhea, dysmenorrhea, menopause* and *uterine tumors,* as its "blood-moving" properties can purge stagnant blood out of the uterus.

Myrrh has also been recommended to help *toothache* pain, and can be used in liniment for *bruises, aches* and *sprains.*

It is most commonly used in Chinese medicine for *rheumatic, arthritic* and *circulatory problems.* It is combined with such herbs as *notoginseng, safflower stamens, Angelica sinensis, cinnamon* and *Salvia miltiorrhiza,* usually in alcohol, and used both internally and externally.

Myrrh is used more frequently in Ayurveda, Unani medicine and Western herbalism, which ascribe to it tonic and rejuvenative properties. A related species, known as *guggul* in Ayurvedic medicine is considered one of the best substances for the treatment of circulatory problems, nervous system disorders and rheumatic complaints. Myrrh (Daindhava) is used in many rasayana formulas in Ayurveda.

However rasayana herbs have special processing. Outside of this form myrrh is said to be contraindicated for pregnant women or women with excessive uterine bleeding, and not be used with evidence of kidney dysfunction or stomach pain.

MODERN USAGE

In pharmacy, myrrh is used as an *antiseptic* and is most often used in mouthwashes, gargles and toothpastes for prevention and treatment of *gum disease.* Myrrh is currently used in some liniments and healing salves that may be applied to abrasions and other minor skin ailments. It is also used in the production of Fernet.

NEEM

Botanical Name	:	*Azadirachta indica*
Family	:	Meliaceae
Parts Used	:	Every parts
Common Name	:	Neem

HABITAT

Neem tree is found in abundance in tropical and semi-tropical regions like Burma. It cannot grow in extreme cold climate, though it can survive without much rainfall.

Neem tree is found throughout India. It is a popular village tree. Although it is also widely grown in Ranthambore National Park, Bandhavgarh National Park, Mrugavani National Park, Bannerghata National Park, Sariska Wildlife Sanctuary and Guindy National Park.

DESCRIPTION

It is a tall evergreen tree with the small bright green leaves. It is up to 100 feet tall. It blossoms in spring with the small white flowers. It has a straight trunk. Its bark is hard rough and scaly, fissured even in small trees. The colour of the bark is brown grayish. The leaves are alternate and consists of several leaflets with serrated edges. Its flowers are small and white in colour.

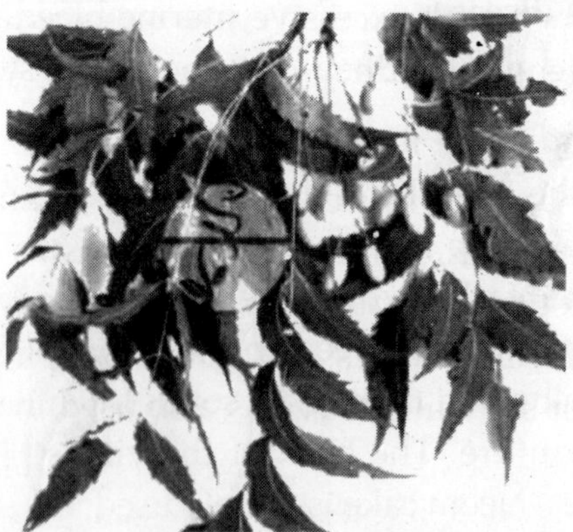

Fig. 19.3: Neem

It is popularly known as the *miracle tree*. It is known as *Nimba* in India. The Sanskrit name of Neem is *Arishtha* meaning the reliever of the sickness. *A. juss, A. azedarac* are the other related species of Neem tree.

CULTIVATION

Neem tree can easily be grown in the dry, stony, shallow and clayey soils. It needs very little water and plenty of sunlight. It grows slowly during the first year of planting. It can be propagated through the seeds and cuttings. Young neem tree can not tolerate excessive cold.

MEDICINAL USES

The indigenous people of Nilgiris consume the dried and powered tubulers of the terrestrial orchids as an energizing tonic. Neem also holds medicinal value. Each part of neem is used in the medicines. It has been used in Ayurvedic medicines for more than 4000 years. Neem oil extracted from its seeds is used in medicines, pest control and cosmetics etc. Its leaves are used in the treat Chickenpox. According to the Hindus, it is believed that the *Goddess of the chickenpox*. Neem tea is usually taken to reduce the headache and fever. Its flowers are used to cure intestinal problems. Neem bark acts as an analgesic and can cure high fever as of malaria. Even the skin diseases can be cured from the Neem leaves. Indians even believe that the Neem can even purify diseases.

OTHER USES

People in India use its twigs to brush their teeth. Neem is considered as the useful tree in rehabilitating the waste land areas. Neem seed pulp is useful for methane gas production. It is also useful as carbohydrate which is rich base for other industrial fermentations. Neem bark contains tannins which are used in tanning and dyeing. In south India its wood is used to make the furniture. The bark of the yields the fibre that is woven into ropes. Neem cake is widely used in India as fertilizer for sugarcane, vegetable and other cash crops. Many countries have been consistently growing the Neem tree against the global warming. The worldwide Neem Foundation has helped in making the people aware about the importance of neem and its uses globally.

CULTURAL IMPORTANCE

One can find Neem in almost all the parts of India. It is said that planting Neem tree in the house is a ensured passage to heaven. Its leaves are stung on the main entrance to remain away from the evil spirits. Brides take bath in the water filled with the Neem leaves. Newly born babies are laid upon the Neem leaves to provide them with the protective aura. Neem gives out more oxygen than other trees. The neem tree is also connected with the Sun, in the story of Neembark 'The Sun in the Neem tree'.

CURCUMA LONGA

Botanical Name	:	*Curcuma longa*
Family	:	Zingiberaceae (Ginger Family)
Parts Used	:	Oleo-gum-resin from the stem
Common Name	:	Haldi, Turmeric

HABITAT

Mainly India (especially Andhra Pradesh and Tamil Nadu). India produces 6,00,000 tons of turmeric annually which is 75% of world production of 8,00,000 tons. Trunk — grows to just over 1 metre, Leaves — lengthy and rectangular in shape; Flowers: lengthy white spike flowers, Root System — rhizomes.

CULTIVATION

- Planting with the first monsoon showers; irigation is acceptable;
- Pieces of rhizome are planted;
- Furrows and ridges;
- Well fertilized; and
- Annual crop taking 7-10 months to mature.

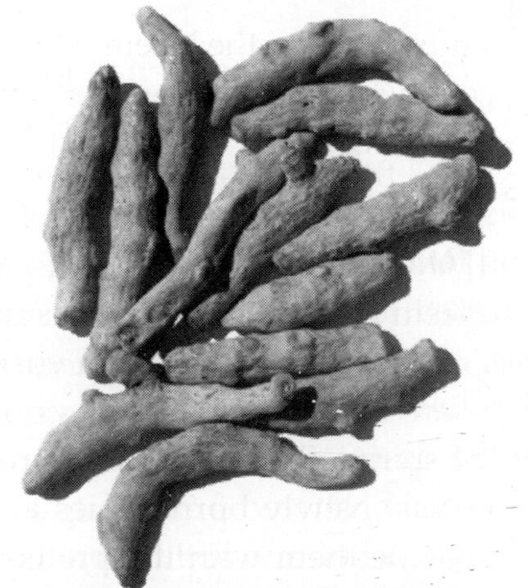

Fig. 19.4: Curcuma Longa

DESCRIPTION OF CURCUMA LONGA EXTRACT

Curcuma longa is a plant native to India and is the source of its culinary spice known as *Turmeric* and its medicinal extract called *Curcumin*.

Curcuma longa extract is a yellow-orange polyphenol. In its usual form it is a dry yellow powder that is oil-soluble in its natural state. The extract is without flavour and aroma. It colors food readily if there is oil present. Its strong anti-oxidant and anti-inflammatory characteristics are its most obvious medicinal properties.

Curcuma longa extract is derived from the root of the Curcuma longa plant first by drying and powdering, then by a solvent extraction. The resulting powder is 18 times stronger in the essential ingredients than is the common spice which is simply a powdered form of the dried root.

Curcuma Longa extract has attracted the interest of researchers in the fields of *Alzheimer's Disease, Memory Deficits, Arthritis, Cancer* and *Diabetes*. In the laboratory, it can significantly reduce the Amyloid-beta polymers of Alzheimer's Disease thus improving memory and mental performance in rodents.

MEDICINAL USES

The rhizome (*root*) of turmeric has long been used in traditional Asian medicine to treat *gastrointestinal* upset, *arthritic* pain. Turmeric has long been used as an *anti-inflammatory*, to treat digestive disorders, *osteoarthritis, atherosclerosis, cancer* and *liver* problems and for the treatment of skin diseases and wound healing. It is believed to strengthen the overall energy of the body, relieve *gas, dispel worms, regulate menstruation, dissolve gallstones*, and relieve *arthritis*. The active components of turmeric reduce the destructive activity of parasites or round-worms. It has also demonstrated in animals a protective effect on the liver, anti-tumor action and ability to reduce inflammation and fight certain infections.

TRADITIONAL AND MODERN USES

In India, Curcuma Longa has been in use as a culinary ingredient since 3000 B.C. It is used as a food coloring for curry and as a preservative for food. As a medicine it is used to treat a wide variety of ailments including stomach ache, skin problems, muscular problems and arthritis. Indians are thought to consume between 80 and 200 mg per day of the extract. India as a whole consumes 4,80,000 tons of turmeric annually.

In China it has been used as a topical analgesic, and for flatulence, colic, hepatitis, ringworm and chest pain.

In Europe it is used in many foods as a coloring in mustard, cheese, margarine, beverages and cakes. In the recent past it has been used for dyspepsia, chronic anterior uveitis and Helicobacter pylori bacteria.

STUDY QUESTIONS

1. Write short notes on the following:
   (a) Myrrh;
   (b) Neem; and
   (c) Curcuma longa.
2. Explain the medicinal uses of Curcuma longa.

■■■

Chapter 20

Antimalarials

CINCHONA

Botanical Name	:	*Cinchona officinals*
Family	:	Rubiaceae
Parts Used	:	Cinchona bark
Common Name	:	Quinine

The plant known as the *cinchona* is a tall evergreen tree that often reaches between fifty to a hundred feet in height when fully mature. The leaves of the cinchona are flat and broad, marked off by large veins running in the lamina which has a shiny green surface. Cinchona flowers are white, pink or red in color and are often elongated; they are also covered all over thickly with silky hairs, giving them a very distinct appearance.

Malaria was a major enemy for the American troops who fought their way from one island to island during the Second

World War. These troops "island hopped" across many places in the South Pacific, where they faced a formidable non-human enemy in the form of the deadly protozoan parasite that causes malaria. In most of the tropical jungles of these islands, the deadly microscopic foes lay for human victims and caused a lot of needless casualties. Malaria is caused by the protozoans belonging to the genus Plasmodium, which when injected into the human blood by way of the needle fine proboscis of a mosquito, will subsequently bring on the debilitating disease of malaria on the unlucky victim.

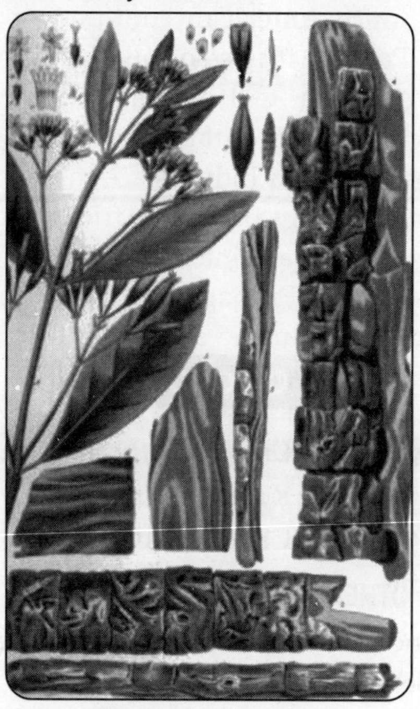

Fig. 20.1: Cinchona

The compound called *quinine* found in the *bark* of the cinchona was the chemical weapon of choice against malaria. Cinchona trees are in fact not an indigenous species to Indonesia. They were introduced to Java by European colonists. These tall and broad leaved evergreen trees are new world plants native to the Americas. Cinchona is a distinctive plant with fragrant clusters of small flowers and was originally found in tropical

America. Spanish priests were the first to collect the plants in the early 17th century from the Andean region of South America. They recognized the curative powers of the bitter tasting cinchona bark in treating malaria – the natives traditionally used the cinchona bark to treat malaria. Cinchona trees thrive in rain forests found at elevations between 3,000 and 11,000 feet in South America, there are at least forty documented cinchona species in South American forests.

HABITAT AND CULTIVATION

The cinchona is indigenous to the mountainous tropical regions of the South American continent, particularly the tropical area of Peru – it is also found in other countries in tropical South America. Cultivation of the cinchona is big business, and cinchona plantations can be found in Asian countries such as India and Indonesia –mainly Java. Cinchona is also cultivated in many parts of Africa. In these areas, the cultivation of the cinchona is intensive and carried out on large commercial tree farms. Propagation of the cinchona trees is done from cutting late in the spring season. Harvest of the product consists of the removal of trunk bark and bark from the branches and the root. The bark is normally only removed from six to eight year old trees, and the collected bark is then subjected to drying in the sun on mats. Annually, approximately 8,000 tons of the bark is harvested from such farms

MEDICINAL AND OTHER USES

The name cinchona reportedly comes from the name of a Spanish Countess, the Countess of Chinchon, who was treated for a fever using a remedy made from the bark while in South America. Upon recovering, the countess had saplings of the plant sent to Europe, where the plant species were subsequently name after her. The curative powers of cinchona bark was initially revealed to Europeans by Jesuit priests who traveled to Peru in the 17th century, the Jesuits found that the native people chewed on the bark of the cinchona to prevent shaking and chills that came after they worked in icy streams for the early

Spanish colonial mines. The native peoples had traditionally used the bark for treating fevers and chills as well as malaria. The Jesuits eventually linked the shaking from cold to the shaking of the body commonly seen during a bout of malarial fever in patients. These Jesuits then went a step further and tried chewing on the bark as a means to treat malarial fevers. The cure worked, however, the Jesuits were not always trusted, and the medication was suspect to some degree as bark from some varieties of cinchona was not potent enough to cure malaria. When it was initially introduced, chewing the bark did not always result in a complete cure from malaria. This was one factor that brought on distrust and persecution of many Jesuits in different European countries.

Cinchona bark remedies have been used in various herbal treatments by the indigenous people of Peru over the centuries. The bark remains a traditional and much utilized herbal remedy for treating all kinds of fevers, various digestive problems, and different types of infections or disorders. Malaria was primarily treated using extracts from the cinchona bark, in particular quinine, till about the World War I and the inter war years. Synthetic quinine became available during the Second World War. The synthetic form of the alkaloid was mainly used. However, from the 1960s onwards, the malarial parasite began to develop resistance to the synthetic medication chloroquinine. This situation brought natural quinine out of the shelves again for use in treating malaria. All kinds of fever induced symptoms and feverish conditions in the body can also be treated using quinine. Cinchona bark also stimulates the secretion of the saliva, moreover this bitter tonic induces digestive secretions and boosts the appetite — aiding the recovery of the weak digestive system. An infusion made from the bark of the cinchona is effectively used as a gargle for treating sore, infected throats and other oral problems. Herbal remedies made from the cinchona plant are used in the treatment of muscular cramps, particularly the muscular cramps that come in the night. Remedies made from the cinchona are also helpful in bringing relief from chronic arthritis and related problems. Cinchona is used in the Indian ayurvedic system of medicine for the treatment of problems such as sciatica and dysentery, in addition to problems connected with kapha and other disorders.

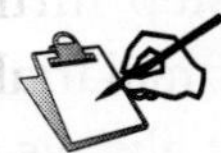

STUDY QUESTIONS

1. Write a detailed note on Cinchona officinals.
2. Explain the medicinal and other uses of Cinchona.

■■■

Chapter 21

Oxytocics

ERGOT

Botanical Name	:	*Claviceps purpurea*
Family	:	Clavicepitaceae
Parts Used	:	Heart Wood, Leaves, Flowers
Common Name	:	Ergot or Ryes, Spurred rye

DESCRIPTION

Rye is a grass that was first cultivated rather late in human history, perhaps as recently as 2000 to 3000 years ago. It is still grown extensively in northern Europe and Asia. It lacks the proteins that make wheat suitable for living, and rye bread is denser and usually darker than the wheat bread, hence called Black Bread.

Ergot is a fungus. It appears as black grain size fungal structures. This is a disease of cereal crops and grasses. The disease causes reduced yield and quality of grains and hay and also causes a livestock disease called *ergotism,* if infected grains or hay are fed. The disease cycle of the ergot fungus was first described in the 1800s, but the connection with ergot and epidemics among people and animals was known several hundred years earlier. Ergot's medicinal applications and animal poisoning properties first called attention to this plant disease. Human poisoning was common in Europe in the Middle Ages when ergoty rye bread was often consumed.

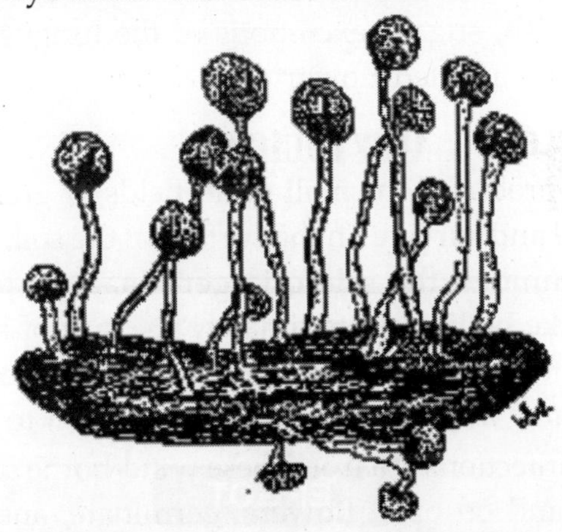

Fig. 21.1: Germinated ergot sclerotium. The rounded heads on these stalks produce spores that infect flowers in summer.

Ergot occurs to some extent every year on cereals and grasses in North Dakota. The disease generally is more prevalent in rye and triticale than in other cereals, but significant losses have also been reported in spring wheat, durum, barley, and other small grains. Although the crop loss caused by this disease is important, the effects of the ergot's alkaloid toxins on man and animals is of much greater significance.

SYMPTOMS AND SIGNS (ERGOT AS A PLANT DISEASE)

The most common sign of ergot is the dark purple to black sclerotia (ergot bodies) found replacing the grain in the heads of cereals and grasses just prior to harvest. The ergot bodies consist of a mass of vegetative strands of the fungus. The interior of the sclerotia is white or tannish-white. In some grains, ergot bodies are larger than the normal grain kernels, while in other grains, such as wheats, grain kernels and the ergot bodies may be similar in size. A larger size separation between the sclerotia and the grain kernel simplifies the removal of ergot bodies during grain cleaning.

Prior to development of the sclerotia bodies, the fungus develops a stage in the open floret (flowering head part) commonly called "honey dew". The "honey dew" consists of sticky, yellowish, sugary excretions of the fungus which form droplets on the infected flower parts.

DISEASE CYCLE

Sclerotia produced in small grain fields or grassy areas fall to the ground and survive on the surface of the soil. In the spring and early summer, the sclerotia germinate to produce tiny mushroom-like bodies approximately the size of a pin. Spores (ascospores) formed by a sexual process in these bodies are shot into the air, and wind currents may carry them to grain heads.

The first infections are from these wind-borne sexual spores. The spores land on open flowers, germinate, and the fungus then invades the embryo of the developing kernel (Fig. 21.2). Soon a yellow-white, sweet, sticky fluid ("honey dew") exudes from the infected flowers. The fluid contains a large number of asexually produced fungus spores (conidia). Many species of

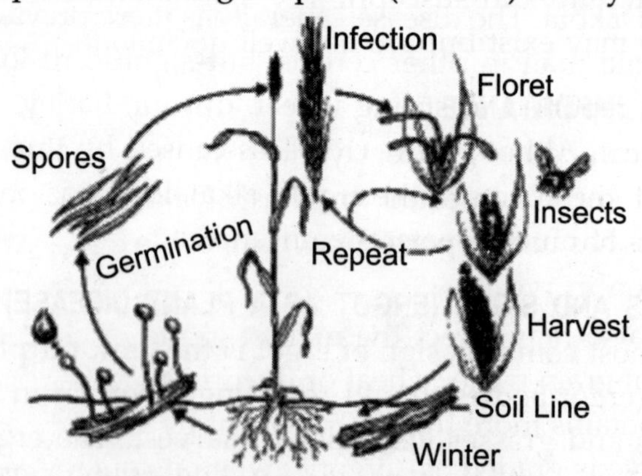

Fig. 21.2: Disease cycle of Ergot

insects visit the "honey dew" and become contaminated with the fungus spores. These insects visit other grass flowers and spread the fungus, in a repeating cycle that continues as long as the florets are open. Spores may be transferred to other grain heads by rain-splash and direct contact, as well.

Once the fungus becomes established in the florets, it grows throughout the embryos and replaces them, later producing the dark sclerotia. Many sclerotia fall to the ground before harvest and overwinter on the soil surface, serving as potential sources of spores the following year.

ENVIRONMENTAL CONDITIONS THAT FAVOUR THE DISEASE

Ergot develops more abundantly during wet seasons. Wet weather and wet soils favor germination of the ergot bodies, and cool, wet weather during flowering favors development of the "honey-dew" stage. Dry weather during flowering is detrimental to spore production and germination. Susceptibility to infection among crops increases with any condition that may prolong flowering or cause sterile florets.

HOST RANGE

The same fungus, Claviceps purpurea, can produce ergot in many hosts. Rye, triticale, wheat, durum, barley, oat, quack grass, crested wheat grass, brome grass, foxtail, rye grass, orchard grass, timothy, wild rye, and other grasses serve as ergot hosts. Differences in susceptibility among cultivars within a grain crop may exist but are not well documented.

ECONOMIC IMPORTANCE

Ergot can cause a direct yield loss in proportion to the number of kernels infected. In North Dakota, as much as 10 percent loss has been reported in wheat, while losses of 5 percent are common in rye.

Ergot also may affect the market grade of a grain. In the commercial grain trade, wheat or durum is graded as "ergoty" when it contains more than 0.05 percent by weight of the ergot sclerotia; rye is graded as "ergoty" when it contains more than

0.3 percent by weight of ergot sclerotia, and triticale, oat, or barley are "ergoty" when they contain more than 0.1 percent.

Most of the sclerotia can be removed from ergoty grain with modern cleaning machinery, unless broken pieces are present or the sclerotia are similar in size to the grain. However, it is costly and often difficult to remove enough sclerotia to meet the legal standards, and traces which have proven toxic to livestock are left.

CONTROL OF ERGOT IS SMALL GRAIN CROPS AND GRASSES

- Rotate cereals and grasses with nonsusceptible crops for one year or longer. The ergot sclerotia usually do not survive in the soil for more than one year. Therefore, summer fallow or crop rotation to a non-cereal crop for at least one year will help reduce ergot.
- Deep-plow fields which have a severe ergot infestation to bury the sclerotia. The ergot sclerotia will not germinate if buried more than 1 inch deep.
- Plant only ergot-free seed to avoid introducing or re-introducing the fungus into the field.
- Eradicate or prevent wild grasses from reaching heading in fields, rocklands, headlands, ditches, and fence rows. Mow wild and escaped grasses and pastures, or graze pastures before they flower, to prevent ergot infections.
- Resistant commercial varieties of wheat, barley, rye or cultivated grasses are not available. However, some differences among varieties may occur, and those with long flowering periods may be more frequently infected.

EFFECT OF ERGOT ON ANIMALS

Ergot is toxic to animals. Animals consume ergot by eating the sclerotia present in contaminated feed. All domestic animals are susceptible, including birds. Cattle seem to be the most susceptible.

Two well known forms of ergotism exist in animals, an acute form characterized by convulsions, and a chronic form characterized by gangrene. A third form of ergotism is characterized by hyperthermia (increased body temperature) in cattle, and a fourth form is characterized by agalactia (no milk) and lack of mammary gland development, prolonged gestations, and early foal deaths in mares fed heavily contaminated feed. Which form of ergotism is manifested depends on the type of ergot consumed and the ratio of major toxic alkaloids present in the ergot: ergotamine, ergotoxine, and ergometrine. *Claviceps purpurea,* the common cause of ergot in North Dakota, is usually associated with gangrenous ergotism. Claviceps paspali, an ergot of *Paspalum spp.* of plants, is most commonly associated with central nervous derangement. Paspalum is a water grass distributed in pastures in southern states, but is not commonly found in North Dakota.

The responses of animals consuming ergot are usually quite variable and are dependent on variations in alkaloid content, frequency of ingesting ergot, quantity of ergot ingested, climatic conditions under which ergot grew, the species of ergot involved, and the influence of other impurities in the feed such as histamine and acetylcholine.

Animals fed large amounts of ergot over time lose portions of their hooves, ears (Fig. 21.3), tails, combs, and wattles. Spontaneous abortion and loss of milk has occurred in cows and sows fed even small amounts of ergot. Ergoty feed should not be fed to breeding females.

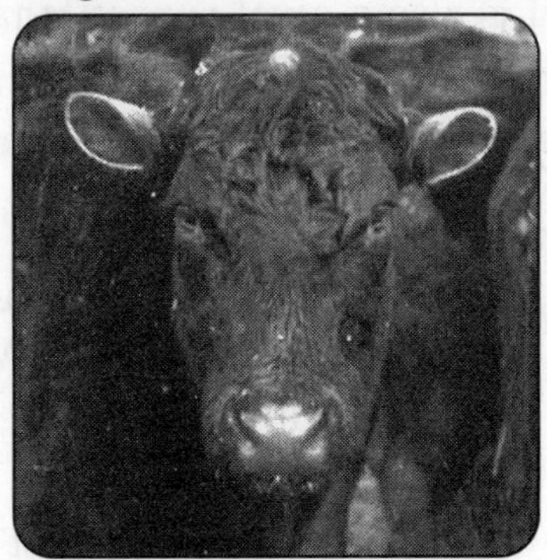

Fig. 21.3: Animals fed large amounts of ergot over time lose portions of their ears or other extremeties.

TREATMENT OF ERGOT POISONING

The only treatment for erotism is to remove the ergot-contaminated feed or remove the animals from the contaminated pasture. If nervous signs are present, call your veterinarian for medical advice and supplemental therapy such as pain control. If dry gangrene is present, the affected portion will be sloughed. There is nothing to reverse this process. If secondary infections or open wounds are present, call your veterinarian for appropriate therapy.

PREVENTION AND CONTROL OF ERGOT POISONING

Prevention is based on feeding feed and forage that are free of ergot. For pastures, graze the infected fields before seed heads begin to flower. The ergot is contained in the ovary of the flower Commercially prepared feeds will rarely contain ergot. Non-commercial grain (home grown) should be screened prior to feeding (and planting to prevent contamination of future crops). Special care should be taken in feeding screenings. If feeding ergoty grain is unavoidable, the amount of sclerotia should be reduced to an amount less than 0.1% (by weight) of the feed through mixing with clean' grain. Again, ergoty feed should not be fed to breeding females.

PHARMACOLOGY

Ergot is a fungus that lives on rye and other grasses and is pathogenic to its host as well as to humans and other animals that ingest it. Ergot is also a great source for the art of healing and the pharmaceutical industry.

Like most great pharmacological resources, ergot is a powerful poison. More specifically, many ergot alkaloids have a poisonous effect on the central nervous system, interfering heavily with neurotransmitter function. And here also lies the great promise of ergot as medicine.

USES IN TRADITIONAL MEDICINE

Ergot is an *old member of the materia medica*. It has been used in traditional medicine and it has been scientifically studied for more than 50 years. Among those studying ergot and its derivatives was the Swiss chemist *Albert Hofman* whose experiments let to the discovery of LSD, an ergot derivative that strongly interferes with the neurotransmitter serotonin.

In the field of conventional medicine, ergot derivatives are nowadays mostly used for their potential to enhance another neurotransmitter, dopamine. A dopamine deficiency is a common grave medical condition, *Parkinson's disease.*

While the ergot derivative LSD is used almost exclusively as recreational drug with practically no use in conventional medicine, dopamine enhancing ergot derivatives are sold in pharmacies around the world. The most common ergot prescription drug is probably Sandoz' Parlodel (bromocriptine by generic name). Even though it's very much a conventional medication, bromocriptine and other dopamine enhancing ergot derivatives have a clear potential as life-style drugs. Not all, but many ergot-based medications for Parkinson's Disease have a profound sexuality enhancing (side) effect.

All dopamine-enhancing medications can be used in the treatment of *Parkinson's Disease,* but not each and every dopamine enhancement produces pro-sexual (side) effects. On a similar level, while many medications used for serotonin enhancement (in the treatment of clinical depression) have *anti-sexual effect,* this anti-sexual effect is not an unavoidable side effect of serotonin enhancement.

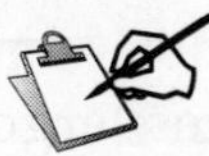

STUDY QUESTIONS

1. Write a detailed note on ergot.
2. What are the uses of ergot in traditional medicine?

■■■

22

CHAPTER

VITAMINS

SHARK LIVER OIL

DESCRIPTION

Shark liver oil is promoted as a complementary or alternative form of treatment for cancer and other diseases. The oil is taken from the liver of cold-water sharks. Shark liver oil is a rich source of alkylglycerols, chemicals that may have anti-cancer properties. Alkylglycerols are also found in human bone marrow and in breast milk. Other chemicals in shark liver oil being studied against cancer are squalamine and squalene.

Shark liver oil is widely used alongside conventional cancer treatment in northern Europe and is sold as a dietary supplement in the United States. Available scientific evidence does not support claims that shark liver oil supplements are effective against cancer in humans. Recent research has focused on certain components of shark liver oil (*alkylglycerols, squalamine,* and *squalene*).

MEDICINAL USE

Shark liver oil is promoted as a dietary supplement used to boost the *immune system,* fight off infections, heal wounds, and to treat cancer and lessen the side effects of conventional cancer treatment.

Most shark liver oil supplements have not been tested to find out if they interact with medicines, foods, or other herbs and supplements. Even though some reports of interactions and harmful effects may be published, full studies of interactions and effects are not often available. Because of these limitations, any information on ill effects and interactions below should be considered incomplete.

Although many people have taken shark liver oil, the issue of potential toxicity at the usual doses has not been well studied. Some mild digestive problems such as nausea, upset stomach, and diarrhea have been reported. may have serious health consequences.

BENEFITS OF SHARK LIVER OIL

Shark liver oil benefits people in the following ways:

- Provides immune system support.
- Contains antioxidant properties.
- Helps in maintenance of healthy skin.
- Supports joint health.
- Aids in healthy digestion.
- Supports healthy energy levels and reduces fatigue.
- Supports respiratory health.
- Aids in wound healing and minimizes scarring.
- Increases energy levels by supplying cells of the body with more oxygen.

EFFECTIVENESS OF SHARK LIVER OIL

Shark liver oil is effective for the following medical conditions:

- Ataxia.
- Ataxia associated with a vitamin E deficiency.
- Vitamin A deficiency.
- Vitamin C deficiency.
- Vitamin E deficiency.

May be effective for the following conditions, though further research is needed:

- Age-related maculopathy.
- Age-related macular degeneration.
- Alzheimer's disease.
- Vascular dementia.
- Anemia.
- Arthritis.
- Cancer.
- Bladder cancer.
- Beta-thalassemia.
- Cancer-related fatigue.
- Cancer chemotherapy side effects.
- Cancer associated anorexia.
- Chemotherapy.
- Cisplatin-induced neurotoxicity.
- Connective tissue diseases and disorders.
- Dysmenorrhea (painful menstruation).
- Eclampsia.
- Huntington's disease.
- Dyspraxia (a wide range of developmental disorders).
- Granuloma annulare (chronic skin condition).
- Infertility.
- Intracranial hemorrhage (brain bleeding).
- Leukemia.

RISKS ASSOCIATED WITH SHARK LIVER OIL

There are certain risk factors which can be directly or indirectly contributed to a person taking shark liver oil supplements. Some of the following conditions can be potentially serious and should be addressed and evaluated by a qualified medical professional.

- **High blood pressure:** there have been multiple human studies done which suggest a small reduction in blood pressure in those who take certain types of omega-3 fatty acids. It may be necessary to take higher doses to experience the healthful benefits and at higher doses shark liver oil can cause an increased risk of bleeding. Therefore it is necessary to consult with a medical professional prior to taking any type of supplement.
- **Hypertriglyceridemia:** scientific studies have shown people who take excessive amounts of shark liver oil experience a worsening in low-density lipoprotein levels, which is the "bad" cholesterol.
- **Secondary cardiovascular disease prevention:** most human studies report that regular consumption of shark liver oil can reduce the risk of non-fatal heart attacks, fatal heart attacks and sudden death. Most people studied were also using standard heart medications and while there are benefits to shark liver oil, there is also an increased risk of side effects from traditional heart medications and therapies.

SAFETY OF SHARK LIVER OIL

The *Food and Drug Administration* does not strictly govern nor regulate herbs or supplements so there is no guarantee of safety, strength or purity and the side effects may vary. There are certain people who may benefit from taking shark liver oil supplements and there are others who should read the product label and consult with a physician prior taking the drug.

People who have allergies or are hypersensitive to fish should not take shark liver oil or omega-3 fatty acid products derived from fish. There have been reported cases of anaphylaxis and skin rash in people who are allergic to nuts or certain alpha linolenic acid or omega-3 fatty acid (both contained in shark liver oil supplements) products that are obtained from nuts they are allergic to.

AMLA

Botanical Name	:	*Emblica officinalis*
Family	:	Euphorbiaceae
Parts Used	:	Fruit
Common Name	:	Indian Gooseberry (Amla), Amalaki

HABITAT

It is found natively in India. Indian gooseberry has been used as valuable ingredient of various medicines in India and abroad.

DESCRIPTION

Amla is one of the most celebrated herbs in the Indian traditional medicine system, Ayurveda. Amla's traditional uses include as a laxative, eye wash, appetite stimulant, restorative tonic, and to treat anorexia, indigestion, diarrhea, anemia, and jaundice. Amla is becoming increasingly well known for its unusually high levels of Vitamin C, which is resistant to storage and heat damage due to cooking.

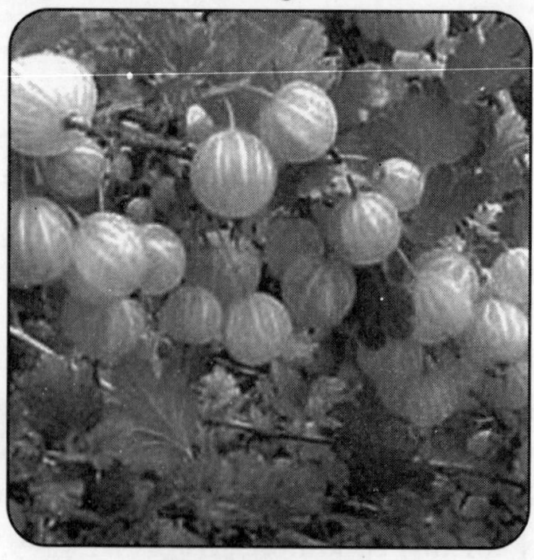

Fig. 22.1: Amla

PHARMACOLOGY

Emblica officinalis is effective in the treatment of amlapitta (*peptic ulcer*)and in dyspepsia. The fruits exhibit hypolipi-adaemic and antiatherosclerotic effects in rabbits and rats. The fruit extract has antimutagenic activity on certain directly acting mutagens in some strains of *Salmonella typhimurium*.The extract of amla also has antimicrobial properties.

Amlaki is an antioxidant with free radical scavenging properties which may be due to the presence of high levels of super oxide dismutase.

MEDICINAL USES

Indian gooseberry is beneficial in the treatment of respiratory disorders. It is especially valuable in tuberculosis of the lungs asthma and bronchitis.

Diabetes

This herb, due to its high vitamin C content, is effective in controlling diabetes. A tablespoon of its juice mixed with a cup of bitter gourd juice, taken daily for two months. Will stimulates the pancreas and enable is to secrete insulin, thus reducing the blood sugar in the diabetes. Diet restrictions should be strictly observed while taking this medicine. It will also prevent eye complication in diabetes.

Heart Disorder

Indian gooseberry is considered an effective remedy for heart disease. It tones up the functions of all the organs of the body and builds up health by destroying the heterogeneous or harmful and disease causes elements. It also renews energy.

Eye Disorder

The juice of Indian Gooseberry with honey is useful in preserving eyesight. It is beneficial in the treatment of conjunctivitis and glaucoma. It reduces intracular tension in a remarkable manner. a cup of juice mixed with honey can be taken twice daily for this condition.

Rheumatism

To treat rheumatism a teaspoon of the powder of the dry fruit mixed with 2 teaspoons of jaggery can be taken twice daily for a month.

Scurvy

As an extremely rich source of vitamin C, Indian gooseberry is one of the best remedy for scurvy. Powder of the dry herb, mixed with an equal quantity of sugar, can be taken in doses of 1 teaspoon, thrice daily with milk.

Ageing

Indian gooseberry has revitalizing effects, as it contains an element which is very valuable in preventing ageing and in maintaining strength in old age. It improves body resistance and protect the body against infection. It strengthens the heart, hair and different gland in the body.

OTHER USES

Hair Tonic

Indian gooseberry is an accepted hair tonic in traditional recipes for enriching hair growth and pigmentation. The fruit, cut into pieces is dried preferably in the shade. These pieces are boiled in coconut oil till the solid matter becomes charres. This darkish oil is excellent in preventing graying .The water is which dried amla pieces are soaked overnight is also nourishing to hair and can be used for the last rinse while washing the hair. Indian gooseberry is used in various ways. The best way to take it with the least loss vitamin C, is to eat it raw with a little salt. It is often used in the form of pickles and it is dried and powdered. The berry may also be used as a vegetable. It is boiled in a small amount of water till soft and taken with a little salt.

STUDY QUESTIONS

1. Write short notes on the following:
   (a) Shark liver oil; and
   (b)Amla.
2. Explain the various medicinal uses of amla.

23 CHAPTER

ENZYMES

INTRODUCTION

Enzymes are very efficient catalysts for biochemical reactions. They speed up reactions by providing an alternative reaction pathway of lower activation energy.

HOW ENZYMES WORK

For two molecules to react they must collide with one another. They must collide in the right direction (orientation) and with sufficient energy. Sufficient energy means that between them they have enough energy to overcome the energy barrier to reaction. This is called the *activation energy*.

Enzymes have an active site. This is part of the molecule that has just the right shape and functional groups to bind to one of the reacting molecules. The reacting molecule that binds to the enzyme is called the substrate.

An enzyme-catalysed reaction takes a different 'route'. The enzyme and substrate form a reaction intermediate. Its formation has a lower activation energy than the reaction between reactants without a catalyst.

TYPES OF ENZYMES

There are three main categories of enzymes—

(i) Metabolic enzymes, which are produced within the body,

(ii) Digestive enzymes, which the body produces also, and

(iii) Food enzymes.

(i) Metabolic Enzymes

Metabolic enzymes are responsible for running the body at the level of the blood, tissues and organs. They are required for the growth of cells and repair and maintenance of all the body's organs and tissues. Metabolic enzymes take protein, fat, and carbohydrates and transfoım them into the proper balance of working cells and tissues. They also remove worn-out material from the cells, keeping them clean and healthy.

(ii) Digestive Enzymes

Digestive enzymes aid in the digestion of food and the absorption and delivery of nutrients throughout the body. The most commonly known digestive enzymes are secreted from the pancreas into the stomach and small intestine. Each enzyme is specific to a particular compound which it breaks or synthesizes. The three most important enzymes for digestion are protease, which digests protein; amylase, which digests carbohydrates; and lipase, which digests fat.

(iii) Food Enzymes

Food enzymes are derived solely from raw fruits, vegetables, and supplemental sources. Like digestive enzymes, they enable the body to digest the food by breaking down the various nutrients — proteins, fats, carbohydrates, and vitamins and minerals — into smallest compounds that the body can absorb. They are absolutely essential in maintaining optimal health.

Overwhelming evidence shows that food enzymes play an important role by predigesting food in the upper stomach. Supplementation of food enzymes is necessary today because so much of the food is processed or cooked.

Most food enzymes are destroyed at the temperatures used to cook and process food. Food enzymes are extremely sensitive to temperatures above 118 °F. When raw foods are processed or heated in any way, they may lose 100% of their enzymes activity and up to 85% of their vitamin content. Unfortunately, even the raw food might be enzyme-deficient if it was grown in nutrient-lacking soil.

COENZYMES

To function properly, food enzymes must also work in tandem with the coenzymes of vitamins and minerals. Unlike the enzymes in raw plant foods, coenzymes are not completely destroyed by cooking. Unless the enzymes from raw food are present, the coenzymes in the food cannot be utilized to their full potential.

For all these reasons, supplementing with enzymes is crucial to achieving a more efficient digestive process and better absorption of food's nutrients.

When an animal has an enzyme deficiency, it develops many health problems. These include digestive disturbances, constipation, gas, bloating, colon problems, excess body fat, and problems as serious as heart disease. Enzyme deficiencies have been linked to premature aging and degenerative diseases as well. In fact, studies have shown that diets deficient in enzymes can cause a 30% reduction in life span. Cancer research has discovered that certain enzymes are absent in the blood and urine of many cancer patients. Lack of enzymes and the resulting malabsorption of nutrients can also cause allergic reactions, poor healing of wounds, and skin problems.

Enzyme supplements help create more energy, promote faster and easier digestion, and encourage superior nutrient absorption. The animal's digestive system works best when enzyme supplements assist in setting the nutrients free for the body to absorb and use.

Other types of enzymes include—

- DNA Repair Enzymes,
- DNA Restriction-Modification Enzymes,
- DNA Catalytic,
- Immobilized Enzymes,
- Holoenzymes,
- Hydrolases,
- Isoenzymes,
- Isomerases,
- Ligases,
- Lyases,
- Multienzyme Complexes,
- Oxidoreductases,
- Penicillin-Binding Proteins,
- Recombinases,
- Catalytic RNA, and
- Transferases.

Classes of Enzymes

Enzymes can be grouped into *functional classes* that perform similar chemical reactions. Each type of enzyme within such a class is highly specific, catalyzing only a single type of reaction. Thus, hexokinase adds a phosphate group to d-glucose but ignores its optical isomer l-glucose; the blood-clotting enzyme thrombin cuts one type of blood protein between a particular arginine and its adjacent glycine and nowhere else, and so on.

There are **six major classes of enzymes**—

- Oxidoreductases,
- Transferases,
- Hydrolases,
- Lyases,
- Isomerases, and
- Ligases.

FUNCTIONAL CLASSES OF ENZYMES

- **ATPases** – Hydrolyze ATP. Many proteins with a wide range of roles have an energy-harnessing ATPase activity as part of their function, for example, motor proteins such as myosin and membrane transport proteins such as the sodium-potassium pump.
- **Hydrolases** – General term for enzymes that catalyze a hydrolytic cleavage reaction.
- **Isomerases** – Catalyze the rearrangement of bonds within a single molecule.
- **Kinases** – Catalyze the addition of phosphate groups to molecules. Protein kinases are an important group of kinases that attach phosphate groups to proteins.
- **Lyases** –Add or remove of groups to form double bonds (not by hydrolysis).
- **Ligases** – Ligate two substrates at the expense of ATP hydrolysis.
- **Nucleases** – Breakdown nucleic acids by hydrolyzing bonds between nucleotides.
- **Oxidoreductases** – General name for enzymes that catalyze reactions in which one molecule is oxidized while the other is reduced. Enzymes of this type are often called oxidases, reductases, and dehydrogenases.
- **Phosphatases** – Catalyze the hydrolytic removal of a phosphate group from a molecule.
- **Polymerases** – Catalyze polymerization reactions such as the synthesis of DNA and RNA.
- **Proteases** – Breakdown proteins by hydrolyzing bonds between amino acids.
- **Transferases** – Remove groups (not including H) from substrates and transfer them to acceptor molecules (not including water).

Enzyme names typically end in "-ase," with the exception of some enzymes, such as pepsin, trypsin, thrombin and lysozyme that were discovered and named before the convention became generally accepted at the end of the nineteenth century. The common name of an enzyme usually indicates the substrate and the nature of the reaction catalyzed. For example, citrate synthase catalyzes the synthesis of citrate by a reaction between acetyl CoA and oxaloacetate.

PAPAYA

Botanical Name	:	*Carica papaya*
Family	:	Caricaceae
Parts Used	:	Leaves, Fruits, Roots
Common Names	:	Papaya, Papita, Paw Paw, Kates, Papaw

HABITAT

Throughout India. Originally from Southern Mexico, Central America and Northern South America, the papaya is now cultivated in most countries with a tropical climate, such as Brazil, India, South Africa, Sri Lanka, Haiti, and Southeast Asia.

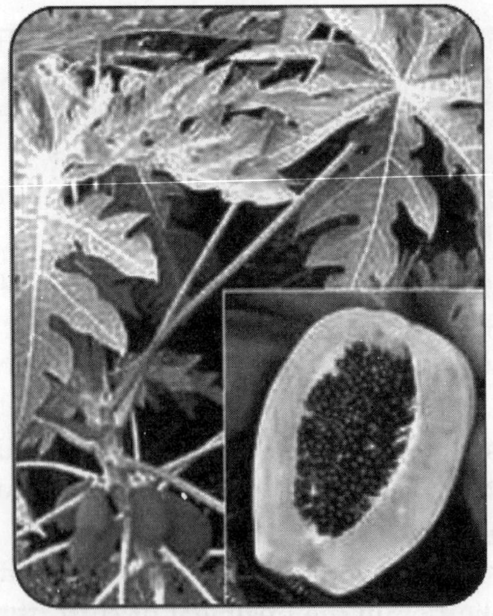

Fig. 23.1: Carica papaya

DESCRIPTION

The *papaya* (from *Carib* via Spanish), is the fruit of the plant Carica papaya, in the genus Carica. It is native to the tropics of the Americas, and was cultivated in Mexico several centuries before the emergence of the Mesoamerican classic cultures.

It is a large *tree-like plant*, the single stem growing from 5 to 10 meters tall, with spirally arranged leaves confined to the top of the trunk; the lower trunk is conspicuously scarred where leaves and fruit were borne.

The *leaves* are large, 50-70 cm diameter, deeply palmately lobed with 7 lobes. The tree is usually unbranched if unlopped.

The *flowers* are similar in shape to the flowers of the Plumeria but are much smaller and wax like. They appear on the axils of the leaves, maturing into the large 15-45 cm long, 10-30 cm diameter fruit.

The *fruit* is ripe when it feels soft (like a ripe avocado or a bit softer) and its skin has attained an amber to orange hue. The fruit's taste is vaguely similar to pineapple and peach, although much milder without the tartness.

USES OF PAPAYA

The ripe fruit is usually eaten raw, without the skin or seeds. The unripe green fruit of papaya can be eaten cooked, usually in curries, salads and stews. It also has a relatively high amount of pectin, which can be used to make jellies.

Green papaya fruit and the tree's latex are both rich in an enzyme called papain, a protease which is useful in tenderizing meat and other proteins. Its ability to breakdown tough meat fibres was utilized for thousands of years by indigenous Americans. It is included as a component in powdered meat tenderizers, and is also marketed in tablet form to remedy digestive problems. Green papaya is used in Thai cuisine, both raw and cooked.

Papain is also popular (in countries where it grows) as a topical application in the treatment of cuts, rashes, stings and burns. Papain ointment is commonly made from fermented papaya flesh, and is applied as a gel-like paste.

The black seeds are edible and have a sharp, spicy taste. They are sometimes ground up and used as a substitute for black pepper. In some parts of Asia the young leaves of papaya are steamed and eaten like spinach.

MEDICINAL USES

The juice has been seen to have an antiproliferative effect on liver cancer cells cultured in the laboratory, probably due to its component of lycopene. Papaya has been used for digestive problems and intestinal worms.The softening and disintegrating qualities of papain (generally in alkaline combination, as with borax or potassium carbonate), have been taken advantage of in the treatment of warts, corns, sinuses, and chronic forms of scaly eczema, cutaneous tubercles, and other hardness of the skin, produced by irritation, etc., and injected into indolent glandular tumors to promote their absorption. Green fruits are used to treat high blood pressure and also used as an aphrodisiac. It is useful in round worm infestation, stomachalgia, dyspepsia, constipation, amenorrhoea, skin diseases and general debility.

USE OF PAPAIN

Carica papaya contains an enzyme known as ***papain***, present in the fruit, stem and leaves. Papain is a *cysteine protease* hydrolase enzyme present in papaya (Carica papaya) and mountain papaya (*Vasconcellea cundinamarcensis*). Its utility is in breaking down tough meat fibers and has been utilized for thousands of years in its native South America. It is sold as a component in powdered meat tenderizer available in most supermarkets.

Papain, in the form of a meat tenderizer such as Adolph's, made into a paste with water, is also a home remedy treatment for jellyfish, bee, yellow jacket (wasps) stings, mosquito bites, and possibly stingray wounds, breaking down the protein toxins in the venom.

Papain is used to dissociate cells in the first step of cell culture preparations. A 10-minute treatment of small tissue pieces (less than 1 mm cubed) will allow papain to begin breaking down the extracellular matrix molecules holding the cells together. After 10 minutes, the tissue should be treated with a protease inhibitor solution to stop the protease action (if left untreated papain's activity will lead to complete lysis of the cells). The tissue must then be triturated (passed quickly up and down through a Pasteur pipette) in order to break up the pieces of tissue into a single cell suspension.

It is also used as an ingredient in various enzymatic debriding preparations, notably Accuzyme. These are used in the care of some chronic wounds to clean up dead tissue.

It can also be found as an ingredient in some toothpastes or mints as teeth-whitener. Its whitening effect in toothpastes and mints however is minimal, because the papain is present in low concentrations, and will be quickly diluted by saliva. It would take several months of using the whitening product to have noticeably whiter teeth.

Papain is the main ingredient of Papacarie, a gel used for chemomechanical dental caries removal. Besides the advantage of avoiding the use of rotary cutting tools, it does not interfere in the bond strength of restorative materials to dentin.

Papain also is used to treat *arthritis*. The level of the compounds vary in the fruit, latex, leaves, and roots.

IMMUNOGLOBULINS

An antibody digested by papain yields three fragments: two 50 kDa Fab fragments and one 50 kDa Fc fragment. The papain-digested antibody is unable to promote agglutination, precipitation, opsonization, and lysis.

AMYLASE (DIASTASE)

Diastase is one of the principles of the digestive fluids of the animal body. It appears during the fermentation of starchy substances—grains. It is one of the enzymes capable of being classed with pepsin and pancreatin of the digestive group, Its especial function is the conversion of the starch molecule into a sugar molecule.

Amylase (diastase) is supplied as a clear yellow/brown liquid. It is a form of α-amylase that acts on starch (amylose and amylopectin) and breaks it down to simple sugars such as maltose and dextrins. Many organisms, including humans, use amylase to render dietary starch soluble so it can be absorbed during digestion.

Amylase (diastase) is free of reducing sugars, so the progress of the reaction can be monitored in two ways. First, by using the iodine test to check for loss of the starch substrate. Second, by using Benedict's solution to check for the appearance of reaction product (sugars).

Reducing Sugars

Reducing sugars have a carbonyl group (—CO) that can be oxidised in certain conditions. Examples of reducing sugars include glucose, fructose and maltose. Note, ordinary cane sugar, sucrose, is not a reducing sugar.

Iodine Test (MC26.1)

The iodine test is used to detect the presence of starch, specifically amylose. A solution of iodine in potassium iodide (MC26.1, I/KI, 1.5%/3%) forms an intense blue-black colour when it comes into contact with amylose.

Benedict's Solution (MC4.1)

Benedict's Solution (MC4.1) is based on copper sulphate, CuSO4, which is a clear transparent blue colour in solution. When Benedict's solution is heated in the presence of a reducing sugar, the sugar is oxidised and the Cu^{2+} is reduced to Cu^{+}, forming a characteristic red-orange precipitate of $Cu^{2}O$. A colour change from blue to orange confirms the presence of reducing sugars.

Malt Diastase

Malt diastase is a carbohydrolytic enzyme useful for digestive support and general nutrition support. Malt diastase is characterized by the ability to breakdown amylose and other polysaccharides. The enzyme works with amylase and glucoamylase to digest carbohydrate rich foods such as grains as well as malt, maltose, and sugars. Malt diastase is also known as maltase. It is produced by the cells lining the small intestine.

Malt Extract

Malt extract is produced by mashing malt, removing the solids, and then using an evaporator to concentrate the aqueous fraction. The resulting product is a thick syrup containing sugars, vitamins, and minerals.

Taka Diastase

Taka diastase is a form of diastase which results from the growth, development, and nutrition of a distinct microscopic fungus known as *Aspergillus oryzae* (Koji). Taka diastase is named after Jokichi Takamine, who developed the method first used for its extraction. Two grains of Takadiastase is the usual dose, although five grains is often given. The dose is usually given in a capsule during or at the end of the meal, In liquid form one dram contains two grains.

YEAST

Yeasts are eukaryotic micro-organisms classified in the kingdom Fungi, with about 1,500 species currently described; they dominate fungal diversity in the oceans. Most reproduce asexually by budding, although a few do so by binary fission. Yeasts are unicellular, although some species with yeast forms may become multicellular through the formation of a string of connected budding cells known as *pseudohyphae*, or false hyphae as seen in most molds. Yeast size can vary greatly depending on the species, typically measuring 3–4 μm in diameter, although some yeasts can reach over 40 μm.

GROWTH AND NUTRITION

Yeasts are *chemoorganotrophs* as they use organic compounds as a source of energy and do not require sunlight to grow. The main source of carbon is obtained by hexose sugars such as glucose and fructose, or disaccharides such as sucrose and maltose. Some species can metabolize pentose sugars like ribose, alcohols, and organic acids. Yeast species either require oxygen for aerobic cellular respiration (obligate aerobes), or are anaerobic but also have aerobic methods of energy production (facultative anaerobes). Unlike bacteria, there are no known yeast species that grow only anaerobically (obligate anaerobes). Yeasts grow best in a neutral or slightly acidic pH environment.

Yeasts will grow over a temperature range of 10°C (50°F) to 37°C (99°F), with an optimal temperature range of 30°C (86°F) to 37°C (99°F), depending on the type of species (*S. cerevisiae*) works best at about 30°C (86°F). Above 37 °C (99°F) yeast cells become stressed and will not divide properly. Most yeast cells die above 50°C (122°F). If the solution reaches 105°C (221°F) the yeast will disintegrate. There is little activity in the range of 0°C (32°F)—10°C (50°F). The cells can survive freezing under certain conditions, with viability decreasing over time.

Yeasts are very common in the environment, but are usually isolated from sugar-rich material. Some good examples include naturally occurring yeasts on the skins of fruits and berries (such as grapes, apples or peaches), and exudates from plants (such as plant saps or cacti). Some yeasts are found in association with soil and insects. Yeast are generally grown in the laboratory on solid growth media or liquid broths.

Common media used for the cultivation of yeasts include—Potato Dextrose Agar (PDA) or potato dextrose broth, Wallerstien Laboratories Nutrient agar (WLN), Yeast Peptone Dextrose agar (YPD), and Yeast Mould agar or broth (YM). The antibiotic cycloheximide is sometimes added to yeast growth media to inhibit the growth of Saccharomyces yeasts and select for wild/indigenous yeast species. This will change the yeast process.

USES

The useful physiological properties of yeast have led to their use in the field of biotechnology. Fermentation of sugars by yeast is the oldest and largest application of this technology. Many types of yeasts are used for making many foods: Baker's yeast in bread production, brewer's yeast in beer fermentation, yeast in wine fermentation and for xylitol production. Yeasts are also one of the most widely used model organisms for genetics and cell biology.

Alcoholic Beverages

Alcoholic beverages are defined as beverages that contain ethanol (C_2H_5OH). This ethanol is almost always produced by fermentation — the metabolism of carbohydrates by certain species of yeast under anaerobic or low-oxygen conditions. Beverages such as wine, beer, or distilled spirits all use yeast at some stage of their production.

Beer

A mixture of diatomaceous earth and yeast after filtering beer. Brewer's yeast (also known as brewing yeast) can mean any live yeast used in brewing. It can also mean yeast obtained as a by-product of brewing, dried and killed, and used as a dietary supplement for its B vitamin content.

Baking

Yeast, most commonly *Saccharomyces cerevisiae,* is used in baking as a leavening agent, where it converts the fermentable sugars present in the dough into carbon dioxide. This causes the dough to expand or rise as the carbon dioxide forms pockets or bubbles. When the dough is baked it "sets" and the pockets remain, giving the baked product a soft and spongy texture. The use of potatoes, water from potato boiling, eggs, or sugar in a bread dough accelerates the growth of yeasts. Salt and fats such as butter slow down yeast growth. The majority of the yeast used in baking is of the same species common in alcoholic fermentation.

Nutritional Supplements

Yeast is used in nutritional supplements popular with vegans and the health conscious, where it is often referred to as "nutritional yeast". It is a deactivated yeast, usually saccharomyces cerevisiae. It is an excellent source of protein and vitamins, especially the B-complex vitamins, whose functions are related to metabolism as well as other minerals and cofactors required for growth. It is also naturally low in fat and sodium. Some brands of nutritional yeast, though not all, are fortified with vitamin B_{12}, which is produced separately from bacteria. Nutritional yeast, though it has a similar appearance to brewer's yeast, is very different and has a very different taste.

Brewer's Yeast

Brewer's yeast is a type of fungus formally known as Saccharomyces cervisiae. Along with other saccharomyces species, brewer's yeast is used to brew beer and bake some breads, and can also be used as a nutritional supplement in an inactive form. Like other yeasts, brewer's yeast will ferment carbohydrates when it comes into contact with them, forming a froth of carbon dioxide which can ferment grains into beer and cause bread to rise. When used as a dietary supplement, brewer's yeast can provide the body with a number of essential vitamins and minerals including vitamin B. While brewer's yeast can be used to bake bread, most bakers use baker's yeast specifically, a sweet and less bitter culture of sacchraomyces.

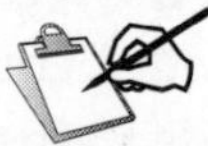

STUDY QUESTIONS

1. Write short notes on the following:
   (a) Enzymes;
   (b) Yeast;
   (c) Papaya; and
   (d) Amylase.
2. Discuss the medicinal uses of papaya.

■■■

CHAPTER 24

PERFUMES AND FLAVOURING AGENTS

PEPPERMINT OIL

Botanical Name	:	*Mentha piperita*
Family	:	Lamiaceae/Labiatae
Parts Used	:	Leaves, whole herb
Common Names	:	Peppermint, hortela, mint, menta, mentha montana, menthe

HABITAT

The plant, indigenous to Europe, is now widespread in cultivation throughout all regions of the world. It is found wild occasionally with its parent species.

DESCRIPTION

Peppermint or *Mentha piperita* is also known as *Mentha balsamea* Willd. It is a hybrid mint, a cross between the water-mint (Mentha aquatica) and spearmint (Mentha spicata).

Mentha piperita, a perennial herb of the mint family (Lamiaceae/Labiatae) grown for its essential oil, distilled for use in medicine and as a flavouring.

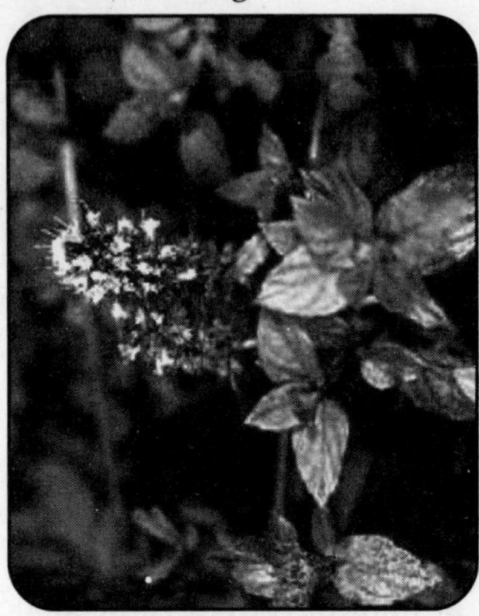

Fig. 24.1: Mentha piperita

It is a herbaceous rhizomatous perennial plant growing to 30–90 cm (12–35 inch) tall, with smooth stems, square in cross section. The *rhizomes* are wide-spreading, fleshy, and bare fibrous roots.

The *leaves* are from 4–9 cm (1.6–3.5 inch) long and 1.5–4 cm (0.59–1.6 inch) cm broad, dark green with reddish veins, and with an acute apex and coarsely toothed margins. The leaves and stems are usually slightly hairy.

The *flowers* are purple, 6–8 mm (0.24–0.31 inch) long, with a four-lobed corolla about 5 mm (0.20 inch) diameter; they are produced in whorls (verticillasters) around the stem, forming thick, blunt spikes. Flowering is from mid to late summer.

CULTIVATION

Peppermint generally thrives in shade and expands quickly by underground stolons. If you choose to grow peppermint, it is advisable to plant it in a container, otherwise it can rapidly take over a whole garden. It needs a good water supply, and is ideal for planting in part-sun to shade areas.

The leaves and flowering tops are the usable portion of the plant. They are collected as soon as the flowers begin to open and then are carefully dried. The wild form of the plant is less suitable for this purpose, with cultivated plants having been selected for more and better oil content. Seeds sold at stores labelled peppermint generally will not germinate into true peppermint, but into a particularly poor-scented spearmint plant. The true peppermint might rarely produce seeds, but only by fertilization from a spearmint plant, and contribute only their own spearmint genes.

MEDICINAL USES

Peppermint has a high menthol content, and is often used as a flavouring in tea, ice cream, confectionery, chewing gum, and toothpaste. The oil also contains menthone and menthyl esters, particularly menthyl acetate. It is the oldest and most popular flavour of mint-flavoured confectionery. Peppermint can also be found in some shampoos and soaps, which give the hair a minty scent and produce a cooling sensation on the skin.

There are 25-30 species of Peppermint. It is a stimulant, a tonic, and helps digestive system disorders. Studies have found that it is effective for the treatment of conditions such as dysentery. It is an anti-diarrheal agent, a vermifuge (a substance that works well against worms) working especially well against hookworms, and it is often used to stimulate bile flow.

Peppermint's antispasmodic properties have produced a total and immediate resolution of blockage of Oddi's sphincter (located in the intestinal tract) in animal studies. Because of its anti-inflammatory properties, Peppermint is used to treat rheumatism. Laboratory research studies with Peppermint have found antiviral, antifungal and antibacterial activity.

Peppermint works on the salivary glands, the first process in digestion. It acts as a sedative to the stomach and helps strengthen the bowels. Peppermint strengthens and soothes the bowels, helping to avoid cramping.

Peppermint oil is the most extensively used of all the volatile oils, both medicinally and commercially. The characteristic anti-spasmodic action of the volatile oil is more marked in this than in any other oil, and greatly adds to its power of relieving pains arising in the alimentary canal. From its stimulating, stomachic and carminative properties, it is valuable in certain flatulence and colic.

Peppermint, increases stomach acidity. Irritates mucous membranes and the gastrointestinal tract. It is use for chills, colic, fever, nausea, diarrhea, heart trouble, rheumatism, convulsions, spasms, and headaches.

These (peppermints) relax the muscles of the digestive tract and stimulate bile flow, so are useful for indigestion, flatulence, colic, and similar conditions. They reduce nausea and can be helpful for travel sickness; they also promote sweating in fevers and influenza.

Peppermint is used medicinally to treat indigestion and intestinal colic, as well as colds, fever, and headache. The pharmacology of peppermint focuses almost entirely on its menthol components. Peppermint and menthol possess carminative, antispasmodic, and choleretic properties, and are also used as an external analgesic and nasal decongestant. The mechanism behind peppermint oil's antispasmodic effects has recently been determined. Researchers believe that peppermint oil's inhibition of isolated smooth muscle contractions occurs via blockage of calcium influx into the muscle cells.

The pharmacological effects of peppermint and peppermint oil are useful in a number of clinical situation; the most notable include irritable bowel syndrome, intestinal colic, gallstones, musculoskeletal pain, and the common cold.

MENTHOL

Menthol is an organic compound made synthetically or obtained from peppermint or other mint oils. It is a waxy, crystalline substance, clear or white in color, which is solid at room temperature and melts slightly above. Menthol has local anesthetic and counterirritant qualities, and it is widely used to relieve minor throat irritation.

HABITAT

Mentha arvensis is the primary species of mint used to make natural menthol crystals and natural menthol flakes. This species is primarily grown in the Uttar Pradesh region in India.

MEDICINAL USES

Most of menthol's uses are related to its stimulation of the skin's cold receptors. This property makes menthol produce a cooling effect when inhaled or applied to the skin.

Because of its cooling effect, menthol is used in products meant to relieve skin irritation, sore throat, or nasal congestion.

It may be used to treat sunburn, fever, or muscle aches as well. In traditional Asian medicine, menthol may be prescribed for *nausea, diarrhea, indigestion, headache, cold,* or *sore throat*.

Products that commonly contain menthol include *toothpaste*, cough drops, lip balm, *mouthwash, gum,* and *cigarettes*.

Practitioners of *homeopathic medicine* believe that menthol can interfere with the efficacy of homeopathic remedies, and some even go so far as to advise against the use of mint toothpaste.

Menthol has very low toxicity, although menthol poisoning is possible if large quantities are consumed. However, any ill effects from the use of menthol are extremely rare. Many people around the world enjoy the cooling sensation of menthol in gum, candy, lip gloss, and other products.

LEMON OIL

Botanical Name	:	*Citrus limonum*
Family	:	Rutaceae
Parts Used	:	Peel
Common Name	:	Lemon essential oil, Citrus lemon, Nimbo

DESCRIPTION

The lemon is the common name for *Citrus limon*. The reproductive tissue surrounds the seed of the angiosperm lemon tree. Lemon is a small, straggling tree about 11 feet high, irregularly branched, the bark varying in colour from clear grey on the trunk, green on the younger branches to a purplish colour on the twigs. The evergreen leaves are ovate-oval. The well-known fruit is an ovoid berry, about three inches long, nipple-shaped at the end, smooth, bright yellow, indented over the oil-glands, having an acid, paleyellow pulp. About forty-seven varieties are said to have been developed during the centuries of cultivation.

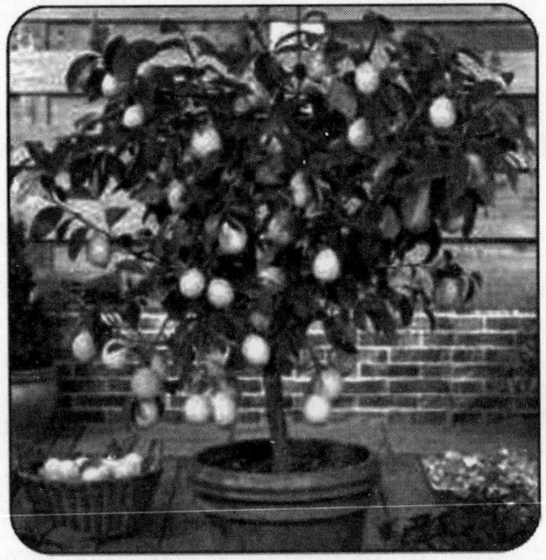

Fig. 24.2: Citrus lemon

The lemon is used for both culinary and nonculinary purposes throughout the world. The fruit is used primarily for its juice, though the pulp and rind (zest) are also used, primarily in cooking and baking.

Lemon juice is about 5% (approximately 0.3 mole per liter) citric acid, which gives lemons a tart taste, and a pH of 2 to 3. This makes lemon juice an inexpensive, readily available acid for use in educational science experiments. Because of the tart flavour, many lemon-flavored drinks and candies are available on the market, including lemonade.

OIL EXTRACTION

The commercial production of lemon oil was initiated in the regions of Spain, Florida, Portugal, Italy, Israel and California. Earlier, the Romans used the oil for stomach upsets and to sweeten the breath. The extraction of lemon oil is done from the fresh rind of the fruit (Citrus limonum or Citrus limon) of the Lemon tree (of the Rutaceae family). During the process, the oil is expressed through cold pressing from the fruits.

MEDICINAL USES

The major properties of this essential oil are being *antibacterial, antiviral, antihistamine, antifungal, antiseptic* and much more to cure several ailments. The major benefits that can be availed from this wonder oil are enumerated as:

Carrying along an extremely calming nature, lemon oil helps in *removing mental fatigue, exhaustion, dizziness, anxiety, nervousness, and nervous tension.*

The carminative nature of lemon oil comes to perfect use when the oil is applied to treating various stomach problems including indigestion, acidity, stomach upsets, cramps, etc.

With its distinctively refreshing aroma, the lemon oil comes out to be a good ingredient for *perfumes*. Even many scented candles and potpourris contain lemon oil.

ORANGE OIL

Botanical Name	:	*Citrus aurantium*
Family	:	Rutaceae
Parts Used	:	Fruit, Flowers, Peel
Common Name	:	Citrus vulgaris, Citrus Bigaradia, Citrus aurantium amara, Nagaranga, Bigarade Orange, Bitter Orange, Seville Orange (Sweet) Portugal Orange.

HABITAT

It is found in India, China, Spain and Madeira, etc.

CULTIVATION

The evergreen tree of orange has dark green leaves, beautiful white flowers and bright orange round fruits. Being native to the regions of China, these trees are now cultivated extensively in America and other regions of the world. Since old times, orange oil has been used in many Curacao type liqueurs and for the flavouring of food, drink and confectionery items. On addition to furniture polish, the oil helps to protect against damage from insects.

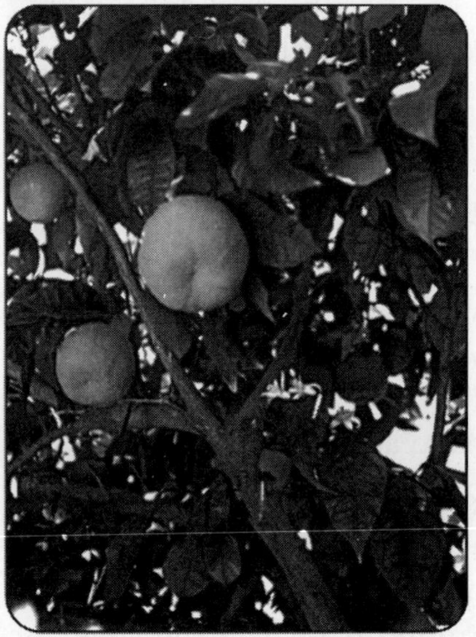

Fig. 24.3: Citrus aurantium

DESCRIPTION

It is a small tree with a smooth, greyish brown bark and branches that spread into a fairly regular hemisphere. The oval, alternate, evergreen leaves, 3 to 4 inches long, have sometimes a spine in the axil. They are glossy, dark green on the upper side, paler beneath. The calyx is cup-shaped and the thick, fleshy petals, five in number, are intensely white, and curl back.

The fruit is earth-shaped, a little rougher and darker than the common, sweet orange: the flowers are more strongly scented and the glands in the rind are concave instead of convex.

The small, immature fruits are sometimes used under the name of Orange berries for flavouring Curaçoa (peel from the sour orange). They are the size of a cherry and dark greyish-brown in colour. Formerly an essence was extracted from them.

The peel is used both fresh and dried. Much is imported from Malta, cut more thinly than that prepared in England.

The volatile oil of the *bitter orange peel* is known as *Oil of Bigarade*, and *sweet orange oil* as *Oil of Portugal.*

Orange oil is one of the most difficult to preserve, the most satisfactory method being to add 10 per cent of its volume of olive oil.

The flowers yield by distillation an essential oil known as *Neroli*, which forms one of the chief constituents of *Eau-de-Cologne*. A pomade and an oil are also obtained from them by maceration.

The oil from Sweet Orange blossoms is found in commerce under the name of *Neroli petalae.* Being far less fragrant it only fetches half the price of neroli oil and on that account is frequently used to adulterate the true neroli oil.

OIL EXTRACTION

The essential orange oil is extracted from the orange peels through the process of cold pressing. The yield becomes somewhere around 0.3-0.5%. The shelf life of this thin in consistency essential oil is usually 6 months. The fruits are botanically known as *Citrus sinensis* (also known as *Citrus aurantium var. dulcis* and *C. aurantium var. sinensis*) of the Rutaceae family, and are also known as *Portugal* or *China oranges.*

MEDICINAL USES

This essential oil is having rich sources of various therapeutic properties, enumerated as *antiseptic, anti-depressant, anti-spasmodic, anti-inflammatory, carminative, diuretic, chola-gogue, sedative,* and *tonic.*

The essential oil of orange assures to give quick and effective *relief from inflammations* (internal or external) and caused by any reason such as over intake of spices, fever, infections, side effects of antibiotics, gas, ingestion of toxic substances, narcotics, etc.

One can be reminded of the happy moments with *rejuvenated thought in mind,* merely by smelling orange oil.

Having mild *aphrodisiac properties,* systematic and regular usage of orange oil can cure problems such as frigidity, erectile problems, impotence, loss of interest in sex, etc.

Being a carminative agent, the oil helps in *removal of gases from the intestines.* Thus, it provides remedy from chest pains, indigestion and uneasiness, raised blood pressure, heart attack and acute stomach aches.

It promotes *secretions from all glands,* exocrine or endocrine. Thus it is seen to promote menstruations, flow of milk from breasts, digestive juices and bile, hormones, and enzymes.

LEMON GRASS OIL

Botanical Name	:	*Cymbopogon citratus*
Family	:	Poaceae (Gramineae)
Common Name	:	Lemon grass, Fever grass, Sereh, Citroengrass

HABITAT

Lemon grass essential oil is extracted from *Cymbopogon citratus.* It is also known as *Andropogon citratus, A. schoenathus* —West Indian, Madagascar or Guatemala lemon grass; Andropogon flexuosus, Cymbopogon flexuosus - East Indian, Cochin, British India or native lemon grass), of the *Poaceae* family.

DESCRIPTION

It is a perennial fast-growing aromatic grass, tropical grass with clumped, bulbous stems that ultimately become leaf blades. growing to about 1 meter (3 feet) high with long, thin leaves and originally was growing wild in India. It produces a network of roots and rootlets that rapidly exhaust the soil.

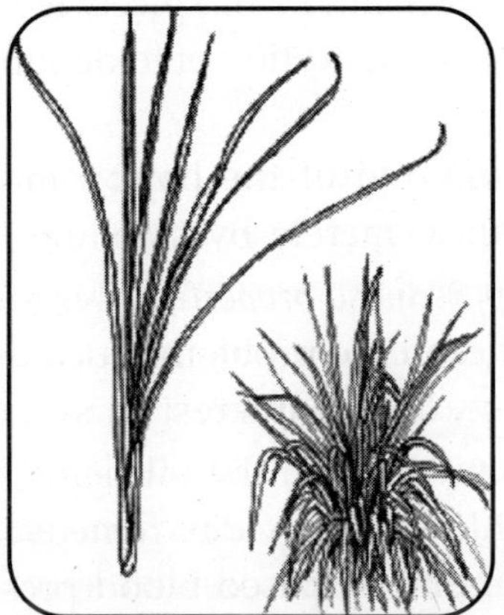

Fig. 24.4: Cymbopogon citratus

Lemon grass is in the same grass family as citronella and palmarosa; it has a lemon flavour. It has a branched cluster of stalked flowers and grows in clumps up to 6 inch tall; when crushed the fragrance resembles the scent of lemon.

Lemon grass oil is a yellow or amber liquid that is antiseptic; it can be used to treat athlete's foot (tinea pedia).

In India it is known as "choomana poolu" and is also referred to as *Indian Verbena* or *Indian Melissa oil* and used in Ayurvedic medicine to help bring down fevers and treat infectious illnesses. It is a valuable ingredient in perfumes and citrus-type soaps and is also an insect deterrent.

It is a fresh smelling oil that can be used with success for fighting jet lag, cellulite, revitalizing a tired body and mind, as well as keeping the family pet free of fleas and ticks.

EXTRACTION

Lemongrass oil is extracted from the fresh or partly dried leaves by steam distillation.

THERAPEUTIC PROPERTIES

The therapeutic properties of lemon grass oil are analgesic, anti-depressant, antimicrobial, antipyretic, antiseptic, astringent, bactericidal, carminative, deodorant, diuretic, febrifuge, fungicidal, galactagogue, insecticidal, nervine, nervous system sedative and tonic.

MEDICINAL USES

Lemon grass oil revitalizes the body and relieves the symptoms of jetlag, clears headaches and helps to combat nervous exhaustion and stress-related conditions.

It is a great overall tonic for the body and it boosts the parasympathetic nervous system, which is a boon when recovering from illness, as it also stimulates glandular secretions.

It is useful with respiratory infections such as sore throats, laryngitis and fever and helps prevent spreading of infectious diseases. It is helpful with colitis, indigestion and gastro-enteritis.

Lemon grass oil helps tone the muscles and tissue, relieves muscle pains by making the muscle more supple. It helps with correcting poor circulation and as an insect repellant. It helps to keep pets clean of fleas, ticks and lice.

It also is used for clearing up oily skin and acne, as well as athlete's foot. It alleviates excessive perspiration.

SANDALWOOD OIL

Botanical Name	:	*Santalum album*
Family	:	Santalaceae (Sandalwood family)
Common Name	:	Chandan, Sandalwood

DESCRIPTION

Sandalwood is an evergreen tree, growing up to 4-9 m tall. The trees have a long life, and may live up to one hundred years of age. The tree is variable in habit, usually upright to sprawling, and may intertwine with other species. The plant parasitises the roots of other tree species, but without major detriment to its hosts. The reddish or brown bark can be almost black and is smooth in young trees, becoming cracked with a red reveal. The heartwood is pale green to white as the common name indicates. The oval leaves are thin, oppositely arranged.

Smooth surface is shiny and bright green, with a glaucous (bluish-grey or green) pale underside. Fruit is produced after three years, viable seeds after five. These seeds are distributed by birds. Sandalwood has made its presence felt in the perfumery industry due to its excellent fragrance.

Sandalwood is an evergreen tree that boasts of its gorgeous small purple flowers. It is predominantly grown in Southern Tropical Asia.

Extracting oil from the sandalwood plant is not easy, as it the plant takes a minimum of 30 years to mature. The aroma of sandalwood is sweet, delicate, balsamic and floral. The consistency of sandalwood varies between medium and thick.

The colour of sandalwood essential oil is usually clear with a yellowish touch.

The method employed for *oil extraction* is steam *distillation*.

MEDICINAL USES

Sandalwood oil was used traditionally to treat skin diseases, acne, dysentery, gonorrhea, and a number of other conditions.

It is extremely beneficial in curing bronchitis, depression, stretch marks, leucorrhea, scars, laryngitis etc. It is also considered valuable in *meditative yoga practices*. The fragrance of sandalwood usually lasts for quite a longer period of time.

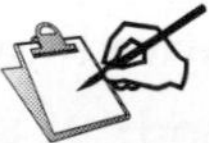

STUDY QUESTIONS

1. Write short notes on the following:
   (a) Menthol;
   (b) Lemon Oil;
   (b) Sandalwood Oil;
   (d) Peppermint Oil; and
   (e) Lemon Grass Oil.
2. Explain the medicinal uses of Peppermint Oil and Sandalwood Oil.

■■■

25

CHAPTER

Pharmaceutical Aids

HONEY

Honey is a sweet aliment produced by honey bees (and some other species) and derived from the nectar of flowers. Honey gets its sweetness from the monosaccharides fructose and glucose and has approximately the same relative sweetness as that of granulated sugar (97% of the sweetness of sucrose, a disaccharide). Honey has attractive chemical properties for baking, and a distinctive flavour which leads some people to prefer it over sugar and other sweeteners.

Honey, a most assimilable carbohydrate compound, is a singularly acceptable, practical and most effective aliment to generate heat, create and replace energy, and furthermore, to form certain tissues. Honey, besides, supplies the organism with substances for the formation of enzymes and other biological ferments to promote oxidation. It has distinct germicidal properties and in this respect greatly differs from milk which is an exceptionally good breeding-ground for bacteria. Honey is a most valuable food, which today is not sufficiently appreciated. Its frequent if not daily use is vitally important.

NUTRITION

Honey is a mixture of sugars and other compounds. With respect to carbohydrates, honey is mainly fructose (about 38.5%) and glucose (about 31.0%), making it similar to the synthetically produced inverted sugar syrup which is approximately 48% fructose, 47% glucose, and 5% sucrose. Honey's remaining carbohydrates include maltose, sucrose, and other complex carbohydrates. Honey contains trace amounts of several vitamins and minerals. As with all nutritive sweeteners, honey is mostly sugars and is not a significant source of vitamins or minerals. Honey also contains tiny amounts of several compounds thought to function as poisons, including—sodium cyanide, pinobanksin (*antioxidant bioflavonoid),* vitamin C, catalase, and pinocembrin (It is a flavanone, and an antioxidant found in honey and propolis). The specific composition of any batch of honey depends on the flowers available to the bees that produced the honey.

FORMATION

Honey is created by bees as a food source. In cold weather or when food sources are scarce, bees use their stored honey as their source of energy. By contriving for bee swarms to nest in artificial hives, people have been able to semi-domesticate the insects, and harvest excess honey. In the hive there are *three* types of bee—a single female *queen* bee, a seasonally variable number of *male* drone bees to fertilize new queens, and some 20,000 to 40,000 female *worker* bees. The worker bees raise larvae and collect the nectar that will become honey in the hive. Leaving the hive, they collect sugar-rich flower nectar and return. In the process, they release Nasonov pheromones. These pheromones lead other bees to rich nectar sites by 'smell'. Honeybees also release Nasonov pheromones at the entrance to the hive, which enables returning bees to return to the proper hive.

In the hive the bees use their "honey stomachs" to ingest and regurgitate the nectar a number of times until it is partially digested. The bees work together as a group with the regurgitation and digestion until the product reaches a desired quality. It is then stored in honeycomb cells. After the final regurgitation, the honeycomb is left unsealed. However, the nectar is still high in both water content and natural yeasts which, unchecked, would cause the sugars in the nectar to ferment. The process continues as bees inside the hive fan their wings, creating a strong draft across the honeycomb which enhances evaporation of much of the water from the nectar. This reduction in water content raises the sugar concentration and prevents fermentation. Ripe honey, as removed from the hive by a beekeeper, has a long shelf life and will not ferment if properly sealed.

HONEY IN MODERN THERAPEUTICS

Honey plays an insignificant part in our modern Materia Medial, though strained, clarified, borated and rose honey are listed in many pharmacopoeias. The mel depuratum (clarified honey) is rather an inadequate substance because it is subjected to heating and is filtered through cloth which also robs it of some mineral elements. Honey is today a more popular nostrum than the medical profession would surmise. Physicians, with few exceptions, grin broadly at the mere mention of the medicinal and food merits of honey. The diuretic effect of honey which was well known in antiquity, is still employed in kidney and bladder involvements. In pyelitis (inflammation of the renal pelvis) honey increases the amount of urine and exerts a decided antiseptic effect. The patients quickly improve; the urine clears and loses its putrid odor. The laxative effect of honey in these cases is also of advantage. Antioxidants in honey have even been implicated in reducing the damage done to the colon in colitis. Honey has also been used for centuries as a treatment for sore throats and coughs. The antibacterial and antiseptic properties of honey aid in healing sore throats and laryngitis.

Honey produced from the flowers of rhododendrons, mountain laurels, sheep laurel, and azaleas may cause honey intoxication.

Symptoms include dizziness, weakness, excessive perspiration, nausea, and vomiting. Less commonly, low blood pressure, shock, heart rhythm irregularities, and convulsions may occur, with rare cases resulting in death.

Honey intoxication is more likely when using "natural" unprocessed honey and honey from farmers who may have a small number of hives. Commercial processing, with pooling of honey from numerous sources generally dilutes any toxins.

PRESERVATION

Because of its unique composition and the complex processing of nectar by the bees which changes its chemical properties, honey is suitable for long term storage and is easily assimilated even after long preservation. History knows examples of honey preservation for decades, and even centuries. The main goal is to prevent the fermentation of the honey. Honey should also be protected from oxidation.

The ideal example is the natural process of bees sealing of the honey in honeycomb cells with wax caps. The best honey is in the uncut honey combs. After being removed from the comb, honey is very vulnerable, and the main losses of quality take place during preservation and distribution.

ARACHIS HYPOGAEA

Botanical Name	:	*Arachis hypogaea*
Family	:	Fabaceae (Leguminosae)
Parts Used	:	Seed
Common Name	:	Peanut, or Groundnut

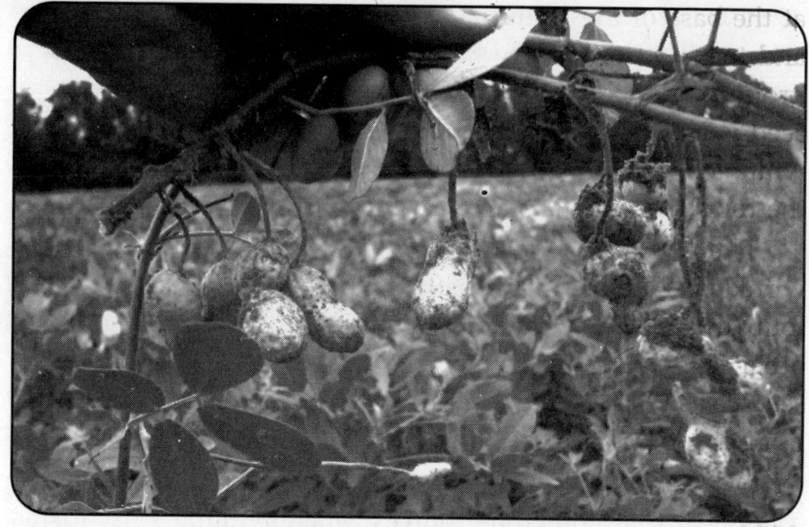

Fig. 25.1: Arachis hypogaea

DESCRIPTION

The *peanut*, or *groundnut* (Arachis hypogaea), is a species in the legume family (*Fabaceae*) native to South America, Mexico and Central America. It is an annual herbaceous plant growing to 30 to 50 cm (1 to 1.5 ft) tall. The leaves are opposite, pinnate with four leaflets (two opposite pairs; no terminal leaflet), each leaflet 1 to 7 cm (3/8 to 2¾ inch) long and 1 to 3 cm (3/8 to 1 inch) broad. The flowers are a typical peaflower in shape, 2 to 4 cm (¾ to 1½ inch) across, yellow with reddish veining. After pollination, the fruit develops into a legume 3 to 7 cm (1 to 2 inch) long, containing 1 to 4 seeds, which forces its way underground to mature.

Peanuts are also known as earthnuts, groundnuts, goobers, goober peas, pindas, jack nuts, pinders, manila nuts, g-nuts, and monkey nuts; the last of these is often used to mean the entire pod.

CULTIVATION

The orange veined, yellow petaled, pea-like flower of the Arachis hypogaea is borne in auxiliary clusters above ground. Following self-pollination, the flowers fade and wither. The stalk at the base of the ovary, called the pedicel, elongates rapidly, and turns downward to bury the fruits several inches in the ground, where they complete their development. When the seed is mature, the seed coat (mesocarp) changes colour from white to a reddish brown. The entire plant, including most of the roots, is removed from the soil during harvesting.

The pods act in nutrient absorption. The fruits have wrinkled shells that are constricted between pairs of the one to four (usually two) seeds per pod. The mature seeds resemble other legume seeds such as beans, but they have paper-thin seed coats, rather than the usual, hard legume seed coats.

USES

Peanuts are found in a wide range of grocery products. Edible peanuts account for two-thirds of the total peanut use in the United States. Popular confections include salted peanuts, peanut butter (sandwiches, candy bars, and cups), peanut brittle, and shelled nuts (plain/roasted). Salted peanuts are usually roasted in oil and packed in retail size, plastic bags or hermetically sealed cans. Dry roasted, salted peanuts are also marketed in significant quantities. The primary use of peanut butter is in the home, but large quantities are also used in the commercial manufacture of sandwiches, candy, and bakery products.

MEDICINAL USES

Peanuts are a rich source of protein (roughly 30 grams per cup after roasting). Peanuts are a significant source of resveratrol, a chemical studied for potential anti-aging effects and also associated with reduced cardiovascular disease and reduced cancer risk. Peanuts are a source of Coenzyme Q_{10} along with oily fish, beef, soyabeans and spinach.

Although many people enjoy foods made with peanuts, some people have mild to severe allergic reactions. For people with peanut allergy, exposure can cause fatal anaphylactic shock. For these individuals, eating a single peanut or just breathing the dust from peanuts can cause a fatal reaction. An allergic reaction also can be triggered by eating foods that have been processed with machines that have previously processed peanuts, making the avoidance of such food difficult.

ARACHIS OIL

Peanut oil (arachis oil) is an organic material oil derived from peanuts, noted to have the slight aroma and taste of its parent legume. In the U.K. it is marketed as "groundnut oil".

It is often used in Chinese, South Asian and Southeast Asian cuisine much as olive oil is used in the Mediterranean. Peanut oil is appreciated for its high smoke point relative to many other cooking oils. Its major component fatty acids are oleic acid (56.6%) and linoleic acid (26.7%). The oil also contains some palmitic acid, arachidic acid, arachidonic acid, behenic acid, lignoceric acid and other fatty acids.

It is also used as the main ingredient in some ear-wax removing products along with almond oil. Peanut oil is also used as a fecal softener.

Peanut oil is most commonly used when frying foods, particularly french fries and chicken. Chick-fil-A fries chicken in peanut oil.

Peanut oil is a monounsaturated fat. As such it may be substituted into a diet to reduce the negative health effects of eating trans fat and saturated fat.

STARCH

Starch or *amylum* is a polysaccharide carbohydrate consisting of a large number of glucose units joined together by glycosidic bonds. Starch is produced by all green plants as an energy store and is a major food source for humans. Pure starch is a white, tasteless and odourless powder that is insoluble in cold water or alcohol. It consists of two types of molecules: the linear and helical amylose and the branched amylopectin. The cereal grains (wheat, rice, corn, oats, barley) as well as tubers such as potatoes are rich in starch.

Starch can be separated into two fractions—amylose and amylopectin. Natural starches are mixtures of amylose (10-20%) and amylopectin (80-90%).

Amylose forms a colloidal dispersion in hot water whereas amylopectin is completely insoluble. The structure of amylose consists of long polymer chains of glucose units connected by an alpha acetal linkage.

Chemical Test for Starch or Iodine

Amylose in starch is responsible for the formation of a deep blue colour in the presence of iodine. The iodine molecule slips inside of the amylose coil.

Iodine–KI Reagent

Iodine is not very soluble in water, therefore the iodine reagent is made by dissolving iodine in water in the presence of potassium iodide. This makes a linear triiodide ion complex with is soluble. The triiodide ion (I^{+3}) slips into the coil of the starch causing an intense blue-black colour.

Starch Test

Add Iodine–KI reagent to a solution or directly on a potato or other materials such as bread, crackers, or flour. A blue-black colour results if starch is present. If starch amylose is not present, then the colour will stay orange or yellow. Starch amylopectin does not give the colour, nor does cellulose, nor do disaccharides such as sucrose in sugar.

Iodine Test

When following the changes in some inorganic oxidation reduction reactions, iodine may be used as an indicator to follow the changes of iodide ion and iodine element. Soluble starch solution is added. Only iodine element in the presence of iodide ion will give the characteristic blue black colour. Neither iodine element alone nor iodide ions alone will give the colour result.

Energy Store of Plants

In photosynthesis, plants use light energy to produce glucose from carbon dioxide. The glucose is stored mainly in the form of starch granules, in plastids such as chloroplasts and especially amyloplasts. Toward the end of the growing season, starch accumulates in twigs of trees near the buds. Fruit, seeds, rhizomes, and tubers store starch to prepare for the next growing season.

Glucose is soluble in water, hydrophilic, binds much water and takes up much space; glucose in the form of starch, on the other hand, is not soluble and can be stored much more compactly.

Uses of Starch

Starch can be used as a thickening, stiffening or gluing agent when dissolved in warm water, giving wheatpaste. As an additive for food processing, food starches are typically used as thickeners and stabilizers in foods such as puddings, custards, soups, sauces, gravies, pie fillings, and salad dressings, and to make noodles and pastas.

Medicinal Uses

Starch ingestion occurs when someone accidentally or intentionally swallows starch.

Cooking and *laundry starch* are both made from vegetable products, most commonly—

- Corn.
- Potatoes.
- Rice.
- Wheat.

Both are usually considered nonpoisonous (nontoxic), but some older laundry starches may contain:

- Borax.
- Magnesium salts.
- Polishing agents.

For *cooking starch*:

- Gastrointestinal;
  - Intestinal blockage.
  - Stomach area pain.

For *laundry starch* (with very long-term use):

- Bladder and kidneys;
  - Significantly decreased urine output (or none).
- Eyes, ears, nose, and throat
  - Jaundice (eyes become yellow).
- Gastrointestinal;
  - Diarrhoea.
  - Vomiting.
- Heart and blood;
  - Convulsions.
  - Collapse.
  - Fever.
  - Low blood pressure.
- Skin
  - Blisters.
  - Bluish skin, lips, or fingernails.
  - Flaking skin.
  - Yellow skin.
- Nervous system
  - Coma.
  - Drowsiness.
  - Twitching of the arms, hands, legs, or feet.
  - Twitching of the facial muscles.

RICE STARCHES

Rice starches are the little known secret of the starch world, comprising a very small percentage of the total starch usage. Do not be fooled by the fact that rice starches are not as common as the other starch sources. They have many unique attributes that make them some of the most interesting starches in the food industry.

WHEAT STARCH

Triticum aestivum (bread wheat) is by far the most important of all wheat species, the highest yielding and the widest ranging as well as the one most suited to bread making. Its centre of origin is thought to be somewhere south of the Caspian Sea but its rise to prominence came only after wheat cultivation had spread to more humid areas. During the last two thousand years it has come to replace almost all other species and has spread to almost all parts of the world where wheat can be grown.

Wheats are freely tillering, usually robust grasses 60-120 cm tall. All species are annuals. Leaves are usually softly hairy with two prominent hairy auricles. The leaf blades are narrow with approximately 12 veins. The inflorescence is a typical spike with a single spikelet at each node. Each spikelet consists of a pair of stiff glumes and from one to nine florets borne on a very short rachilla. The upper one or two florets are sterile. The glumes are about the same size as the lemmas, are asymmetrical and with the side away from the rachis being larger. The lemmas are thinner than the glumes, awned or awnless.

Starch is one of the most abundant natural raw materials in nature and is consumed as a component of bread, pasta, rice, breakfast cereals, cakes, biscuits and potatoes. A large proportion is also consumed after conversion to ethanol in beverages. Starch is a polymer of α-D-glucose that can be chemically or physically modified, it can also undergo hydrolysis to yield a range of derivatives from glucose syrups to polyols.

Starch is produced by the Martin process or Slurry process. Raw starch milk streams are freed from insolubles (small gluten particles, fibres and insoluble pentosans) by rotating screens or jet refiners. These are used as slurry for feeding or are concentrated or dried together with concentrated solubles and bran as wheat gluten feed.

Wheat starch grains are bimodal in size, B-starch (15-20%) is 2-15 mm diameter and the larger A-starch granules (80-85%) are 20-35 mm. B-starch is always highly contaminated with pentosans, fine fibres, lipids and protein, and for this reason the two fractions are worked up separately and recombined after washing and concentration, the resulting concentrated starch milk is then ready for further processing.

POTATO STARCH

Potato starch is made through an extensive process of washing, sometimes cooking, and then separating the starch present in potato cell walls so that it can be made into powdered or liquid form. In cooking, potato starch is often considered a substitute thickener for cornstarch or white flour. However, it has a higher heat point than cornstarch, so it may be superior for certain foods that require high temperatures.

Another benefit to potato starch, especially as compared to wheat flour as a thickener, is that it is gluten free. This means folks who want nice thick gravy, or soups or stews, but have not been able to achieve this with flour due to gluten intolerance, can use potato starch instead with excellent results. Like cornstarch, you generally have to dissolve the potato starch in a little bit of water before adding it as a thickener so it will blend easily with other ingredients. Many people especially prefer starch made from potatoes or corn when thickening sauces because it can help the sauces remain translucent; whereas flour creates a more muddied appearing sauce.

KAOLINITE

Kaolinite, which is named for its type locality, Kao-Ling, Jianxi, China; is a common phyllosilicate mineral. It lends it name to the *kaolinite group*, members of which also belong to the larger general group known as the *Clays*. Kaolinite's structure is composed of silicate sheets (Si_2O_5) bonded to aluminum oxide/hydroxide layers [$Al_2(OH)_4$] called gibbsite layers. Gibbsite is an aluminum oxide mineral that has the same structure as these aluminum layers in kaolinite. The silicate and gibbsite layers are tightly bonded together with only weak bonding existing between these silicate/gibbsite paired layers (called *s-g layers*). The weak bonds between these s-g layers causes the cleavage and softness of this mineral. The structure is very similar to the Serpentine Group and at times the two groups are combined into a Kaolinite-serpentine Group.

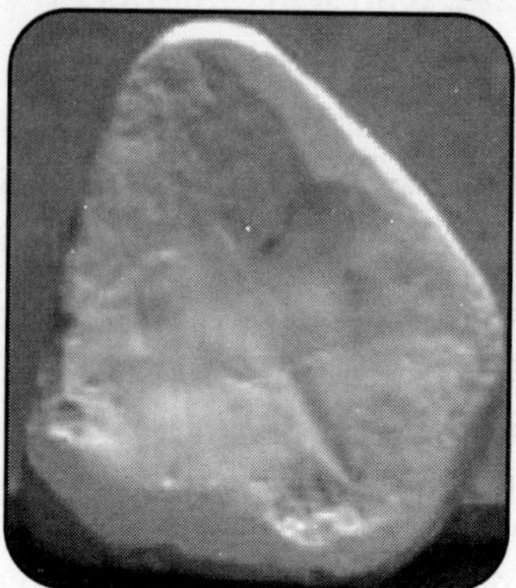

Fig. 25.2: Kaolinite (Clay)

Kaolinite shares the same chemistry as the minerals halloysite, dickite and nacrite. The four minerals are polymorphs; meaning they have the same chemistry, but different structures. All four minerals form from the alteration (mostly weathering) of aluminum rich silicate minerals such as feldspars. Kaolinite is by far the most common and most clay deposits contain at least some kaolinite. In fact, clay deposits will frequently be nearly 100% kaolinite pure!

Kaolinite is important to the production of ceramics and porcelain. It is also used as a filler for paint, rubber and plastics since it is relatively inert and is long lasting. But the greatest demand for kaolinite is in the paper industry to produce a glossy paper such as is used in most magazines.

PHYSICAL CHARACTERISTICS

- Colour is usually white, colourless, greenish or yellow.
- Luster is earthy.
- Crystals are translucent.
- Crystal System is triclinic.
- Crystal habits include foliated and earthy masses. Crystals of any size are quite rare, usually microscopic.
- Cleavage is perfect in one direction.

- Fracture is earthy.
- Hardness is 1.5-2 (can leave marks on paper).
- Specific gravity is 2.6 (average).
- Streak is white.
- Clay like properties when water is added.
- Associated minerals include fluorite, microcline, pyrite, hemimorphite, augite, dickite, halloysite, montmorillonite, quartz, muscovite and other clays.

USES

Kaolin is used in ceramics, medicine, coated paper, as a *food additive*, in *toothpaste*, as a light diffusing material in white incandescent light bulbs, and in cosmetics. It is generally the main component in porcelain.

It is also used in paint to extend titanium dioxide (TiO_2) and modify gloss levels; in rubber for semi-reinforcing properties; and in adhesives to modify rheology. A folk medicine use is to soothe an upset stomach, similar to the way parrots (and later, humans) in South America originally used it. In traditional Chinese medicine, it is used for restricting leakage from intestines and stopping diarrhea, blood containment and stopping bleeding, wounds healing.

PECTIN

Pectin is a natural part of human diet, but does not contribute significantly to nutrition. The daily intake of pectin from fruit and vegetables can be estimated to be around 5 g (assuming consumption of approximately 500 g fruit and vegetable per day).

Pectin is a long chain of pectic acid and pectinic acid molecules. Because these acids are sugars, pectin is a polysaccharide. It is prepared from citrus peels and the remains of apples after they are squeezed for juice.

In the plant, pectin is the material that joins the plant cells together. When fungus enzymes breakdown the pectin in fruit, the fruit gets soft and mushy. It is produced commercially as a white to light brown powder, mainly extracted from citrus fruits, and is used in food as a gelling agent particularly in jams and jellies. It is also used in fillings, sweets, as a stabilizer in fruit juices and milk drinks and as a source of dietary fibre.

USES

Pectin is a thickener in many products. If there is sufficient sugar in the mixture, pectin forms a firm gel.

Jams and jellies are thickened with pectin. Pectin binds water, and thus keeps products from drying out. It stabilizes emulsions.

Pectin combines with the calcium and whey proteins of milk, stabilizing foams and gels made with cream or milk.

In human digestion, pectin goes through the small intestine more or less intact. Pectin is thus a soluble dietary fiber.

Consumption of pectin has been shown to reduce blood cholesterol levels. The mechanism appears to be an increase of viscosity in the intestinal tract, leading to a reduced absorption of cholesterol from bile or food. In the large intestine and colon, microorganisms degrade pectin and liberate short-chain fatty acids that have positive influence on health (prebiotic effect).

In medicine, pectin increases viscosity and volume of stool so that it is used against constipation and diarrhoea. Pectin is also used in throat lozenges as a demulcent. In cosmetic products, pectin acts as stabilizer. Pectin is also used in wound healing preparations and specialty medical adhesives, such as colostomy devices.

SOURCES AND PRODUCTION

Apples, quince, plums, gooseberries, oranges and other citrus fruits contain much pectin, while soft fruits like cherries, grapes and strawberries contain little pectin.

Typical levels of pectin in plants are (fresh weight):

- Apples, 1–1.5%
- Apricot, 1%
- Cherries, 0.4%

- Oranges 0.5–3.5%
- Carrots approx. 1.4%
- Citrus peels, 30%.

The main raw-materials for pectin production are dried citrus peel or apple pomace, both by-products of juice production. Pomace from sugar-beet is also used to a small extent.

From these materials, pectin is extracted by adding hot dilute acid at pH-values from 1.5–3.5. During several hours of extraction, the protopectin loses some of its branching and chain-length and goes into solution. After filtering, the extract is concentrated in vacuum and the pectin then precipitated by adding ethanol or isopropanol. An old technique of precipitating pectin with aluminium salts is no longer used (apart from alcohols and polyvalent cations; pectin also precipitates with proteins and detergents).

CITRUS PECTIN

Citrus pectin is a plant fibre obtained from the rind and peel of citrus fruits such as lemons, grapefruits, oranges and tangerines. Structurally, pectin is classified as a water soluble, complex polysaccharide, rich in the sugar-galactose. At a molecular level, pectin is a strong binding agent, which directly relates to its tremendous detoxification and cholesterol lowering properties.

Citrus pectin is very bioavailable and has a galactose rich make-up, giving it the ability to deliver the following extra-ordinary benefits:

- Removes heavy metals and toxins
- Promotes cardiovascular health
- Promotes normal cell growth.

Cilantro and Garlic have been included in the Pectin Plus® formula because they both support cardiovascular health, while also supporting detoxification, particularly heavy metal detoxification. In fact both cilantro and garlic greatly add to the efficiency of citrus pectin's detoxification action.

Together, acting with very different biochemical mechanisms, Citrus Pectin, Cilantro and Garlic work synergistically in detoxifying the body, promoting "normal" cell growth and cardiovascular health. Pectin Plus® is a Powerful detoxifier

In today's world, more than ever, we are exposed to a wide variety of toxins: They are in our air, food and water, in the workplace and at home. We even generate toxins within our own bodies. Our bodies are designed to be self-cleansing and self-healing. The internal detoxification process is an automatic daily procedure of the major detoxification organs. Toxins, however produce irritation and inflammation, adding to the burden of our digestive system. When our digestive system becomes overwhelmed, it is no longer able to adequately perform detoxification functions. This is a condition called *"toxic overload"*.

Exposure to toxins results in an increased production of free radicals which over time damage or age our body tissues. Long term "toxic overload" may result in metabolic and genetic alternations that can affect cell growth, behaviour and immune response. This is because the molecular structures of toxins are carcinogenic as they interact with human DNA.

OLIVE OIL

Olive oil is a fruit oil obtained from the olive (*Olea europaea*; family *Oleaceae*), a traditional tree crop of the Mediterranean Basin. The wild olive tree originated in Asia minor and spread from there as far as Southern Africa, Australia, Japan and China. It is commonly used in cooking, cosmetics, pharmaceuticals, and soaps and as a fuel for traditional oil lamps. Olive oil is used throughout the world, but especially in the Mediterranean.

CONSTITUENTS

Olive oil is composed mainly of the mixed triglyceride esters of oleic acid and palmitic acid and of other fatty acids, along with traces of squalene (up to 0.7%) and sterols (about 0.2%

phytosterol and tocosterols). The composition varies by cultivar, region, altitude, time of harvest, and extraction process.

Olive oil contains a group of related natural products with potent antioxidant properties which give extra-virgin unprocessed olive oil its bitter and pungent taste and which are esters of tyrosol and hydroxytyrosol, including oleocanthal and oleuropein.

TYPES OF OLIVE OIL

Generally, olive oil is extracted by pressing or crushing olives. Olive oil comes in different varieties, depending on the amount of processing involved. Varieties include:

(i) **Extra virgin.** Considered the best, least processed, comprising the oil from the first pressing of the olives.

(ii) **Virgin.** From the second pressing.

(iii) **Pure.** Undergoes some processing, such as filtering and refining.

(iv) **Extra light.** Undergoes considerable processing and only retains a very mild olive flavour.

USES

Olive oil is a natural juice which preserves the taste, aroma, vitamins and properties of the olive fruit. Olive oil is the only vegetable oil that can be consumed as it is freshly pressed from the fruit. The beneficial health effects of olive oil are due to both its high content of monounsaturated fatty acids and its high content of antioxidative substances.

The higher the temperature to which the olive oil is heated, the more one should prefer the use of refined olive oils. When extra-virgin olive oil is heated above 350°C (662°F), the unrefined particles within the oil get burned. This leads to deteriorated taste and even toxicity.

Olive oil can be used as an effective shaving oil to shave facial and other body hair giving results that are equivalent to expensive commercial products.

MEDICINAL USE

Olive oil is good for *high blood pressure, weight loss, migraine, headache, earache, ear wax* and many other diseases.

Like olive oil, onion juice is also very helpful in lowering cholesterol. It's a blood purifier.

Application of olive oil on the pelvis helps to resolve *Menstrual Pain* or *Dysmenorrhea*.

Olive oil is very well tolerated by the stomach. In fact, olive oil's protective function has a beneficial effect on *ulcers* and *gastritis*. Olive oil activates the secretion of bile and pancreatic hormones much more naturally than prescribed drugs.

Olive oil is unlikely to cause *allergic* reactions, and as such is used in preparations for lipophilic drug ingredients. It does have demulcent properties, and mild laxative properties, acting as a stool softener. It is also used at room temperature as an ear wax softener.

There is a large body of clinical data to show that consumption of olive oil can provide heart health benefits such as favourable effects on *cholesterol* regulation and *LDL cholesterol oxidation,* and that it exerts *anti inflammatory, antithrombotic, anti hypertensive* as well as *vasodilatory* effects both in animals and in humans.

Olive oil helps to build a more healthy balance between omega-6 fats and omega-3 fats.

LANOLIN

Lanolin also called *Adeps Lanae,* wool wax, wool fat, anhydrous wool fat or wool grease, is a greasy yellow substance secreted by the sebaceous glands of wool-bearing animals, with the vast majority of it used by humans coming from domestic sheep.

Chemically akin to wax, it can be used as a skin ointment or water-proofing wax, and is also sometimes used as a raw material in the manufacture of such products as shoe polish. Lanolin's ability to act as a waterproofing wax aids sheep in shedding water from their coats.

Certain breeds of sheep produce large amounts of lanolin, and the extraction can be performed by squeezing the sheep's harvested wool between rollers. Most or all of the lanolin is removed from wool when it is processed into textiles, such as yarn or felt.

MEDICINAL AND OTHER USES

Lanolin is used commercially in many products ranging from rust-preventative coatings to cosmetics to lubricants. Some sailors use lanolin to create a slippery surface on their propellers and stern gear to which barnacles cannot adhere. The water-repellent properties make it valuable as a lubricant grease where corrosion would otherwise be a problem, particularly on stainless steel, which becomes more vulnerable to corrosion when starved of oxygen.

Medical grade lanolin is used as a cream to soothe skin, as it is hypoallergenic and bacteriostatic. In this form it is used by some breastfeeding mothers on sore and cracked nipples. This grade of lanolin can also be used to treat chapped lips, diaper rash, dry skin, itchy skin, rough feet, minor cuts, minor burns and skin abrasions. Many varieties of shaving cream contain lanolin. As an ointment base, it is readily absorbed through skin, facilitating absorption of the medicinal chemicals it carries. Some folk medicine traditions use lanolin in the nose, in small amounts, to treat head colds.

The emulsifying agent Eucerit in *Nivea* is made from lanolin, and is the key to NIVEA Creme's unique properties.

Using cosmetic products which contain impure lanolin can result in an allergic reaction in some people. Lanolin is often used as a raw material for producing vitamin D_3.

Lanolin is often used by baseball players to soften and break in their gloves (shaving cream that contains lanolin is popularly used for this).

Anhydrous lanolin is also used as a lubricant for brass instrument tuning slides.

Lanolin is a grease that is secreted from wool-bearing animals, such as sheep. Because it is hypoallergenic and impedes the growth of bacteria, medical grade lanolin is used as a cream to soothe skin. It has also been used to treat chapped lips, diaper rash, and various cuts and abrasions of the skin.

Lanolin provides a moist healing environment. The advantage of moist wound healing is that it prevents evaporation of internal moisture, thereby preventing the formation of scabs on the nipple. It is also possible that the gliding nature of lanolin eases abrasive rubbing from clothing on the nipples.

BEESWAX

Beeswax is a natural wax produced in the bee hive of honey bees of the genus Apis. Worker bees (the females) have eight wax-producing mirror glands on the inner sides of the sternites (the ventral shield or plate of each segment of the body) on abdominal segments 4 to 7. The size of these wax glands depends on the age of the worker and after daily flights begin these glands gradually atrophy. The new wax scales are initially glass-clear and colorless, becoming opaque after mastication by the worker bee.

The wax of honeycomb is nearly white, but becomes progressively more yellow or brown by incorporation of pollen oils and propolis. The wax scales are about 3 millimetres (0.12 inch) across and 0.1 millimetres (0.0039 inch) thick, and about 1100 are required to make a gram of wax.

USES

Beeswax is used commercially to make fine candles, cosmetics and pharmaceuticals including bone wax (cosmetics and pharmaceuticals account for 60% of total consumption), in polishing materials (particularly shoe polish and furniture polish) and as a component of modelling waxes. It is commonly used during the assembly of pool tables to fill the screw holes and the seams between the slates.

Squeezebox makers use beeswax as an adhesive, when blended with pine rosin, to attach reed plates to the structure inside an squeezebox. Beeswax candles are preferred in most Eastern Orthodox churches because they burn cleanly, with little or no wax dripping down the sides and little visible smoke.

Beeswax is also prescribed as the material (or at least a significant part of the material) for the Paschal candle ("Easter Candle") and is recommended for other candles used in the liturgy of the Roman Catholic Church.

It is also used as a coating for cheese, to protect the food as it ages. While some cheese-makers have replaced it with plastic, many still use beeswax in order to avoid any unpleasant flavours that may result from plastic.

The burning characteristics of beeswax candles differ from those of paraffin. A beeswax candle flame has a "warmer," more yellow colour than that of paraffin, and the colour of the flame may vary depending on the season in which the wax was harvested.

Beeswax is also an ingredient in moustache wax, as well as hair pomades.

As a skin care product a German study found beeswax to be superior to similar "barrier creams" (usually mineral oil based creams, such as petroleum jelly), when used according to its protocol.

MEDICINAL USES

General medicinal uses of *Bee propolis* include treatment of the cardiovascular and blood systems (anemia), respiratory apparatus (for various infections), dental care, dermatology (tissue regeneration, ulcers, eczema, wound healing—particularly burn wounds, mycosis, mucous membrane infections and lesions), cancer treatment, immune system support and improvement, digestive tracts (ulcers and infections), liver protection and support and many others.

ACACIA

Botanical Name	:	*Acacia nilotica*
Family	:	*Fabaceae*
Parts Used	:	Wood
Common Name	:	Babul, Thorn trees, Kikar

Acacia is a genus of shrubs and trees belonging to the subfamily *Mimosoideae* of the family *Fabaceae*. The plants tend to be thorny and pod-bearing, with sap and leaves typically bearing large amounts of tannins. Acacias are also known as *thorntrees*, whistling thorns or wattles, including the yellow-fever acacia and umbrella acacias.

There are roughly 1300 species of Acacia worldwide, about 960 of them native to Australia, with the remainder spread around the tropical to warm-temperate regions of both hemispheres, including Europe, Africa, Southern Asia, and the Americas.

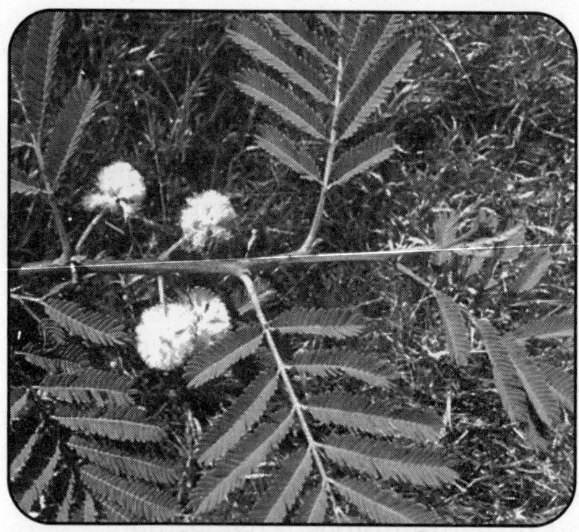

Fig. 25.3: Acacia nilotica

DESCRIPTION

The leaves of acacias are compound pinnate in general. In some species, however, more especially in the Australian and Pacific islands species, the leaflets are suppressed, and the leaf-stalks (petioles) become vertically flattened, and serve the purpose of leaves. These are known as *phyllodes*. The vertical orientation of the phyllodes protects them from intense sunlight, as with their edges towards the sky and earth they do not intercept light so fully as horizontally placed leaves. A few species (such as *Acacia glaucoptera*) lack leaves or phyllodes altogether, but possess instead cladodes, modified leaf-like photosynthetic stems functioning as leaves.

USES

Honey made by bees using the acacia flower as forage is considered a delicacy, appreciated for its mild flowery taste, soft running texture and glass-like appearance. Acacia honey is one of the few honeys which does not crystallize.

Many Acacia species have important uses in *traditional medicine*. Most all of the uses have been shown to have a scientific basis, since chemical compounds found in the various species have medicinal effects. In Ayurvedic medicine, *Acacia nilotica* is considered a remedy that is helpful for treating premature ejaculation. A 19th century Ethiopian medical text describes a potion made from an Ethiopian species of Acacia (known as grar) mixed with the root of the tacha, then boiled, as a cure for rabies. An astringent medicine, called *catechu* or cutch, is procured from several species, but more especially from Acacia catechu, by boiling down the wood and evaporating the solution so as to get an extract.

Ornamental species of acacia are also used by homeowners and landscape architects for home security. The sharp thorns of some species deter unauthorized persons from entering private properties, and may prevent break-ins if planted under windows and near drainpipes. The aesthetic characteristics of acacia plants, in conjunction with their home security qualities, makes them a considerable alternative to artificial fences and walls.

TRAGACANTH

Botanical Name	:	*Astragalus gummifer*
Family	:	Leguminosae
Parts Used	:	Gummy exudation
Common Name	:	Tragacanth

HABITAT

It is found in Asia Minor, Persia and Kurdistan.

DESCRIPTION

The plant is a small branching thorny shrub, the stem of which exudes a gum, vertical slits giving flat ribbon-shaped pieces and punctures giving tears; these have a horny appearance, are nearly colourless or faintly yellow, marked with numerous concentric ridges; the flakes break with a short fracture, are odourless and nearly tasteless; soaked in cold water, they swell and form a gelatinous mass 8 or 10 per cent only dissolving.

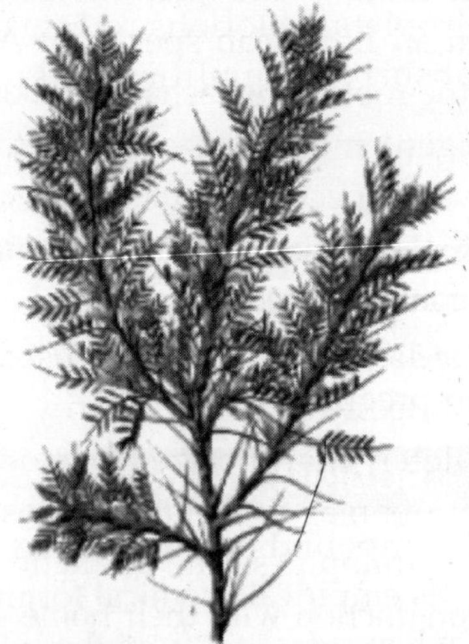

Fig. 25.4: Astragalus gummifer

CONSTITUENTS

The portion soluble in water contains chiefly polyarabinan-trigalaetangeddic acid; the insoluble part is called bassorin.

Tragacanth also contains water, traces of starch, cellulose, and nitrogenous substances, yielding about 3 per cent ash.

MEDICINAL USES

Demulcent, but owing to its incomplete solubility is not often used internally. It is much used for the suspension of heavy, insoluble powders to impart consistence to lozenges, being superior to gum arabic, also in making emulsions, mucilago, etc. Mucilage of Tragacanth has been used as an application to burns; it is also employed by manufacturers for stiffening calico, crape, etc.

Tragacanth has been used as a demulcent in cough and cold preparations and to manage diarrhoea. It also has been shown to moderate the blood sugar level, but this has not been demonstrated consistently. However, limited information is available.

In **folk medicine** it has been used for a laxative, persistent cough, diarrhea, and as an aphrodesiac. Modern pharmaceutical uses include an adhesive agent for pills and tablets, and for emulsifying oil droplets in lotions, creams and pastes. Its superior water absorbing qualities make it an excellent thickening agent.

TOXICOLOGY

Tragacanth is highly susceptible to bacterial contamination, and preparations contaminated with enterobacteria have been reported to have caused fetal deaths when administered intraperitoneally to pregnant mice.

SODIUM ALGINATE

The chemical compound sodium alginate is the sodium salt of alginic acid. Its empirical chemical formula is $NaC_6H_7O_6$. Its form as a gum, when extracted from the cell walls of brown algae, is used by the foods industry to increase viscosity and as an emulsifier. It is also used in indigestion tablets and the preparation of dental impressions. Sodium alginate has no discernible flavour.

Another major use of sodium alginate is reactive dye printing, where it is used in the textile industry.

USES

A major application for sodium alginate is as thickener for reactive dyestuffs (such as the Procion cotton-reactive dyes) in textile screen-printing and carpet jet-printing. Alginates do not react with these dyes and wash out easily, unlike starch-based thickeners.

Sodium alginate is a good chelator for pulling radioactive toxins such as iodine-131 and strontium-90 from the body which have taken the place of their non-radioactive counterparts. It is also used in immobilizing enzymes by inclusion.

As a food additive, sodium alginate is used especially in the production of gel-like foods. For example, bakers "Chellies" are often gelled alginate "jam". Also, the pimento stuffing in prepared cocktail olives is usually injected as a slurry at the same time that the stone is ejected; the slurry is subsequently set by immersing the olive in a solution of a calcium salt which causes rapid gelation by electrostatic cross-linking. Now-a-days it is also used in the biological experiments for the immobilization of cells to obtain important products like alcohols, organic acids,etc.

AGAR-AGAR

Botanical Name	:	*Gelidium amansii*
Family	:	Gelidium (Algae)
Parts Used	:	The mucilage dried, after boiling the seaweed
Common Name	:	Agar-agar, red algae

HABITAT

It is commonly found in the shallow coast of many East and Southeast Asian countries and Japan.

DESCRIPTION

A seaweed gathered on the East Indian coast and sent to China, it is derived from the various species of Sphaerococcus Euchema and Gelidium. It is brownish-white in colour with thorny projections on its branches; the best variety, known as Japanese Isinglass, contains large quantities of mucilage.

The seaweed after collection is spread out on the shore until bleached, and then dried; it is afterwards boiled in water and the mucilaginous solution strained, the filtrate being allowed to harden, and then it is dried in the sun.

The time for collection of the Algae is summer and autumn when the bleaching and drying can take place, but the final preparation of Agar-agar is carried out in winter from November to February. The Japanese variety is derived from several kinds of Algae and comes into European commerce in *two* forms: (i) In transparent pieces 2 feet long, the thickness of a straw, prepared in Singapore by treating it in hot water and (ii) In yellowish white masses about 1 inch wide and 1 foot long.

CONSTITUENTS

Agar-agar contains glose, which is a powerful gelatinizing agent. It is precipitated from solution by alcohol. Acetic, hydrochloric and oxalic acids prevent gelatinization of Agar-agar.

MEDICINAL USES

Agar-agar is widely used as a treatment for constipation, but is usually employed with Cascara when atony of the intestinal muscles is present. It does not increase peristaltic action. Its therapeutic value depends on the ability of the dry Agar to absorb and retain moisture. Its action is mechanical and analogous to that of the cellulose of vegetable foods, aiding the regularity of the bowel movements. It is sometimes used as an adulterant of jams and jellies.

DOSAGE AND PREPARATIONS

It is usually administered in small shreds mixed with fruit, milk or any convenient vehicle. It is not wise to give it in powder, as this gives rise to irritation in some cases. Half to one ounce may be taken at a time. One ounce to a pint of boiling water makes a suitable jelly for invalids and may be flavoured with lemon.

OTHER SPECIES

Sri lanka Agar-agar, or Agal agal, which is the native name of *Gracillaria lichenoides*, is largely used in the East for making soups and jellies. *Gigartina speciosa,* a variety found on the Swan River, was erroneously supposed to have formed the edible swallow's nest, but it has been ascertained that this delicacy comes from a peculiar secretion in the birds themselves. Malaysia Agar-agar comes from the straits between Borneo and Celebes and consists of impure *Euchema Spinolum* incrusted with salt.

GUAR GUM

Guar gum, also called *guaran*, is a *galactomannan*. It is primarily the ground endosperm of guar beans. The guar seeds are dehusked, milled and screened to obtain the guar gum. It is typically produced as a free flowing, pale, off-white coloured, coarse to fine ground powder.

The guar plant, also known as a *cluster plant*, grows primarily in Pakistan and the northern regions of India. It thrives on the drought/monsoon cycles present in those areas.

The plants are harvested after the monsoon season and the seeds are allowed to dry in the sun.

The seeds are then manually or mechanically separated and processed into a flour or sold as split seeds. Guar gum is an important cash crop for the Indian and Pakistani economies.

While consumers may balk at such "exotic" ingredients as locust bean gum, carageenan and guar gum, the truth is many of our ice creams, puddings and canned sauces would be fairly inedible without them.

Guar gum is not just a thickening agent, but a binder and plasticizer as well. When untreated ice cream melts and refreezes, grainy ice crystals often form. Guar gum has the natural ability to bind with water molecules, preventing them from forming the unwanted crystals. Processed foods with creamy textures are primarily held together with binders such as guar gum. Without a binder, the individual ingredients might separate into a watery mess.

Guar gum is a water-soluble fibre that acts as a bulk forming laxative, and as such, it is claimed to be effective in promoting regular bowel movements and relieve constipation and chronic related functional bowel ailments such as diverticulosis, Crohn's disease, colitis and irritable bowel syndrome, among others. The increased mass in the intestines stimulates the movement of waste and toxins from the system, which is particularly helpful for good colon health, because it speeds the removal of waste and bacteria from the bowel and colon.

In addition, because it is soluble, it is also able to absorb toxic substances (bacteria) that cause infective diarrhea. Guar gum is also capable of reducing the absorbability of dietary minerals (other than calcium), when foods and/or *nutritional supplements* containing them are consumed concomitantly with it. However, this is less of a concern with guar gum than with various nonsoluble dietary fibres. It also functions as an adjuvant for diabetic drugs that are sometimes employed for the treatment of noninsulin dependent diabetes. The effect is to help lower blood glucose levels. Thus, *diabetic patients* who are taking drugs should consult their doctors before supplementing with guar gum.

GELATIN

Gelatin is a translucent, colourless, brittle, nearly tasteless solid substance, derived from the collagen inside animals skin and bones. It is commonly used as a gelling agent in food, pharmaceuticals, photography, and cosmetic manufacturing. Substances containing gelatin or functioning in a similar way are called *gelatinous*.

Gelatin is a protein produced by partial hydrolysis of collagen extracted from the bones, connective tissues organs, and some intestines of animals such as domesticated cattle, pigs, and horses. The natural molecular bonds between individual collagen strands are broken down into a form that rearranges more easily. Gelatin melts when heated and solidifies when cooled again. Together with water, it forms a semi-solid colloid gel. Gelatin forms a solution of high viscosity in water, which sets to a gel on cooling, and its chemical composition is, in many respects, closely similar to that of its parent collagen.

Gelatin solutions show viscoelastic flow and streaming birefringence. If gelatin is put into contact with cold water, some of the material dissolves. The solubility of the gelatin is determined by the method of manufacture. Typically, gelatin can be dispersed in a relatively concentrated acid. Such dispersions are stable for 10–15 days with little or no chemical changes and are suitable for coating purposes or for extrusion into a precipitating bath.

Gelatin is also soluble in most polar solvents. Gelatin gels exist over only a small temperature range, the upper limit being the melting point of the gel, which depends on gelatin grade and concentration and the lower limit, the ice point at which ice crystallizes. The mechanical properties are very sensitive to temperature variations, previous thermal history of the gel, and time.

USES

Probably best known as a gelling agent in cooking, different types and grades of gelatin are used in a wide range of food and non-food products.

Common examples of foods that contain gelatin are gelatin desserts, trifles, aspic, marshmallows, and confectioneries such as Peeps, gummy bears and jelly babies. Gelatin may be used as a stabilizer, thickener, or texturizer in foods such as jams, yoghurt, cream cheese, and margarine; it is used, as well, in fat-reduced foods to simulate the mouthfeel of fat and to create volume without adding calories.

Gelatin is used for the clarification of juices, such as apple juice, and of vinegar. Isinglass, from the swim bladders of fish, is still used as a fining agent for wine and beer. Beside hartshorn jelly, from deer antlers (hence the name "hartshorn"), Isinglass was one of the oldest sources of gelatin. Gelatine was used for hardening paper in Colonial times.

TECHNICAL USES

- Capsules made of gelatin.
- Certain professional lighting equipment uses color gels to change the beam colour. These used to be made with gelatin, hence the name colour gel.
- Gelatin typically constitutes the shells of pharmaceutical capsules in order to make them easier to swallow. Hypromellose is a vegan-acceptable alternative to gelatin, but is more expensive to produce.
- Animal glues such as hide glue are essentially unrefined gelatin.
- It is used to hold silver halide crystals in an emulsion in virtually all photographic films and photographic papers. Despite some efforts, no suitable substitutes with the stability and low cost of gelatin have been found.
- Used as a carrier, coating or separating agent for other substances; for example, it makes beta-carotene water-soluble thus imparting a yellow colour to any soft drinks containing beta-carotene.
- Gelatin is closely related to bone glue and is used as a binder in match heads and sandpaper.
- Cosmetics may contain a non-gelling variant of gelatin under the name hydrolyzed collagen.
- As a surface sizing, it smooths glossy printing papers or playing cards and maintains the wrinkles in *crêpe paper*.

OTHER USES

- Blocks of ballistic gelatin simulate muscle tissue as a standardized medium for testing firearms ammunition.
- Gelatin is used by synchronized swimmers to hold their hair in place during their routines as it will not dissolve in the cold water of the pool. It is frequently referred to as "knoxing", a reference to Knox brand gelatin. Though commonly used, the owners of the trademark object to the genericized use of the term.
- When added to boiling water and cooled, unflavoured gelatin can make a home-made hair styling gel that is cheaper than many commercial hair styling products, but by comparison has a shorter shelf life (about a week) when stored in this form (usually in a refrigerator). After being applied to scalp hair, it can be removed with rinsing and some shampoo.
- It is commonly used as a biological substrate to culture adherent cells.
- Also used by those who are sensitive to tannins (which can irritate the stomach) in teas, soups or brews.
- It may be used as a medium with which to consume LSD. LSD in gelatin form is known as "windowpane" or "gel".
- Gelatin is used to make the shells of paintballs, similar to the way pharmaceutical capsules are produced.

MEDICAL AND NUTRITIONAL PROPERTIES

Although gelatin is 98-99% protein by dry weight, it has less nutritional value than many other protein sources. Gelatin is unusually high in the non-essential amino acids glycine and proline (i.e., those produced by the human body), while lacking certain essential amino acids (i.e., those not produced by the human body). It contains no tryptophan and is deficient in isoleucine, threonine, and methionine. The approximate amino acid composition of gelatin is: glycine 21%, proline 12%, hydroxyproline 12%, glutamic acid 10%, alanine 9%, arginine 8%, aspartic acid 6%, lysine 4%, serine 4%, leucine 3%, valine

2%, phenylalanine 2%, threonine 2%, isoleucine 1%, hydroxylysine 1%, methionine and histidine <1% and tyrosine <0.5%. These values vary, especially the minor constituents, depending on the source of the raw material and processing technique.

Gelatin is one of the few foods that cause a net loss of protein if eaten exclusively. In the 1960s, several people died of malnutrition while on popular liquid protein diets.

STUDY QUESTIONS

1. Write short notes on the following:
   (a) Honey;
   (b) Beeswax;
   (c) Kaolinite;
   (d) Agar-agar;
   (e) Olive Oil;
   (f) Lanolin; and
   (g) Gelatin.
2. Discuss the medical and nutritional properties of Gelatin.
3. Write a detailed note on starch.
4. Explain the medicinal an other uses of Beeswax.

■■■

26

CHAPTER

Miscellaneous Drugs

LIQUORICE

Botanical Name	:	*Glycyrrhiza glabra*
Family	:	Leguminosae
Parts Used	:	Root
Common Name	:	Mulethi

DESCRIPTION

Liquorice is a tall, erect herb with compound leaves, lilac or light violet flowers and flat fruit. The plant grows up to about 1.5 meters in height. It is a popular flavouring agent. It is densely covered with small spinous outgrowths.

The dried roots and underground stems or rhizomes of the plant constitute the drug. The root of the plant is a laxative and expectorant. When externally used it has a soothing effect on the skin. Powdered liquorice is very popular in allopathic medicine. The herb contains glycyrrhizin, glycyrrhizic acid and glycyrrhetinic acid.

HABITAT

The Liquorice plants are shrubs, natives of South-east Europe and South-west Asia, as far as Persia, the *G. glabra* ranging more especially to the westward, the *G. glandulifera* more to the eastward and being the source of the Eastern Liquorice root of commerce.

The Liquorice of medicine and commerce is derived from the sweet root of various species of Glycyrrhiza, a genus which contains about fourteen species, natives of warmer temperate countries in both the New and Old Worlds, ten of them having roots more or less sweet, but most of them not sufficiently so to be of use.

Hundreds of tons of Liquorice for commercial and medicinal purposes are imported annually from Spain, Russia, Germany, France and the East, most of our supply coming from Spain and Italy.

CONSTITUENTS

The chief constituent of Liquorice root, to which its sweet taste is due, is Glycyrrhizin (6 to 8 per cent), obtainable in the form of a sweet, white crystalline powder, consisting of the calcium and potassium salts of glycyrrhizic acid. The drug also contains sugar, starch (29 per cent), gum, protein, fat (0.8 per cent), resin, asparagin (2 to 4 per cent), a trace of tannin in the outer bark of the root, yellow colouring matter, and 0.03 of volatile oil.

The amount of Glycyrrhizin present in Extract of Liquorice varies from 5 to 24 per cent, and the amount of moisture from 8 to 17 per cent. Upon ignition, the extract yields from 5 to 9 per cent of ash.

The roots of *G. glandulifera* and echinata also contain in addition, Glycyrmarin, a bitter principle occurring mostly in the bark.

Glycyrrhizin, or a similar substance, has been obtained from other plants, viz. from the rhizome of Polypodium vulgare, the leaves of Myrrhis odorata, and the bark of Lucuma glycyphloea.

MEDICINAL USES

Liquorice is a valuable remedy for relieving *pain*, discomfort and other symptoms caused by acrid matter in the stomach. It should be taken in powder form.

- Lubricating the *throat* with a decoction of liquorice mixed with honey brings relief in dry cough.
- It is an effective home remedy for *sore throat*. A small piece of raw liquorice if chewed or sucked provides relief by soothing the inflammation.
- Liquorice is useful in treating pain due to *stomach ulcers*, as it soothes the irritation caused by acids. Pieces of the dried root soaked overnight in water and the infusion taken with rice gruel helps in the cure of ulcer. Even allopathic physicians use liquorice for treating ulcers.
- Liquorice alleviates *muscular pains*. Taking an infusion of the roots soaked overnight relieves any chronic joint problems.
- The powder of the herb mixed with butter or ghee and honey can be applied on *cuts* and *wounds* with good results. The leaves of the plant, applied as a poultice is a useful remedy in scalds of the head and body.
- It is used in the treatment of *myopia*. Half a teaspoon of the powder of the root, mixed with an equal amount of honey and half the quantity of ghee, can be given twice daily with milk on an empty stomach in this case.
- It *heals corns* which are just appearing. A paste of liquorice sticks mixed with sesame or mustard oil, if rubbed into the hardened skin at bed time softens the skin and the corn decreases in size.
- It is also used as a laxative in constipation. Its powder is taken with jaggery and water in this condition.

- The sticks of dried rhizomes are soaked in water and the infusion used as a gargle brings quick relief in oral inflammations. Tiny bits of the stick with sugar candy can also be sucked.
- Liquorice is beneficial in treating patchy baldness. Small pieces of the root are ground in milk with a pinch of saffron to a paste. When this paste is applied over the bald patches at bedtime regularly, hair growth is seen within a few weeks. This prescription is very effective in the initial stages of baldness, excessive hair loss and dandruff.

PRECAUTIONS

Continuous and uninterrupted use of liquorice in the treatment of stomach ulcer is not advisable as it may cause increase in weight and puffiness of body. It should also be avoided in pregnancy and in heart and kidney conditions.

TOXICITY

Excessive consumption of liquorice or liquorice candy is known to be toxic to the liver and cardiovascular system, and may produce hypertension and oedema. There have been occasional cases where blood pressure has increased with excessive consumption of liquorice tea, but such occasions are rare and reversible when the herb is withdrawn. Most cases of hypertension from liquorice were caused by eating too much concentrated liquorice candy. Doses as low as 50 grams (2 oz) of liquorice daily for two weeks can cause a significant rise in blood pressure.

GARLIC

Botanical Name	:	*Allium sativum*
Family	:	Liliaceae
Parts Used	:	Flowers; Leaves; Root; Seed, Bulb - raw or cooked
Common Name	:	Lehsun, garlic.

DESCRIPTION

Allium sativum, commonly known as garlic, is a species in the onion family Alliaceae. Its close relatives include the onion, shallot, leek, and chive. Garlic has been used throughout recorded history for both culinary and medicinal purposes. It has a characteristic pungent, spicy flavour that mellows and sweetens considerably with cooking. A bulb of garlic, the most commonly used part of the plant, is divided into numerous fleshy sections called cloves. Single clove garlic (also called Pearl garlic or Solo garlic) also exists—it originates in the Yunnan province of China. The cloves are used as seed, for consumption (raw or cooked), and for medicinal purposes. The leaves, stems (scape), and flowers (bulbils) on the head (spathe) are also edible and are most often consumed while immature and still tender. The papery, protective layers of "skin" over various parts of the plant and the roots attached to the bulb are the only parts not considered palatable.

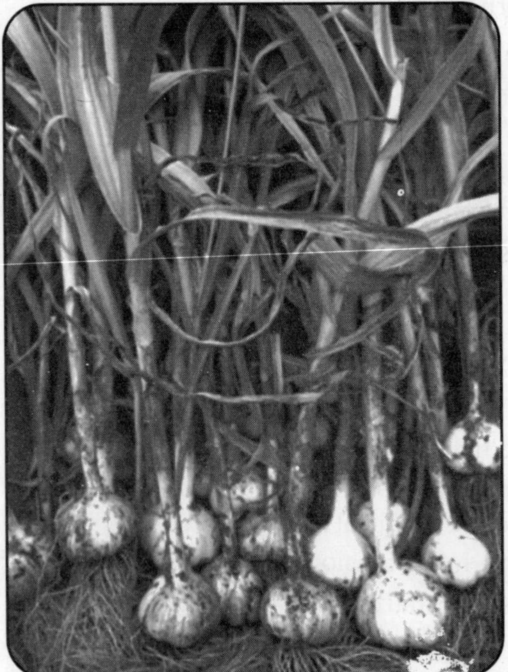

Fig. 26.1: Garlic

HABITAT

Allium sativum grows in the wild in areas where it has become naturalised; it probably descended from the species Allium longicuspis, which grows wild in southwestern Asia. The "wild garlic", "crow garlic", and "field garlic" of Britain are the species *Allium ursinum, Allium vineale,* and *Allium oleraceum,* respectively.

In North America, *Allium vineale* (known as "wild garlic" or "crow garlic") and *Allium canadense,* known as "meadow garlic" or "wild garlic" and "wild onion", are common weeds in fields. One of the best-known "garlics", the so-called elephant garlic, is actually a wild leek (*Allium ampeloprasum*).

CULTIVATION

Garlic is easy to grow and can be grown year-round in mild climates. In cold climates, cloves can be planted in the ground about six weeks before the soil freezes and harvested in late spring. Garlic plants are not attacked by pests. They can suffer from pink root, a disease that stunts the roots and turns them pink or red. Garlic plants can be grown close together, leaving enough room for the bulbs to mature, and are easily grown in containers of sufficient depth.

There are different types or subspecies of garlic, most notably hardneck garlic and softneck garlic. It is important to get the right kind of garlic for your latitude, as garlic can be day-length sensitive. Hardneck garlic is generally grown in cooler climates; softneck garlic is generally grown closer to the equator.

MEDICINAL USES

During the ages Garlic has been a valued natural healer. It has been used to promote the body's energy and strength. Garlic is used in today's natural medicines to help prevent heart disease, strokes, and hypertension.

Garlic's essential oil has a powerful disinfectant that is known for killing tough germs. Garlic has a powerful active ingredient called allicin that is responsible for it's powerful odor.

In preventing heart disease and strokes, garlic decreases the cholesterol levels that can cause heart attacks and stokes and promotes better blood circulation through the heart.

Garlic does have some offending characteristics when eaten; garlic's essential oils are passed through the skin and respiratory system. So when eaten may cause bad breathe and body odour.

Garlic is widely known today for several reasons. It is used as a spice and is an accepted herbal medicine as well. It targets several illnesses including those which affect the heart and liver. It is used for common colds too. It is quite surprising to think that the usual content we mix with our meals contains some substances that can help bring cure to many illnesses.

GARLIC AND THE IMMUNE SYSTEM

By eating raw, boiled or steamed garlic, our body can help fight illnesses. It has an immune boosting capacity which prevents our system from being susceptible to certain diseases. Eating garlic daily can help strengthen your immune resistance despite the presence of stress.

ANTIBACTERIAL AND ANTIFUNGAL PROPERTY OF GARLIC

Garlic also has an antibacterial property. It helps people get cured form bacteria-induced infections. It is also known as an effective treatment of fungal infections. Crushed garlic that is spread over burned areas can help fight infection. Ringworm can also be effectively reduced by rubbing garlic over the affected site. Itching will also be relieved through Garlic use.

GARLIC AND HEART DISEASE

Garlic is best known to treat heart problems. It is a worldwide accepted herbal remedy for those with high blood pressure. Eating garlic daily can help reduce your cholesterol in significant levels. It also lowers blood pressure in time. Garlic is widely known to prevent detrimental heart conditions. Because it lowers the level of bad cholesterol in the body, it also reduces the risk of heart attack and other associated problems.

OTHER USES

Garlic may also be used for diphtheria. It effectively reduces the inflammation in the membranes when chewed. Garlic is eaten when you travel or when you are exposed to heavy pollution. It is also taken as a common colds remedy and a treatment to some digestive problems.

Garlic definitely works in many ways. Who could have ever thought that the simple spice we mix with our meals can bring all these types of cure? Garlic is truly a good remedy that helps heal almost all kinds of illnesses experienced by the body.

PICRORHIZA

Botanical Name	:	*Picrorhiza kurroa*
Family	:	Scrophulariaceae
Parts Used	:	Rhizome
Common Name	:	Kutki and Kuru, Katuka, Kuru and Kadu

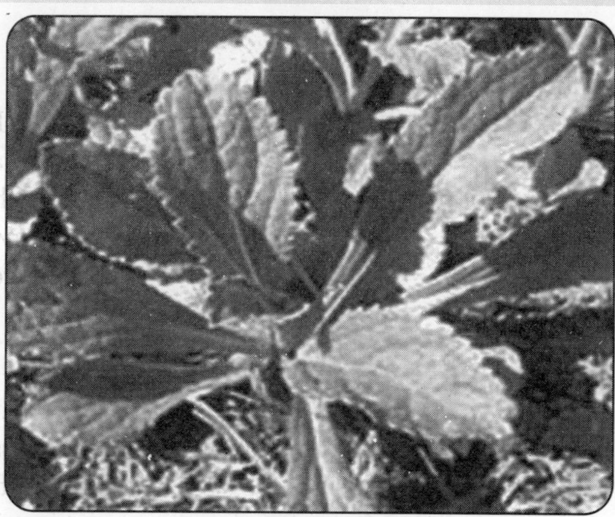

Fig. 26.2: Picrorhiza

DESCRIPTION

It is a small perennial herb from the Scrophulariaceae family. The rhizome of Picrorhiza has been traditionally used to treat worms, constipation, low fever, scorpion sting, asthma and ailments affecting the liver. Current research on Picrorhiza kurroa has focused on its hepatoprotective, anticholestatic, antioxidant, and immune-modulating activity.

HABITAT

Picrorhiza kurroa also known as kutki is found in the North-Western Himalayan region from Kashmir to Kumaun and Garhwal regions in India and Nepal.

CONSTITUENTS

The major constituents in picrorhiza are the glycosides picroside, kutkoside, and rosin, and apocynin. They have been shown in animal studies to be antiallergic, to inhibit platelet-activating factor, and to decrease joint inflammation. According to test tube and animal studies, picrorhiza has antioxidant actions, particularly in the liver. Picroliv has been shown to have an immuno inspiring effect in hamsters, helping to prevent infections.

Picrorhiza increases bile production in the liver, according to rat studies. It has also been shown to protect animals from damage by several potent liver toxins, offering protection as good as or better than silymarin (the flavonoids found in milk thistle). However, it does not have the amount of human research as silymarin.

Picrorhiza kurroa is a well-known herb in the Ayurvedic system of medicine and has traditionally been used to treat disorders of the *liver* and *upper respiratory tract, reduce fevers,* and to treat *dyspepsia, chronic diarrhea,* and *scorpion sting*. It is a small perennial herb from the Scrophulariaceae family, found in the Himalayan region growing at elevations of 3,000-5,000 metres. Picrorhiza kurroa has a long, creeping rootstock that is bitter in taste, and grows in rock crevices and moist, sandy soil. The leaves of the plant are flat, oval, and sharply serrated.

The *flowers,* which appear June through August, are white or pale purple and borne on a tall spike; manual harvesting of the plant takes place October through December. The active constituents are obtained from the root and rhizomes. The plant is self-regenerating but unregulated over-harvesting has caused it to be threatened to near extinction. Current research on Picrorhiza kurroa has focused on its *hepatoprotective, anti-cholestatic, antioxidant,* and *immune-modulating activity.*

SIDE EFFECTS

Loose stools and indigestion have been reported when unprepared picrorhiza rhizomes are used as medicine. However, extracts in alcohol have shown much less tendency to cause such effects. No other adverse effects have been reported with picrorhiza. Although the use of the herb is not discouraged in India during pregnancy and breast-feeding, there is little information to determine the safety of the herb during these times. Certain medicines may interact with picrorhiza.

PHARMACOLOGY

Alcohloic extract of the plant and kutkin possess hepato-protective activity. Plant is a potent immunostimulant of both cell mediated and humoral immunity and exhibits choleretic activity in dogs. Picrorhiza kurroa is also benefical in the management of bronchial asthma.

DOSAGE

Three to four gram of drug is generally given as antiperiodic and 0.6-1.2 gm as bitter tonic. Typical adult dosage is 400 to 1500 mg/day, with dosages up to 3.5 gm/day sometimes being recommended for fevers.

DIOSCOREA

Botanical Name	:	*Dioscorea*
Family	:	Dioscoreaceae
Common Name	:	Chinese yam, Sha yao

There are several herbs derived from species of Dioscorea used in Chinese herb formulas, though only two are used with some frequency. By far the most common is Dioscorea opposita (= Dioscorea batatas), for which the rhizome (tuber) is used; it is called *shan yao* (mountain herb). This is in the "yam" family, and the herb is sometimes simply referred to as "Chinese yam."

DESCRIPTION

They are tuberous herbaceous perennial lianas, growing to 2-12 m or more tall.

The *leaves* are spirally arranged, mostly broad heart-shaped.

The *flowers* are individually inconspicuous, greenish-yellow, with six petals; they are mostly dioecious, with separate male and female plants, though a few species are monoecious, with male and female flowers on the same plant.

The *fruit* is a capsule in most species, a soft berry in a few species.

SPECIES OR VARIETIES

Yam is the common name for some species in the genus *Dioscorea* (family *Dioscoreaceae*). These are perennial herbaceous vines cultivated for the consumption of their starchy tubers in Africa, Asia, Latin America and Oceania. There are hundreds of cultivars among the cultivated species.

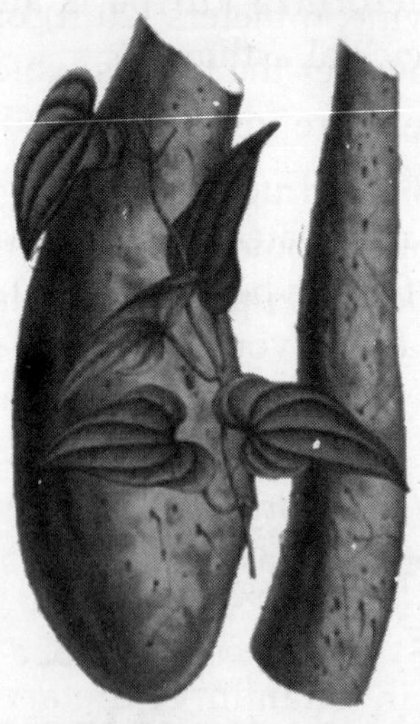

Fig. 26.3: Dioscorea

The *sweet potato* (*Ipomoea batatas*) has traditionally been referred to as a "yam" in parts of the southern United States and Canada, but it is not part of the Dioscoreaceae family.

Shan yao is used extensively in formulas for tonifying the kidney, often combined with rehmannia and cornus for that purpose. Like rehmannia, dioscorea nourishes yin; like cornus, it is an essence astringent.

Dioscorea alata, called "water yam", "winged yam" and "purple yam", was first cultivated in Southeast Asia. Although not grown in the same quantities as the African yams, it has the largest distribution world-wide of any cultivated yam, being grown in Asia, the Pacific islands, Africa, and the West Indies. In the United States it has become an invasive species in some Southern states.

Dioscorea opposita, "Chinese yam", is native to China. The Chinese yam plant is somewhat smaller than the African, with the vines about 3 meters (10 feet) long. It is tolerant to frost and can be grown in much cooler conditions than other yams. It is now grown in China, Korea, and Japan.

Dioscorea bulbifera, the "air potato", is found in both Africa and Asia, with slight differences between those found in each place. It is a large vine, 6 meters (20 ft) or more in length. It produces tubers; however the bulbils which grow at the base of its leaves are the more important food product. They are about the size of potatoes.

Some varieties can be eaten raw while some require soaking or boiling for detoxification before eating. It is not grown much commercially since the flavour of other yams is preferred by most people. However, it is popular in home vegetable gardens because it produces a crop after only four months of growth and continues producing for the life of the vine, as long as two years. Also the bulbils are easy to harvest and cook.

NUTRITIONAL VALUE

Yams are high in Vitamin C, dietary fibre, Vitamin B_6, potassium, and manganese; while being low in saturated fat and sodium. Vitamin C, dietary fibre and Vitamin B6 may all promote good health. Furthermore, a product that is high in potassium and low in sodium is likely to produce a good potassium-sodium balance in the human body, and so protect against osteoporosis and heart disease. Having a low level of saturated fat is also helpful for protection against heart disease.

LINSEED

Botanical Name	:	*Linum usitatissimum*
Family	:	Linaceae
Parts Used	:	Seed
Common Name	:	Alsi

HABITAT

Linseed (*Linum usitatissimum* L.) belongs to the family *Linaceae* and the genus Linum which has 100 species. It has been grown from ancient times for fibre (flax) and for its seed which is rich in oil. The oldest regions of cultivated flax are reported to be in Asia and on the Mediterranean coast.

DISCRIPTION

Linseed is a bushy annual plant, with erect, slender stems that grows up to 30 cm in height. It has alternate, stalkless leaves and blue flowers in loose clusters. The fruits are roundish and 10 celled. Each cell contains one seed which is oval, smooth, shining and usually brown coloured.

Linseed is grown both for its seed oil and for its fibres. It is one of the first crops to be cultivated for its oil bark *fibre* and *flax*. Linseed oil is a yellowish drying oil extracted from the dried ripe seeds of the linseed plant.

AREA AND DISTRIBUTION

Linseed is extensively grown in the countries of the temperate zone as well as in those of the tropical zone. The major linseed-growing countries are Argentina, the U.S.S.R., India, the U.S.A., Canada, Pakistan and Australia. India accounts for about 1.9 million hectares, with a seed production of 4.98 lakhs of tonnes and occupies the third rank among the linseed-producing countries. Australia and Canada have the highest productivity of about 7 quintals per hectare, whereas India averages 255 kg per hac. This yield is the lowest in the world.

In India, Madhya Pradesh leads in yield and acreage, followed by Uttar Pradesh and Maharashtra, Bihar, Rajasthan, Karnataka and West Bengal also grow linseed in large areas. Madhya Pradesh and Uttar Pradesh together contribute to the national linseed production to the extent of about 70 per cent.

CLIMATE AND SOIL

Linseed is grown in the range of latitudes between the 10th and 65th parallels, both north and south. Its cultivation is confined to low elevations, but it can he successfully grown up to 770 metres. Areas with the annual rainfall ranging from 45-75 cm are best suited for its cultivation. The seed crop does well under moderate cold, but the fibre crop grows best in cool moist climates. In India, the crop is grown in the *rabi season* from September-October to February-March.

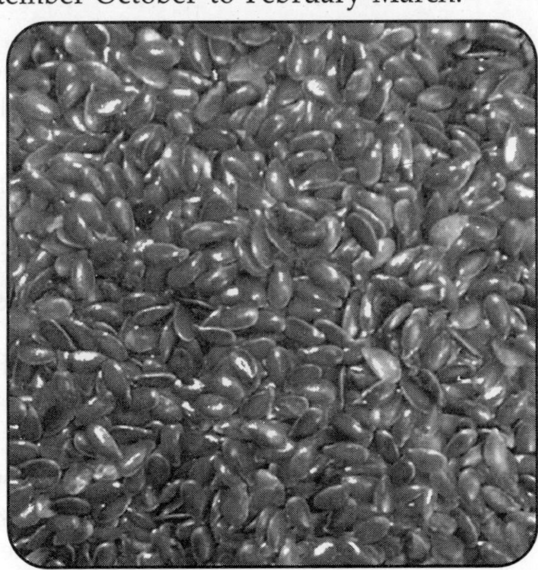

Fig. 26.4: Linseed

Linseed can be grown on different kinds of soils, except the sandy and badly drained heavy clays or clay loams. It does well on the deep clayey black soils of central and peninsular India and on the alluvium loams of the Indo-Gangetic plains.

CULTIVATION

The main season for sowing linseed is October to November, depending upon the cessation of the rains. The crop is grown either broadcast or is drilled in lines 20 to 30 cm apart. In the case of broadcasting, which includes utera sowing also, the seed-rate is kept at 40 kg per ha. For line-sowing, the seed-rate varies from 20 to 510 kg per ha, depending upon the seed size. Thin sowing gives a good number of tillers, but for fibre and weed, thick sowing is desirable.

The deep placement of fertilizer at sowing in the case of the rainfed crop gives better results. Under irrigated conditions, nitrogen is applied in two splits, half the dose as basal and the other half at the first irrigation, 40 to 50 days after sowing. The utera crop is fertilized at the rate of 10 kg of N per ha applied at the time of sowing. The rainfed crop generally requires no interculture. When the crop is irrigated, one weeding becomes essential.

MEDICINAL USES

Linseed oil is an excellent herbal oil that can be applied externally or taken internally as a medicine. Linseed oil is an excellent herbal oil that can be applied externally or taken internally as a medicine. Linseed oil contains Omega-3 fatty acids that help in curing disease like cancer.

It is also helpful in treating arthritis, coronary heart diseases and stroke, hypertension and inflammatory and autoimmune disorders, asthma. If used continuously this oil provide complete relieve in premenstrual syndrome. Oil of linseed is also used as a laxative. It is also used in many medicinal preparation along with other herbs.

SHATAVARI

Botanical Name	:	*Asparagus racemosus*
Family	:	Liliaceous
Part Used	:	Roots
Common Name	:	Satavari

DESCRIPTION

Asparagus racemosus, commonly known as *Satavari* in India is a climbing plant from *liliaceous* family. It widely grows in low forest areas throughout India.

A tall climber with thin leaves. Roots are white, long and tapering at both ends. These roots come out in bunches and spread in the earth. Older plants have longer and thicker roots. Small white and fragrant flowers appear on this plant in the beginning of the rainy season. Fruits in the shape of small berries appear in the autumn.

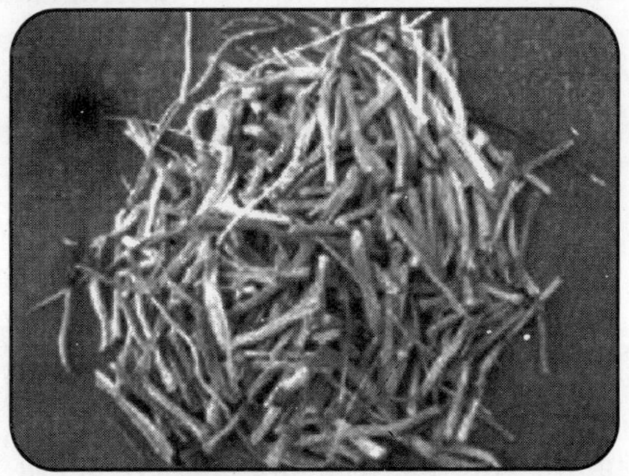

Fig. 26.5: Satavari

CHEMICAL CONSTITUENTS

The plant contains *triterpene saponins* - Shatavarin I - IV, which are phytoestrogen compounds. The plant's action as a galactagogue has been reported. In a study it was shown that in the estrogen—primed rats, Asparagus racemosus could cause both increase in the weight of mammary lobulo - alveolar tissue and the milk yield. Antioxytocic and anti ADH activity in the saponin fractions isolated from the roots of Asparagus racemosus has been observed. A study on the plant was shown to posses anabolic properties viz. growth promotion. The plant is also considered as an adaptogenic substance. Clinical efficacy of root powder evaluated in patients with duodenal ulcer.

MEDICINAL USES

In Ayurveda this amazing herb is known as the "*Queen of Herbs*" because it promotes love and devotion Shatavari has a strong rejuvenating, nurturing, and stabilizing effect on excessive *air, gas, dryness* and agitation in the *body* and *mind*. As such it is traditionally used for *nervousness, anorexia, insomnia,* hyperactive children, and people who are *underweight*.

It is known as the Indian *Female Rejuvenative*, as it is helpful in cases of low milk production, low sex drive, menopause, PMS, and infertility. It helps to balance hormonal system of women and regulates menstruation and ovulation.

It promotes positive emotions while calming airy sensitivity and the fiery emotions such as irritability, anger, jealousy, resentment, and hatred. It also helps with *pain, agitated sleep, disturbing dreams,* and those who have weak emotional and physical heart.

Asparagus racemosus is a potent *immunostimulant;* well-established pharmacological properties of *Asparagus racemosus* include adaptogenic, *antioxidant, antiallergic, immuno-stimulation, uterine relaxation, anticancer, antiulcer, antimicrobial.*

Preclinical studies investigating the effect of *Asparagus racemosus* against the *myelosuppressive* effects of single and multiple doses of cyclophosphamide in mice shows that *Asparagus racemosus* prevented, to a significant degree, leucopenia produced by cyclophosphamide.

In Ayurvedic system of medicine Shatavari is indicated as *brain tonic,* epilepsy and for Vata disorders.

It also indicated in Ayurveda for general weakness due to prolong illnesses. Improves immunity and protects heart, brain and other vital organs of body.

SHANKPUSHPI

Botanical Name : *Convolvulus pluricaulis*
Family : Convolvulus
Common Name : Shankpushpi

DESCRIPTION

Shankhapushpi or scientifically known as *Convolvulus pluricaulis*. Shankhpushpi is a prostrate, spreading, perennial, wild herb commonly found on sandy or rocky ground under xerophytes conditions in northern India.

Shankhpushpi's flowers are blue in colour and the leaves, which are elliptic in shape, are located at alternate positions with branches or flowers.

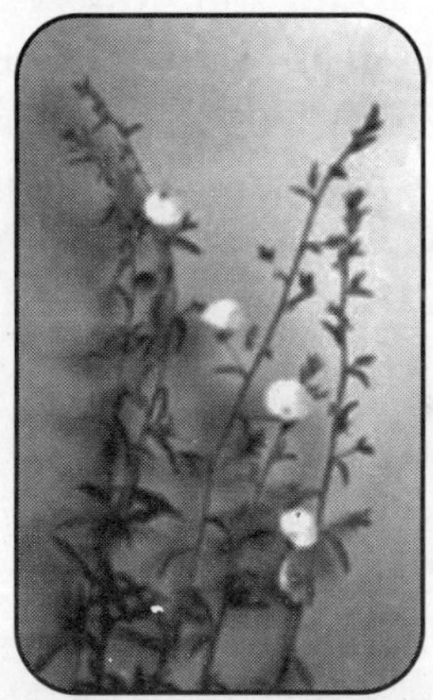

Fig. 26.6: Convolvulus pluricaulis

MEDICINAL USES

The extract of the plant helps in *reducing cholesterol levels* in blood including triglycerides, phospholipids and fatty acids. The whole herb is used medicinally in the form of decoction with cumin and milk in fever, *nervous weakness, loss of memory,* also in *syphilis* and *scrofula.*

Shankhpushpi is used as a *brain tonic.* The plant is reported to be a *prominent memory improving drug.* It is used as a *psycho stimulant* and *tranquilizer.*

PYRETHRUM

Botanical Name	:	*Chrysanthemum*
Family	:	Compositae
Parts Used	:	Root
Common Name	:	Pyrethrum

Pyrethrum is regarded as a section of the genus *Chrysanthemum*, family *Compositae*. Besides their ornamental importance, pyrethrum flowers have been widely used as a source material for preparation of insecticides. Being non-poisonous to man pyrethrum is particularly adapted for controlling household insects, however its use for preparing horticultural dusts and sprays, and livestock sprays is no less popular.

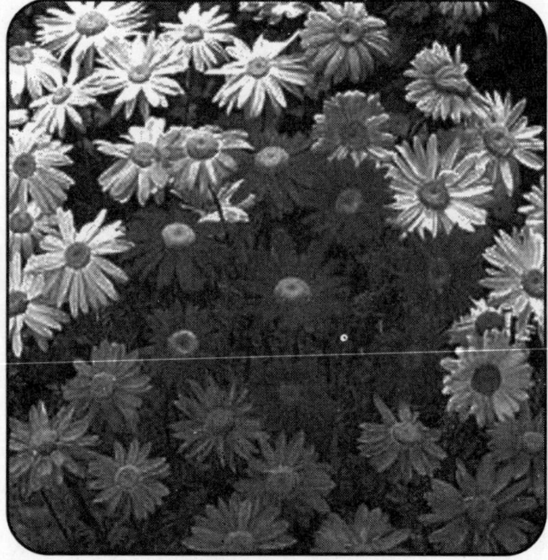

Fig. 26.7: Pyrethrum

Pyrethrum refers to several Old World plants of the genus *Chrysanthemum* (e.g., *C. coccineum*) which are cultivated as ornamentals for their showy flower heads. It is also the name of a natural insecticide made from the dried flower heads of *C. cinerariifolium* and *C. coccineum*. Pyrethrum was used for centuries as an insecticide and as a lice remedy in the Middle East.

C. cinerariifolium is called the *Dalmatian chrysanthemum,* denoting its origin in that region of the Balkans (Dalmatia). It looks more like the common daisy than other pyrethrums. Its flowers, typically white with a yellow center, grow from numerous fairly rigid stems. Plants have blue-green leaves and grow to between 45 to 60 cm in height. The plant is economically important as a natural source of insecticide. The flowers are pulverized and the active components called pyrethrins, contained in the seed cases, are extracted and sold in the form of an oleoresin. This is applied as a suspension in water or oil, or as a powder. Pyrethrins attack the nervous systems of all insects, and inhibit female mosquitoes from biting. When not present in amounts fatal to insects, they still appear to have an insect repellent effect. They are harmful to fish, but are far less toxic to mammals and birds than many synthetic insecticides and are non-persistent, being biodegradable and also breaking down easily on exposure to light. They are considered to be amongst the safest insecticides for use around food. Kenya produced 90% (over 6,000 tonnes) of the world's pyrethrum in 1998, called py for short. Production in Tanzania and Ecuador is also significant.

C. coccineum, the *Persian chrysanthemum,* is native to Caucasus and looks somewhat like a daisy. It produces large white, pink or red flowers.

The *leaves* resemble those of ferns, and the plant grows to between 30 and 60 cm in height.

The *flowering period* is June to July in temperate climates (Northern hemisphere). *C. coccineum* also contains insecticidal pyrethrum substances but it is a poor source compared to *C. cinerariifolium.*

Other species such as *C. balsamita* and *C. marshalli* also contain insecticidal substances, but are less effective than the two species mentioned above.

Pyrethroids are synthetic insecticides based on natural pyrethrum (pyrethrins); one common example is permethrin.

A common formulation of pyrethrin is in preparations containing the synthetic chemical piperonyl butoxide: this has the effect of enhancing the toxicity to insects and speeding the effects when compared with pyrethrins used alone. These formulations are known as *synergized pyrethrins*.

TOBACCO

Botanical Name	:	*Nicotiana tobaccum*
Family	:	Solanaceae
Parts Used	:	Leaf and Stem
Common Name	:	Tobacco, Tamakhu

DESCRIPTION

The *Nicotiana tobaccum* plant (smoking tobacco) comes from the kingdom *Plantae,* and subkingdom *Tracheobionta* (vascular plants).It is also a Spermatophyte which mean "seed plant" and is also considered a Magnoliophyte (flowering plant). Its subclass is Asterides, and comes from the *Solanaceae* family (potato family). The plants genus is *Nicotiana* (tobacco) and similarly its species is the *Nicotiana tabacum* (cultivated tobacco).

Tobacco is related to many other plants which include; vegetables, flowers, weeds, and poisonous herbs like potatoes, tomatoes, eggplant, and petunias. The plant family is *Solanceae* and the genus, Nicotiana contains about 100 different species, however only two of them have been heavily cultivated.

The Nicotiana tobaccum plant is an annual herb that ranges from 0.9-2 m tall. The leaves are elliptic in shape; the flowers grow in clusters at the end of each branch and range from white to light red in colour and form globular seeds. The plant itself is a stalk with large leaves drooping off the main stem. It also has a short root that branches into a very dense root system. The crop can take between 2-5 months before it is ready to be harvested.

Tobaccum is quite sensitive to temperature, air and ground humidity, as well as the type of land. A temperature of 20-30 degrees Celsius is best and for best growth, a humidity of 80-85% and soil without a high level of nitrogen are also needed.

The plant is native to tropical and subtropical American conditions, but is now grown commercially worldwide. The plant is mostly grown in the eastern United States, Brazil, and Argentina. And is often found on dry grasslands, clearings, and along the edges of forests and roads in natural form as well as in cultivated areas.

PLANT PRODUCTS

The nicotine in the tobacco can be used as an effective insecticide, as it is completely biodegradable. Tobacco is also used in enemas for the treatment is intestinal worms or constipation. And lastly, the most common use is the dried tobacco leaves used for chewing, snuffing, or smoking (cigarettes). There are also many other products that use nicotine to help people stop smoking (Patches, gum, etc.).

PROPERTIES

The most valuable part of the plant used is the nicotine, which is found in all parts except the seed. The concentration of nicotine increases with the age of the plant. A mature plant has about 64% nicotine in the leaves, 18% in the stem, 13% in the root, and 5% in the flowers. The chemical structure of nicotine consists of pyridine and pyrrolidine ring. Another chemical property is Anabaseine, an alkaloid similar to nicotine. The physical properties are also very distinct. Nicotine is colourless to pale yellow, very oily and has an unpleasant odour and sharp burning taste. It also slowly becomes brown after it is exposed to light or air. It is soluble in water, alcohol, chloroform, ether, kerosene, and some fixed oils. It should be stored in an airtight container and protected from light.

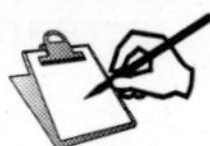

STUDY QUESTIONS

1. Write short notes on the following:
   (a) Dioscorea;

(b) Shatavari;
(c) Linseed; and
(d) Pyrethrum.

2. Write down the antibacterial and antifungal property of Garlic.
3. Discuss the medicinal properties of linseed oil.

27

CHAPTER

Collection and Preparation of Crude Drugs for the Market

COLLECTION AND PREPARATION OF MATERIAL

The first step in the collection of medicinal plants is to acquaint oneself with the market demands. Dealers in crude botanical drugs usually publish lists of the plants they handle and indicate the general range of prices. With such information at hand, and with the aid of this publication, the prospective collector should be able to determine which plants found in his locality offer the best opportunity for profit.

It frequently happens that after gathering considerable quantities of some plant the collector finds that the market is fully supplied at the time and either there is no sale for it or it can be sold only at a price that will not compensate him for his labor. Such a situation may usually be avoided by first submitting representative samples of the material to be collected, together with a statement of the approximate quantity that can be furnished, to a number of reliable dealers. This will generally bring information concerning the market possibilities and the returns that may be expected. Such procedure is especially recommended in the case of plants that are liable to deteriorate in a relatively short time, making it inadvisable to hold them until market conditions improve. Some of the dealers in crude drugs are willing to cooperate in this way with collectors, in order to prevent loss through overcollection and to encourage the collection of adequate supplies of the most-needed plants.

The medicinal value of botanical drugs depends to a large extent on the time of their collection. Roots from annual plants should generally be dug just before the flowering period; those of biennial and perennial plants should be gathered late in the fall or early in the spring, because during the growing season they are deficient in their active constituents and are of poorer quality generally. Barks also should preferably be collected during the dormant season when the sap is not flowing. Leaves and herbs are of most value when collected during the flowering period or just before they have finished growing. Flowers should always be gathered when they first open. Wherever definite information on these points has been available it has been included in the discussion of the various plants.

The proper preparation of the collected material is of the utmost importance. If the material contains dirt or other foreign matter, or if it is moldy or has an undesirable colour or odour, it may be rejected by the dealers or purchased only at a reduced price. Roots should be thoroughly freed from adhering soil and other dirt. Fibrous roots, or rootstocks with numerous small roots or rootless, require careful washing to remove such foreign matter. The larger stems of herbs and leaves should be discarded, as they possess little or no value, and leaves that are partly dried from age or that are discoloured or injured by disease or insects should be excluded if the best price is to be obtained.

The material must be carefully dried. All plant material, in whatever form, is easily spoiled in both appearance and value if improper methods are used to remove the large quantity of moisture that is usually present. Fleshy roots dry very slowly and frequently become moldy unless they are sliced across or lengthwise to permit more rapid evaporation of the moisture. In the drug market such roots occur in various forms, and information on this point should be secured from the dealers or from experienced collectors so that the dried material may conform to market requirements. Leaves readily lose their green colour while drying and sometimes become brown or even black. They should, therefore, be spread out in a well-ventilated room, especially in cloudy weather, and dried as rapidly as possible. Exposure to direct bright sunlight is undesirable because it frequently causes bleaching of the leaves. Fruits, particularly those that are juicy, are especially difficult to handle on account of their tendency to become sour or moldy. They should preferably be spread out in thin layers on wire or cloth screens that will permit a thorough circulation of air end on which they can be frequently stirred. Seeds must be thoroughly cured; even ripe seeds that appear to be dry will frequently heat and spoil if stored without having been spread out and allowed to dry for at least several days.

The best way to store the dried material is to pack it in clean bags or boxes. If, however, the material is likely to be injured by exposure to air or light, or if it is subject to the attack of insects, it should be placed in tightly closed cans or other receptacles and marketed at the earliest opportunity.

COLLECTION AND PREPARATION OF CRUDE DRUGS FROM MARKET

A pharmaceutical drug, also referred to as medicine, medication or medicament, can be loosely defined as any chemical substance intended for use in the medical diagnosis, cure, treatment, or prevention of disease. Medications can be classified in various ways, such as by chemical properties, mode or route of administration, biological system affected, or therapeutic effects. An elaborate and widely used classification system is the *Anatomical Therapeutic Chemical Classification System* (ATC system).

In the fields of medicine, biotechnology and pharmacology, drug discovery is the process by which drugs are designed. In the past most drugs have been discovered either by identifying the active ingredient from traditional remedies or by serendipitous discovery. A new approach has been to understand how disease and infection are controlled at the molecular and physiological level and to target specific entities based on this knowledge.

The process of drug design involves the identification of candidates, synthesis, characterization, screening, and assays for therapeutic efficacy. Once a compound has shown its value in these tests, it will begin the process of drug development prior to clinical trials.

Despite advances in technology and understanding of biological systems, drug discovery is still a lengthy, "expensive, difficult, and inefficient process" with low rate of new therapeutic discovery. Information on the human genome, its sequence and what it encodes has been hailed as a potential windfall for drug discovery, promising to virtually eliminate the bottleneck in therapeutic targets that has been one limiting factor on the rate of therapeutic discovery. However, data indicates that "new targets" as opposed to "established targets" are more prone to drug discovery project failure in general. This data corroborates some thinking underlying a pharmaceutical industry trend beginning at the turn of the twenty-first century and continuing today which finds more risk aversion in target selection among multi-national pharmaceutical companies.

SCREENING AND DESIGN

The process of finding a new drug against a chosen target for a particular disease usually involves High-Throughput Screening (HTS), wherein large libraries of chemicals are tested for their ability to modify the target. For example, if the target is a novel GPCR, compounds will be screened for their ability to inhibit or stimulate that receptor: if the target is a protein kinase, the chemicals will be tested for their ability to inhibit that kinase.

Another important function of HTS is to show how selective the compounds are for the chosen target. The ideal is to find a molecule which will interfere with only the chosen target, but not other, related targets. To this end, other screening runs will be made to see whether the "hits" against the chosen target will interfere with other related targets this is the process of cross-screening. Cross-screening is important, because the more unrelated targets a compound hits, the more likely that off-target toxicity will occur with that compound once it reaches the clinic.

It is very unlikely that a perfect drug candidate will emerge from these early screening runs. It is more often observed that several compounds are found to have some degree of activity, and if these compounds share common chemical features, one or more pharmacophores can then be developed. At this point, medicinal chemists will attempt to use Structure-Activity Relationships (SAR) to improve certain features of the lead compound:

- increase activity against the chosen target.
- reduce activity against unrelated targets.
- improve the "drug-like" or ADME properties of the molecule.

This process will require several iterative screening runs, during which, it is hoped, the properties of the new molecular entities will improve, and allow the favoured compounds to go forward to in vitro and in vivo testing for activity in the disease model of choice.

While HTS is a commonly used method for novel drug discovery, it is not the only method. It is often possible to start from a molecule which already has some of the desired properties. Such a molecule might be extracted from a natural product or even be a drug on the market which could be improved upon (so-called "me too" drugs). Other methods, such as virtual high throughput screening, where screening is done using computer-generated models and attempting to "dock" virtual libraries to a target, are also often used.

Another important method for drug discovery is drug design, whereby the biological and physical properties of the target are studied, and a prediction is made of the sorts of chemicals that might fit into an active site. Novel pharmacophores can emerge very rapidly from these exercises.

Once a lead compound series has been established with sufficient target potency and selectivity and favourable drug-like properties, one or two compounds will then be proposed for drug development. The best of these is generally called the lead compound, while the other will be designated as the "backup".

CHEMICAL DIVERSITY OF NATURAL PRODUCTS

As above mentioned, combinatorial chemistry was a key technology enabling the efficient generation of large screening libraries for the needs of high-throughput screening. However, now, after two decades of combinatorial chemistry, it has been pointed out that despite the increased efficiency in chemical synthesis, no increase in lead or drug candidates has been reached. This has led to analysis of chemical characteristics of combinatorial chemistry products, compared to existing drugs and/or natural products. The chemoinformatics concept chemical diversity, depicted as distribution of compounds in the chemical space based on their physicochemical characteristics, is often used to describe the difference between the combinatorial chemistry libraries and natural products. The synthetic, combinatorial library compounds seem to cover only a limited and quite uniform chemical space, whereas existing drugs and particularly natural products, exhibit much greater chemical diversity, distributing more evenly to the chemical space. The most prominent differences between natural products and compounds in combinatorial chemistry libraries is the number of chiral centers (much higher in natural compounds), structure rigidity (higher in natural compounds) and number of aromatic moieties (higher in combinatorial chemistry libraries). Other chemical differences between these two groups include the nature of heteroatoms (O and N enriched in natural products, and S and halogen atoms more often present in synthetic compounds), as well as level of non-aromatic unsaturation (higher in natural products). As both structure rigidity and chirality are both well-established factors in medicinal chemistry known to enhance compounds specificity and efficacy as a drug, it has been suggested that natural products compare favourable to today's combinatorial chemistry libraries as potential lead molecules.

STRUCTURAL ELUCIDATION

The elucidation of the chemical structure is critical to avoid the re-discovery of a chemical agent that is already known for its structure and chemical activity. Mass spectrometry, often used to determine structure, is a method in which individual compounds are identified based on their mass/charge ratio, after ionization. Chemical compounds exist in nature as mixtures, so the combination of Liquid Chromatography and Mass Spectrometry (LC-MS) is often used to separate the individual chemicals. Databases of mass spectras for known compounds are available. Nuclear Magnetic Resonance Spectroscopy (NMRS) is another important technique for determining chemical structures of natural products. NMRS yields information about individual hydrogen and carbon atoms in the structure, allowing detailed reconstruction of the molecule's architecture.

Drug development is a blanket term used to define the entire process of bringing a new drug or device to the market. It includes drug discovery/product development, pre-clinical research (micro-organisms/animals) and clinical trials (on humans). Few people still refer to the drug developent as mere preclinical development.

Drug development is required to establish the physicochemical properties of the NCE: its chemical makeup, stability, solubility. The process by which the chemical is made will be optimized so that from being made at the bench on a milligram scale by a synthetic chemist, it can be manufactured on the kilogram and then on the ton scale. It will be further examined for its suitability to be made into capsules, tablets, aeresol, intramuscular injectable, subcuteneous injectable, or intravenous formulations. Together these processes are known in *preclinical development* as Chemistry, Manufacturing and Control (CMC).

Many aspects of drug development are focused on satisfying the regulatory requirements of drug licensing authorities. These generally constitute a number of tests designed to determine the major toxicities of a novel compound prior to first use in man. It is a legal requirement that an assessment of major organ toxicity be performed (effects on the heart and lungs, brain, kidney, liver and digestive system), as well as effects on other parts of the body that might be affected by the drug (e.g., the skin if the new drug is to be delivered through the skin). While, increasingly, these tests can be made using in vitro methods (e.g., with isolated cells), many tests can only be made by using experimental animals, since it is only in an intact organism that the complex interplay of metabolism and drug exposure on toxicity can be examined.

The process of drug development does not stop once an NCE begins human clinical trials. In addition to the tests required to move a novel drug into the clinic for the first time it is also important to ensure that long-term or chronic toxicities are determined, as well as effects on systems not previously monitored (fertility, reproduction, immune system, etc.). The compound will also be tested for its ability to cause cancer (carcinogenicity testing).

PHARMACEUTICAL MARKETING

Pharmaceutical marketing is the business of advertising or otherwise promoting the sale of pharmaceuticals or drugs. The marketing of medication has a long history. The sale of miracle cures, many with little real potency, has always been common. Marketing of legitimate non-prescription medications, such as pain relievers or allergy medicine, has also long been practiced. Mass marketing of prescription medications was rare until recently, however. It was long believed that since doctors made the selection of drugs, mass marketing was a waste of resources; specific ads targeting the medical profession were thought to be cheaper and just as effective.This would involve ads in professional journals and visits by sales staff to doctor's offices and hospitals. An important part of these efforts was marketing to medical students.

DIRECT AND INDIRECT MARKETING TO HEALTH CARE PROVIDERS

Physicians are perhaps the most important component in pharmaceutical sales. They write the prescriptions that determine which drugs will be used by the patient. Influencing the physician is the key to pharmaceutical sales. Historically, this was done by a large pharmaceutical sales force. A medium-sized pharmaceutical company might have a sales force of 1000 representatives. The largest companies have tens of thousands of representatives around the world. Sales representatives called upon physicians regularly, providing information and free drug samples to the physicians. This is still the approach today; however, economic pressures on the industry are causing pharmaceutical companies to rethink the traditional sales process to physicians.

Pharmaceutical companies are developing processes to influence the people who influence the physicians. There are several channels by which a physician may be influenced, including self-influence through research, peer influence, direct interaction with pharmaceutical companies, patients, and public instruments that can be used to determine the influencers and buying motives of physicians. There are a number of firms that specialize in data and analytics for pharmaceutical marketing.

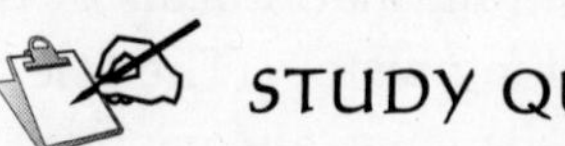

STUDY QUESTIONS

Write short notes on the following:

(a) Collection and preparation of crude drugs from the market; and

(b) Pharmaceutical marketing.

28

CHAPTER

Fibres, Surgical Dressing an Sutures

FIBRE

Fibre, also spelled fibre, is a class of materials that are continuous filaments or are in discrete elongated pieces, similar to lengths of thread. They are very important in the biology of both plants and animals, for holding tissues together. Human uses for fibres are diverse. They can be spun into filaments, string or rope, used as a component of composite materials, or matted into sheets to make products such as paper or felt. Fibres are often used in the manufacture of other materials. Synthetic fibres can be produced very cheaply and in large amounts compared to natural fibres, but natural fibres enjoy some benefits, such as comfort, over their man-made counterparts.

CLASSIFICATION OF FIBRE

Natural Fibres

Natural fibres include those produced by plants, animals, and geological processes. They are biodegradable over time. They can be classified according to their origin:

- **Vegetable fibres** are generally based on arrangements of cellulose, often with lignin: examples include cotton, hemp, jute, flax, ramie, and sisal. Plant fibres are employed in the manufacture of paper and textile (cloth), and dietary fibre is an important component of human nutrition.
- **Wood fibre**, distinguished from vegetable fibre, is from tree sources. Forms include groundwood, thermo-mechanical pulp (TMP) and bleached or unbleached kraft or sulfite pulps. Kraft and sulfite, also called sulphite, refer to the type of pulping process used to remove the lignin bonding the original wood structure, thus freeing the fibres for use in paper and engineered wood products such as fibre board.
- **Animal fibres** consist largely of particular proteins. Instances are spider silk, sinew, catgut, wool and hair such as cashmere, mohair and angora, fur such as sheepskin, rabbit, mink, fox, beaver, etc.
- **Mineral fibres** comprise asbestos. Asbestos is the only naturally occurring long mineral fibre. Short, fibre-like minerals include wollastonite, attapulgite and halloysite.

1. HUMAN-MADE FIBRES

Synthetic or man-made fibres generally come from synthetic materials such as petrochemicals. But some types of synthetic fibres are manufactured from natural cellulose, including rayon, modal, and the more recently developed Lyocell. Cellulose-based fibre s are of two types, regenerated or pure cellulose such as from the cupro-ammonium process and modified cellulose such as the cellulose acetates.

Fibre classification in reinforced plastics falls into two classes:

(i) Short Fibres

It is also known as *discontinuous fibres*, with a general aspect ratio (defined as the ratio of fibre length to diameter) between 20 to 60.

(ii) Long Fibres

It is also known as *continuous fibres*, the general aspect ratio is between 200 to 500.

2. CELLULOSE FIBRES

Cellulose fibres are a subset of man-made fibres, regenerated from natural cellulose. The cellulose comes from various sources. Modal is made from beech trees, bamboo fibre is a cellulose fibre made from bamboo, soya silk is made from soyabeans, sea cell is made from seaweed, etc.

3. MINERAL FIBRES

Fibre glass, made from specific glass, and optical fibre, made from purified natural quartz, are also man-made fibres that come from natural raw materials.

Metallic fibres can be drawn from ductile metals such as copper, gold or silver and extruded or deposited from more brittle ones, such as nickel, aluminum or iron.

Carbon fibres are often based on carbonised polymers, but the end product is pure carbon.

4. POLYMER FIBRES

Polymer fibres are a subset of man-made fibres, which are based on synthetic chemicals (often from petrochemical sources) rather than arising from natural materials by a purely physical process. These fibres are made from:

- Polyamide nylon,
- PET or PBT polyester
- Phenol-formaldehyde (PF)
- Polyvinyl alcohol fibre (PVA)
- Polyvinyl chloride fibre (PVC)
- Polyolefins (PP and PE).
- **Acrylic polyesters,** pure polyester PAN fibres are used to make carbon fibre by roasting them in a low oxygen environment. Traditional acrylic fibre is used more often as a synthetic replacement for wool. Carbon fibres and PF

fibres are noted as two resin-based fibres that are not thermoplastic, most others can be melted.

- **Aromatic polyamids** (aramids) such as Twaron, Kevlar and Nomex thermally degrade at high temperatures and do not melt. These fibres have strong bonding between polymer chains
- **Polyethylene (PE),** eventually with extremely long chains/HMPE (e.g., Dyneema or Spectra).
- **Elastomers** can even be used, e.g., spandex although urethane fibres are starting to replace spandex technology.
- **Polyurethane fibre** Any of a class of very versatile polymers that are made into flexible and rigid foams, fibres, elastomers (elastic polymers), surface coatings, and adhesives. They are produced by reacting a diisocyanate (a compound with two functional groups of the type —NCO) with a diol (a compound with two hydroxyl, or —OH, groups). Foamed polyurethanes, used for insulation and mattress and upholstery filler, are made with organic compounds containing carboxyl groups, causing a reaction that liberates carbon dioxide bubbles throughout the product.
- **Coextruded fibres** have two distinct polymers forming the fibre usually as a core-sheath or side-by-side. Coated fibres exist such as nickel-coated to provide static elimination, silver-coated to provide anti-bacterial properties and aluminum-coated to provide RF deflection for radar chaff. Radar chaff is actually a spool of continuous glass tow that has been aluminum coated. An aircraft-mounted high speed cutter chops it up as it spews from a moving aircraft to confuse radar signals.

5. MICROFIBRES

Microfibres in textiles refer to sub-denier fibre (such as polyester drawn to 0.5 dn or Denier). Denier and Detex are two measurements of fibre yield based on weight and length. If the fibre density is known you also have a fibre diameter, otherwise it is simpler to measure diameters in micrometers. Microfibres in technical fibres refer to ultra fine fibres (glass or meltblown thermo-plastics) often used in filtration. Newer fibre designs include extruding fibre that splits into multiple finer fibres. Most synthetic fibres are round in cross-section, but special designs can be hollow, oval, star-shaped or trilobal. The latter design provides more optically reflective properties. Synthetic textile fibre s are often crimped to provide bulk in a woven, non-woven or knitted structure. Fibre surfaces can also be dull or bright. Dull surfaces reflect more light while bright tends to transmit light and make the fibre more transparent.

Very short and/or *irregular fibres* have been called **fibrils**. Natural cellulose, such as cotton or bleached kraft, show smaller fibrils jutting out and away from the main fibre structure.

GOSSYPIUM HERBACEUM

Botanical Name	:	*Gossypium herbaceum*
Family	:	Malveace
Parts Used	:	Bark, Seeds, Leaves, Flowers and Root bark
Common Name	:	Cotton and Kapas

HABITAT

It is the most widespread of all the species of old world cottons, being distributed throughout the rain-fed savannah areas from Africa, through Arabia and India, to China, Japan and East Indies.

DESCRIPTION

It includes perennial or annual, monopodial or sympodial shrubs, bearing slender trailing branches, which are often purplish in colour.

The *stem*, petiole and leaves are moderately hairy to almost glabrous.

The *leaves* are deeply cut into 3-7 lobes, the lobes are ovate, oblong or curvilinear and acute. The bracteoles are closely investing the bud and flower, triangular, longer than broad, entire or with 3-4 coarse teeth.

The *flowers* are purple, red, yellow or white, with or without red blotch at the base of petals. The capsules are tapering, profusely pitted, usually 3-4 locular, opening widely when ripe. The seeds are small, usually with two coats of hairs. The lint is white, grey or brown fuzz green, grey or white and uniformly distributed over the seed or confined to a tuft at each end.

CONSTITUENTS

Gossypium was isolated from the flowers and gossypetin 8-rhamnoside was isolated from the leaves.

PHARMACOLOGY

Gossypium shows analgesic and anti-inflammatory activity.

TOXICOLOGY

There is no adverse effect reported on the use of this plant as medicine.

INDICATIONS

It is used as aphrodisiac and in male sexual disorders. It is believed to increase the sexual function.

PROPERTIES AND USES

The preparation *Gossypium* is most excellent for diseases of the utero-genital organs. In these diseases it evinces its sole and only virtues, and it ought, on every occasion where it can be procured in its purity, to be used in the stead of ergot, or smut rye, in cases of difficult labor.

The latter will produce uterine inflammation and puerperal fever, while *Gossypium* will achieve the beneficial effects for which ergot is usually administered and leave the system perfectly free from any prejudicial after-results.

The active principle of fresh cotton root forms a most wonderful uterine tonic, and if correctly prepared, will be found invaluable in sterility, vaginitis, whites, menstrual irregularities, green sickness, etc. The seeds are said to possess superior anti-periodic properties.

FLAX

Botanical Name	:	*Linum usitatissimum*
Family	:	Linaceae (Linseed family)
Parts Used	:	Seed, Roots, Flowers and Oil
Common Name	:	Flax or Linseed

HABITAT

It is native to the region extending from the eastern Mediterranean to India and was probably first domesticated in the Fertile Crescent. This is called as *Jawas/Javas* or *Alashi* in Marathi.

CULTIVATION

Flax was extensively cultivated in ancient Egypt. New Zealand flax is not related to flax, but was named after it as both plants are used to produce fibres.

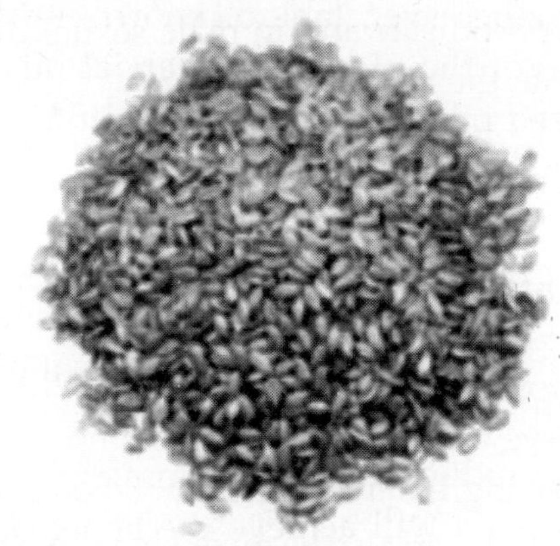

Fig. 28.1: Flex

DESCRIPTION

Flax is an erect annual plant growing to 1.2 m tall, with slender stems. The *leaves* are glaucous green, slender lanceolate, 20–40 mm long and 3 mm broad. The *flowers* are pure pale blue, 15–25 mm diameter, with five petals; they can also be bright red. The *fruit* is a round, dry capsule 5–9 mm diameter, containing several glossy brown seeds shaped like an apple pip, 4–7 mm long.

USES

Flax is grown both for its seeds and for its fibres. Various parts of the plant have been used to make fabric, dye, paper, medicines, fishing nets, hair gels and soap. It is also grown as an ornamental plant in gardens.

FLAX SEEDS

Flax seeds come in two basic varieties, brown and yellow or golden, with most types having similar nutritional values and equal amounts of short-chain omega-3 fatty acids. The exception is a type of yellow flax called **Linola** or *solin*, which has a completely different oil profile and is very low in omega-3. Although brown flax can be consumed as readily as yellow, and has been for thousands of years, it is better known as an ingredient in paints, fibre and cattle feed.

Flax seeds produce a vegetable oil known as *flaxseed* or *linseed oil*, which is one of the oldest commercial oils and solvent-processed flax seed oil has been used for centuries as a drying oil in painting and varnishing.

One hundred grams of ground flax seed supplies about 450 kilo-calories, 41 grams of fat, 28 grams of fibre, and 20 grams of protein.

One tablespoon of ground flax seeds and three tablespoons of water may serve as a replacement for one egg in baking by binding the other ingredients together.

Ground flax seeds can also be mixed in with oatmeal, yogurt, water (similar to Metamucil), or any other food item where a nutty flavour is appropriate. Flax seed sprouts are edible, with a slightly spicy flavour. Excessive consumption of flax seeds can cause diarrhea.

Flax seeds are chemically stable while whole, and milled flax seed can be stored at least four months at room temperature with minimal or no changes in taste, smell, or chemical markers of rancidity. Ground flax seed can go rancid at room temperature in as little as one week. Refrigeration and storage in sealed containers will keep ground flax from becoming rancid for even longer.

POSSIBLE MEDICAL BENEFITS

Flax seeds contain high levels of lignans and Omega-3 fatty acids. Lignans may benefit the heart, possess anti-cancer properties and studies performed on mice found reduced growth in specific types of tumors. Initial studies suggest that flaxseed taken in the diet may benefit individuals with certain types of breast and prostate cancers.

Aside from alpha linolenic acid, flax seed is rich in lignan. Lignan is a type phytoestrogen (antioxidant) and also provides fibre . Researches reveal that lignan in flax seed shows a lot of promise in fighting disease— including a possible role in cancer prevention especially breast cancer. It is thought that lignan metabolites can bind to estrogen receptors, hence inhibiting the onset of estrogen-stimulated breast cancer. Recent studies also showed positive benefits of flax seed oil in IBD (Crohn's Disease and Colitis). Flax seed oil seems to be able to heal the inner lining of the inflamed intestines.

CANNABIS SATIVA

Botanical Name	:	*Cannabis sativa*
Family	:	Cannabaceae
Parts Used	:	Flowers, Leaves, Seeds
Common Name	:	Marijuana

DESCRIPTION

It is an herb that has been used throughout recorded history by humans as a source of fibre, for its seed oil, as food, as a *drug*, as *medicine*, and for *spiritual purposes*. Each part of the plant is harvested differently, depending on the purpose of its use.

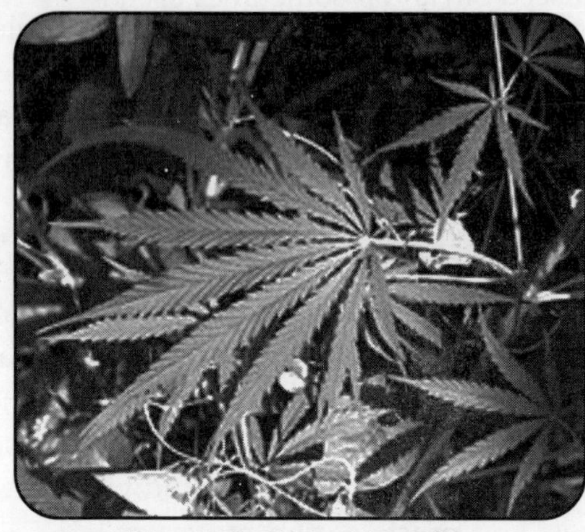

Fig. 28.2: Cannabis sativa

Its seed, chiefly used as caged-bird feed, is a valuable source of protein. The flowers (and to a lesser extent the leaves, stems, and seeds) contain psychoactive and physiologically active chemical compounds known as *cannabinoids* that are consumed for recreational, medicinal, and spiritual purposes.

When so used, preparations of flowers (*marijuana*) and leaves and preparations derived from resinous extract (hashish) are consumed by smoking, vapourizing and oral ingestion. Historically, tinctures, teas, and ointments have also been common preparations.

GENERAL USES

Hemp is used for a wide variety of purposes, including the manufacture of cordage of varying tensile strength, clothing, and nutritional products.

The bast fibre s can be used in 100% hemp products, but are commonly blended with other organic fibre s such as flax, cotton or silk, for apparel and furnishings, most commonly at a 55%/45% hemp/cotton blend.

The inner two fibre s of hemp are more woody, and are more often used in non-woven items and other industrial applications, such as mulch, animal bedding and litter.

The oil from the fruits "seeds") dries on exposure to air (similar to linseed oil) and is sometimes used in the manufacture of oil-based paints, in creams as a moisturizing agent, for cooking, and in plastics. Hemp seeds have been used in bird seed mix. Hempseed is also widely used as a fishing bait.

MEDICINAL USES

Hemp seed oil has *anti-inflammatory* properties. Hemp seed oil has been shown to relieve the symptoms of eczema (a topic dermatitis).

The *Hemp oil* can be used as part of a nutritional programme to maintain and improve good health. With a pleasant nutty flavour, Hemp seed oil is ideal for use in salad dressings, mayonnaise, dips etc. It is not suitable for frying as this reduces the benefits.

Hemp has had a long-standing relationship with humanity; modern science reveals that it contains all the essential amino acids and essential fatty acids necessary for human life, as well as a rare protein known as *globule edestins* that is very similar to the globulin found in human blood plasma.

JUTE

Botanical Name	:	*Corchorus capsularis*
Family	:	Tiliaceae
Parts Used	:	Stem, Leaves, Seeds
Common Name	:	Jute

DESCRIPTION

Jute is a long, soft, shiny vegetable fibre that can be spun into coarse, strong threads. It is produced from plants in the genus Corchorus (*Spp. olitorius, and Capsularis).*

Jute is one of the cheapest natural fibres and is second only to cotton in amount produced and variety of uses. Jute fibres are composed primarily of the plant materials cellulose (major component of plant fibre) and lignin (major components wood fibre). It is thus a ligno-cellulosic fibre that is partially a textile fibre and partially wood. It falls into the bast fibre category (fibre collected from bast or skin of the plant) along with kenaf, industrial hemp, flax (linen), ramie, etc. The industrial term for jute fibre is raw jute. The fibres are off-white to brown, and 1–4 meters (3–12 feet) long.

Jute fibre is often called *hessian*; jute fabrics are also called *hessian cloth* and *jute sacks* are called *gunny bags* in some European countries. The fabric made from jute is popularly known as burlap in North America.

CULTIVATION

Jute matting being used to prevent flood erosion while natural vegetation becomes established. For this purpose, a natural and biodegradable fibre is essential. Jute is a rain-fed crop with little need for fertilizer or pesticides. The production is concentrated in India and Bangladesh. The jute fibre comes from the stem and ribbon (outer skin) of the jute plant. The fibres are first extracted by retting. The retting process consists of bundling jute stems together and immersing them in low, running water. There are two types of retting: stem and ribbon. After the retting process, stripping begins. Women and children usually do this job. In the stripping process, non-fibrous matter is scraped off, then the workers dig in and grab the fibres from within the jute stem.

USES

Jute is the second most important vegetable fibre after cotton; not only for cultivation, but also for various uses. Jute is used chiefly to make cloth for wrapping bales of raw cotton, and to make sacks and coarse cloth. The fibres are also woven into curtains, chair coverings, carpets, area rugs, hessian cloth, and backing for linoleum.

While jute is being replaced by synthetic materials in many of these uses, some uses take advantage of jute's biodegradable nature, where synthetics would be unsuitable. Examples of such uses include containers for planting young trees which can be planted directly with the container without disturbing the roots, and land restoration where jute cloth prevents erosion occurring while natural vegetation becomes established.

The fibres are used alone or blended with other types of fibres to make twine and rope. Jute butts, the coarse ends of the plants, are used to make inexpensive cloth. Conversely, very fine threads of jute can be separated out and made into imitation silk. As jute fibres are also being used to make pulp and paper, and with increasing concern over forest destruction for the wood pulp used to make most paper, the importance of jute for this purpose may increase. Jute has a long history of use in the sackings, carpets, wrapping fabrics (cotton bale), and construction fabric manufacturing industry.

Traditionally jute was used in traditional textile machineries as textile fibres having cellulose (vegetable fibre content) and lignin (wood fibre content). But, the major breakthrough came when the automobile, pulp and paper, and the furniture and bedding industries started to use jute and its allied fibres with their non-woven and composite technology to manufacture nonwovens, technical textiles, and composites. Therefore, jute has changed its textile fibre outlook and steadily heading towards its newer identity, i.e., wood fibre. As a textile fibre, jute has reached its peak from where there is no hope of progress, but as a wood fibre jute has many promising features.

WOOL

Botanical Name	:	*Rubia cardifolia*
Family	:	Rubiaceae
Parts Used	:	Root, Stem and fruit
Common Name	:	Wool, Indian madder

Wool is the fibre derived from the specialized skin cells, called *follicles*, of animals in the *Caprinae* family, principally sheep, but the hair of certain species of other mammals such as goats, llamas, and rabbits may also be called *wool*. Wool has several qualities that distinguish it from hair or fur: it is crimped; it has a different texture or handle; it is elastic; and it grows in staples (clusters).

PROPERTIES

Wool's scaling and crimp make it easier to spin the fleece by helping the individual fibre s attach to each other, so that they stay together. Because of the crimp, wool fabrics have a greater bulk than other textiles, and retain air, which causes the product to retain heat. Insulation also works both ways; Bedouins and Tuaregs use wool clothes to keep the heat out.

The amount of crimp corresponds to the thickness of the wool fibre s. A fine wool like Merino may have up to a hundred crimps per inch, while the coarser wools like karakul may have as few as one to two crimps per inch. Hair, by contrast, has little if any scale and no crimp, and little ability to bind into yarn. On sheep, the hair part of the fleece is called kemp. The relative amounts of kemp to wool vary from breed to breed, and make some fleeces more desirable for spinning, felting, or carding into batts for quilts or other insulating products.

Wool fibre s are hygroscopic, meaning they readily absorb and give off moisture. Wool can absorb moisture almost one-third of its own weight. Wool absorbs sound like many other fabrics. Wool is generally a creamy white colour, although some breeds of sheep produce natural colours such as black, brown, silver, and random mixes.

Wool ignites at a higher temperature than cotton fibre s and some synthetics. It has lower rate of flame spread, low heat release, low heat of combustion, and does not melt or drip; it forms a char which is insulating and self-extinguishing, and contributes less to toxic gases and smoke than other flooring products, when used in carpets. Wool carpets are specified for high safety environments, such as trains and aircraft. Wool is usually specified for garments for fire-fighters, soldiers, and others in occupations where they are exposed to the likelihood of fire.

USES

In addition to clothing, wool has been used for blankets, horse rugs, saddle cloths, carpeting, felt, wool insulation and upholstery. Wool felt covers piano hammers, and it is used to absorb odors and noise in heavy machinery and stereo speakers. Ancient Greeks lined their helmets with felt, and Roman legionnaires used breastplates made of wool felt.

Wool has also been traditionally used to cover cloth diapers. Wool fibre exteriors are hydrophobic (repel water) and the interior of the wool fibre is hygroscopic (attracts water); this makes a wool garment able to cover a wet diaper while inhibiting wicking, so outer garments remain dry. Wool felted and treated with lanolin is water resistant, air permeable, and slightly antibacterial, so it resists the buildup of odor. Some modern cloth diapers use felted wool fabric for covers, and there are several modern commercial knitting patterns for wool diaper covers.

Merino wool has been used in baby sleep products such as swaddle baby wrap blankets and infant sleeping bags, because of its ability to regulate temperature, therefore reducing the risk of overheating and subsequent Sudden Infant Death Syndrome.

SILK

Silk is a natural protein fibre, some forms of which can be woven into textiles. The best-known type of silk is obtained from cocoons made by the larvae of the mulberry silkworm Bombyx mori reared in captivity (sericulture). The shimmering appearance of silk is due to the triangular prism-like structure of the silk fibre which allows silk cloth to refract incoming light at different angles thus producing different colours.

Silks are produced by several other insects, but only the silk of moth caterpillars has been used for textile manufacture. There has been some research into other silks, which differ at the molecular level. Silks are mainly produced by the larvae of insects that complete metamorphosis, but also by some adult insects such as webspinners. Silk production is especially common in the *Hymenoptera* (bees, wasps, and ants), and is sometimes used in nest construction. Other types of arthropod produce silk, most notably various arachnids such as spiders.

PROPERTIES

Silk is one of the strongest natural fibre s but loses up to 20% of its strength when wet. It has a good moisture regain of 11%. Its elasticity is moderate to poor: if elongated even a small amount it remains stretched. It can be weakened if exposed to too much sunlight. It may also be attacked by insects, especially if left dirty.

Silk is a poor conductor of electricity and thus susceptible to static cling.

Unwashed silk chiffon may shrink up to 8% due to a relaxation of the fibre macrostructure. So silk should either be pre-washed prior to garment construction, or dry cleaned. Dry cleaning may still shrink the chiffon up to 4%. Occasionally, this shrinkage can be reversed by a gentle steaming with a press cloth. There is almost no gradual shrinkage or shrinkage due to molecular-level deformation.

USES

Silk's good absorbency makes it comfortable to wear in warm weather and while active. Its low conductivity keeps warm air close to the skin during cold weather. It is often used for clothing such as shirts, blouses, formal dresses, high fashion clothes, negligees, pyjamas, robes, skirtsuits, sun dresses and kimonos.

Silk's elegant, soft luster and beautiful drape makes it perfect for many furnishing applications. It is used for upholstery, wall coverings, window treatments (if blended with another fibre), rugs, bedding and wall hangings. While on the decline now, due to artificial fibres, silk has had many industrial and commercial uses; parachutes, bicycle tires, comforter filling and artillery gunpowder bags. A special manufacturing process which removes the outer irritant sericin coating of the silk makes it suitable as non-absorbable surgical sutures. This process has also recently led to the introduction of specialist silk underclothing for children and adults with eczema where it can significantly reduce itch. Silk cloth is also used as a material on which to write and paint.

VISCOSE RAYON

Rayon is a manufactured regenerated cellulose fibre . Because it is produced from naturally occurring polymers, it is neither a truly synthetic fibre nor a natural fibre, it is a semi-synthetic fibre. Rayon is known by the names *viscose rayon* and art silk in the textile industry. It usually has a high lustre quality giving it a bright shine. Rayon contains the chemical elements carbon, hydrogen, and oxygen.

Rayon is a very versatile fibre and has the same comfort properties as natural fibres. It can imitate the feel and texture of silk, wool, cotton and linen. The fibres are easily dyed in a wide range of colours. Rayon fabrics are soft, smooth, cool, comfortable, and highly absorbent, but they do not insulate body heat, making them ideal for use in hot and humid climates.

The durability and appearance retention of regular rayon are low, especially when wet; also, rayon has the lowest elastic recovery of any fibre. However, HWM rayon is much stronger and exhibits higher durability and appearance retention. Recommended care for regular rayon is dry-cleaning only. HWM rayon can be machine washed.

PRODUCTION METHOD

Regular rayon (or viscose) is the most widely produced form of rayon. This method of rayon production has been utilized since the early 1900s and it has the ability to produce either filament or staple fibres. The process is as follows:

1. **Cellulose.** Production begins with processed cellulose.

2. **Immersion**: The cellulose is dissolved in caustic soda: $(C_6H_{10}O_5)_n$ + nNaOH → $(C_6H_9O_4ONa)_n$ + nH_2O
3. **Pressing.** The solution is then pressed between rollers to remove excess liquid.
4. **White Crumb.** The pressed sheets are crumbled or shredded to produce what is known as "white crumb".
5. **Aging.** The "white crumb" aged through exposure to oxygen.
6. **Xanthation.** The aged "white crumb" is mixed with carbon disulfide in a process known as Xanthation, the aged alkali cellulose crumbs are placed in vats and are allowed to react with carbon disulfide under controlled temperature (20 to 30°C) to form cellulose xanthate:

   $$(C_6H_9O_4ONa)_n + nCS_2 \rightarrow (C_6H_9O_4O\text{-}SC\text{-}SNa)_n.$$

7. **Yellow Crumb.** Xanthation changes the chemical makeup of the cellulose mixture and the resulting product is now called "yellow crumb".
8. **Viscose.** The "yellow crumb" is dissolved in a caustic solution to form viscose.
9. **Ripening.** The viscose is set to stand for a period of time, allowing it to ripen:

$$(C_6H_9O_4O\text{-}SC\text{-}SNa)_n + nH_2O \rightarrow (C_6H_{10}O_5)_n + nCS_2 + nNaOH.$$

10. **Filtering.** After ripening, the viscose is filtered to remove any undissolved particles.
11. **Degassing.** Any bubbles of air are pressed from the viscose in a degassing process.
12. **Extruding.** The viscose solution is extruded through a spinneret, which resembles a shower head with many small holes.
13. **Acid Bath.** As the viscose exits the spinneret, it lands in a bath of sulfuric acid, resulting in the formation of rayon filaments:

   $$(C_6H_9O_4O\text{-}SC\text{-}SNa)_n + ½nH_2SO_4 \rightarrow (C_6H_{10}O_5)_n + nCS_2 + ½nNa_2SO_4.$$

14. **Drawing.** The rayon filaments are stretched, known as drawing, to straighten out the fibres.
15. **Washing.** The fibre s are then washed to remove any residual chemicals.
16. **Cutting.** If filament fibre s are desired the process ends here. The filaments are cut down when producing staple fibres.

High Wet Modulus rayon (HWM) is a modified version of viscose that has a greater strength when wet. It also has the ability to be mercerized like cotton. HWM rayons are also known as "polynosic" or can be identified by the trade name Modal.

High Tenacity rayon is another modified version of viscose that has almost twice the strength of HWM. This type of rayon is typically used for industrial purposes such as tire cord.

Cupramonium rayon has properties similar to viscose but during production, the cellulose is combined with copper and ammonia (Schweizer's reagent).

USES OF RAYON

Some major rayon fibre uses include apparel (e.g., blouses, dresses, jackets, lingerie, linings, scarves, suits, ties, hats, socks), furnishings (e.g., bedspreads, blankets, window treatments, upholstery, slipcovers), industrial uses (e.g., medical surgery products, non-woven products, tire cord), and other uses (e.g., yarn, feminine hygiene products, diapers).

ACETATE RAYON

Acetate rayon or cellulose acetate fibre is one of the earliest synthetic fibres and is based on cotton or tree pulp cellulose ("biopolymers"). These "cellulosic fibres" have passed their peak, as cheap petro-based fibres (nylon and polyester) and have displaced regenerated pulp fibres.

Cellulose acetate is used as a film base in photography, and as a component in some adhesives; it is also used as a synthetic fibre .

PROPERTIES OF ACETATE

Acetate is a very valuable manufactured fibre that is low in cost and has good draping qualities. Properties of acetate have promoted it as the "beauty fibre". Acetate is used in fabrics such as satins, brocades, and taffetas to accentuate luster, body, drape and beauty.

- **Hand.** Soft, smooth, dry, crisp, resilient.
- **Comfort.** Breathes, wicks, dries quickly, no static cling.
- **Drape.** Linings move with the body linings conform to the garment.
- **Colour.** Deep brilliant shades with atmospheric dyeing meet colourfastness requirements.
- **Lustre.** Light reflection creates a signature appearance.
- **Performance.** Colourfast to perspiration staining, colourfast to dry cleaning, air and vapour permeable.
- **Tenacity.** Weak fibre with breaking tenacity of 1.2 to 1.4 g/d; rapidly loses strength when wet; must be dry cleaned.
- **Environmentally friendly.** Made from wood pulp, a renewable resource.
- **Abrasion.** Poor resistance.
- **Heat retention.** Poor thermal retention; no allergenic potential (hypoallergenic).
- **Dyeability.** Cross-dying method where yarns of one fibre and those of another fibre are woven into a fabric in a desired pattern; solution-dying method provides excellent colour fastness under the effects of sunlight, perspiration, air contaminants and washing.

Acetate is derived from cellulose by deconstructing wood pulp into a purified fluffy white cellulose. In order to get a good product special qualities of pulps — dissolving pulps are used. A common problem with these is that the reactivity of the cellulose is uneven, and thereby will the quality of the cellulose acetate sometimes be damaged. The cellulose is then reacted with acetic acid and acetic anhydride in the presence of sulfuric acid. It is then put through a controlled, partial hydrolvsis to remove the sulfate and a sufficient number of acetate groups to give the product the desired properties. The anhydroglucose unit is the fundamental repeating structure of cellulose and has three hydroxyl groups which can react to form acetate esters. The most common form of cellulose acetate fibre has an acetate group on approximately two of every three hydroxyls. This cellulose diacetate is known as secondary acetate, or simply as "acetate".

After it is formed, cellulose acetate is dissolved in acetone into a viscose resin for extrusion through spinnerets (which resemble a shower head). As the filaments emerge, the solvent is evaporated in warm air via dry spinning, producing fine cellulose acetate fibres.

PRODUCTION METHOD

1. Purified cellulose from wood pulp or cotton linters.
2. Mixed with glacial acetic acid, acetic anhydride, and a catalyst.
3. Aged 20 hours-partial hydrolysis occurs.
4. Precipitated as acid-resin flakes.
5. Flakes dissolved in acetone.
6. Solution is filtered.
7. Spinning solution extruded in column of warm air.
8. Filaments are stretched and wound onto beams, cones, or bobbins ready for use.

ACETATE FIBRE CHARACTERISTICS

- Cellulosic and thermoplastic.
- Selective absorption and removal of low levels of certain organic chemicals.
- Easily bonded with plasticizers, heat, and pressure.
- Acetate is soluble in many common solvents (especially acetone and other organic solvents) and can be modified to be soluble in alternative solvents, including water.
- *Hydrophilic*: acetate wets easily, with good liquid transport and excellent absorption; in textile applications, it provides comfort and absorbency, but also loses strength when wet.

- Acetate fibres are hypoallergenic.
- High surface area.
- Made from a renewable resource: wood pulp.
- Can be composted or incinerated.
- Can be dyed, however special dyes and pigments are required since acetate does not accept dyes ordinarily used for cotton and rayon (this also allows cross-dyeing).
- Resistant to mold and mildew.
- Easily weakened by strong alkaline solutions and strong oxidizing agents.
- Can usually be wet cleaned or dry cleaned and generally does not shrink.

MAJOR INDUSTRIAL ACETATE FIBRE USES

- **Apparel.** Linings, blouses, dresses, wedding and party attire, home furnishings, draperies, upholstery and slip covers.
- **Industrial uses.** Cigarette and other filters, ink reservoirs for fibre tip pens.
- **High absorbency products.** Diapers and surgical products.
- **Award Ribbon.** Rosettes for equestrian events, dog/cat shows, corporate awards, advertising and identification products all use cellulose acetate ribbon.

SODIUM ALGINATE

The chemical compound sodium alginate is the sodium salt of alginic acid. Its empirical chemical formula is $NaC_6H_7O_6$. Its form as a gum, when extracted from the cell walls of brown algae, is used by the foods industry to increase viscosity and as an emulsifier. It is also used in indigestion tablets and the preparation of dental impressions. Sodium alginate has no discernible flavour.

USES

A major application for sodium alginate is as thickener for reactive dyestuffs (such as the Procion cotton-reactive dyes) in textile screen-printing and carpet jet-printing. Alginates do not react with these dyes and wash out easily, unlike starch-based thickeners.

Sodium alginate is a good chelator for pulling radioactive toxins such as iodine-131 and strontium-90 from the body which have taken the place of their non-radioactive counterparts. It is also used in immobilizing enzymes by inclusion.

As a food additive, sodium alginate is used especially in the production of gel-like foods. For example, bakers' "Chellies" are often gelled alginate "jam". Also, the pimento stuffing in prepared cocktail olives is usually injected as a slurry at the same time that the stone is ejected; the slurry is subsequently set by immersing the olive in a solution of a calcium salt which causes rapid gelation by electrostatic cross-linking. A similar process can be used to make "chunks" of everything from cat food through "reformed" ham or fish to "fruit" pieces for pies. It has the E-number 401. Now-a-days it is also used in the biological experiments for the immobilization of cells to obtain important products like alcohols, organic acids, etc.

NYLON

Nylon is a generic designation for a family of synthetic polymers known generically as polyamides. Nylon is one of the most commonly used polymers. Nylon is a thermoplastic silky material, first used commercially in a nylon-bristled toothbrush (1938), followed more famously by women's stockings ("nylons"; 1940). It is made of repeating units linked by peptide bonds (another name for amide bonds) and is frequently referred to as polyamide (PA). Nylon was the first commercially successful synthetic polymer. There are two common methods of making nylon for fibre applications. In one approach, molecules with an acid (COOH) group on each end are reacted with molecules containing amine (NH_2) groups on each end. The resulting nylon is named on the basis of the number of carbon atoms separating the two acid groups and the two amines. These are formed into monomers of intermediate molecular weight, which are then reacted to form long polymer chains.

Nylon was intended to be a synthetic replacement for silk and substituted for it in many different products after silk became scarce during World War II. It replaced silk in military applications such as parachutes and flak vests, and was used in many types of vehicle tires.

Nylon fibres are used in many applications, including fabrics, bridal veils, carpets, musical strings, and rope.

Solid nylon is used for mechanical parts such as machine screws, gears and other low- to medium-stress components previously cast in metal. Engineering-grade nylon is processed by extrusion, casting, and injection molding. Solid nylon is used in hair combs. Type 6/6 Nylon 101 is the most common commercial grade of nylon, and Nylon 6 is the most common commercial grade of molded nylon. Nylon is available in glass-filled variants which increase structural and impact strength and rigidity, and molybdenum sulfide-filled variants which increase lubricity.

Aramids are another type of polyamide with quite different chain structures which include aromatic groups in the main chain. Such polymers make excellent ballistic fibres.

Basic Concepts of Nylon Production

The first approach. combining molecules with an acid (COOH) group on each end are reacted with two chemicals that contain amine (NH_2) groups on each end.

This process creates nylon 6,6, made of hexamethylene diamine with six carbon atoms and acidipic acid, as well as six carbon atoms.

The second approach. a compound has an acid at one end and an amine at the other and is polymerized to form a chain with repeating units of $(-NH-[CH_2]n-CO-)_x$. In other words, nylon 6 is made from a single six-carbon substance called *caprolactam*.

NYLON 6,6

- Pleats and creases can be heat-set at higher temperatures.
- More compact molecular structure.
- Better weathering properties; better sunlight resistance.
- Softer "Hand".
- Higher melting point (256°C).
- Superior colourfastness.
- Excellent abrasion resistance.

NYLON 6

- More rapid moisture absorption.
- Easy to dye, more readily fades.
- Greater elasticity and elastic recovery.
- Higher impact resistance.

PRODUCERS OF NYLON

The producers of nylon include: *Honeywell Nylon Inc., Invista, Wellman Inc*. among many others. The *DuPont* Company, is the most famous pioneer of the nylon we know today.

CHARACTERISTICS

- Nylon has the ability to be very lustrous, semilustrous or dull.
- Its high tenacity fibre s are used for seatbelts, tire cords, ballistic cloth and other uses.
- High elongation.
- Excellent abrasion resistance.
- Highly resilient (nylon fabrics are heat-set).
- Paved the way for easy-care garments.
- High resistance to:
  - insects, fungi and animals.
  - molds, mildew, rot.
  - many chemicals.

- Used in carpets and nylon stockings.
- Melts instead of burning.
- Used in many military applications.
- Good specific strength.

USE IN COMPOSITES

Nylon can be used as the matrix material in composite materials, with reinforcing fibres like glass or carbon fibre , and has a higher density than pure nylon. Such thermoplastic composites (25% glass fibre) are frequently used in car components next to the engine, such as intake manifolds, where the good heat resistance of such materials makes them feasible competitors to metals.

SURGICAL DRESSING

A dressing is an adjunct used by a person for application to a wound to promote healing and/or prevent further harm. A dressing is designed to be in direct contact with the wound, which makes it different from a bandage, which is primarily used to hold a dressing in place.

A dressing can have a number of purposes, depending on the type, severity and position of the wound, although all purposes are focused towards promoting recovery and preventing further harm from the wound. Key purposes of are dressing are:

- **Stem bleeding.** Helps to seal the wound to expedite the clotting process.
- **Absorb exudate.** Soak up blood, plasma and other fluids exuded from the wound, containing it in one place.
- **Ease pain.** Some dressings may have a pain relieving effect, and others may have a placebo effect.
- **Debride the wound.** The removal of slough and foreign objects from the wound.
- Protection from infection and mechanical damage.
- Promote healing: through granulation and epithelialisation.

TYPES OF DRESSING

Historically, a dressing was usually a piece of material, sometimes cloth, but the use of cobwebs, dung, leaves and honey have also been described. However, modern dressings include gauzes (which may be impregnated with an agent designed to help sterility or to speed healing), films, gels, foams, hydrocolloids, alginates, hydrogels and polysaccharide pastes, granules and beads. Many gauze dressings have a layer of nonstick film over the absorbent gauze to prevent the wound from adhering to the dressing. Dressings can be impregnated with antiseptic chemicals, as in boracic lint or where medicinal Castor oil was used in the first surgical dressings.

In the 1960s, *George Winter* published his controversial research on moist healing. Previously, the accepted wisdom was that to prevent infection of a wound, the wound should be kept as dry as possible. *Winter* demonstrated that wounds which were kept moist healed faster than those which were left exposed to the air or covered with traditional dressings.

Various types of dressings can be used to accomplish different objectives including:

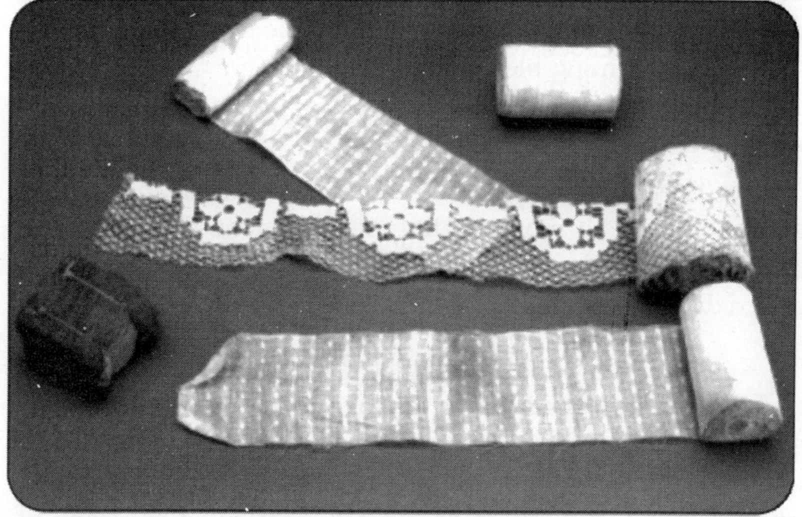

Fig. 28.3: Surgical dressing

- Controlling the moisture content, so that the wound stays moist or dry.
- Protecting the wound from infection.
- Removing slough, and
- Maintaining the optimum pH and temperature to encourage healing.

Occlusive dressings, made from substances impervious to moisture such as plastic or latex, can be used to increase the rate of absorption of certain topical medications into the skin.

USAGE OF DRESSINGS

Applying a dressing is a first aid skill, although many people undertake the practice with no training – especially on minor wounds. Modern dressings will almost all come in a pre-packaged sterile wrapping, date coded to ensure sterility. This is because it will come in to direct contact with the wound, and sterility is required to fulfil the 'protection from infection' aim of a dressing.

Historically, and still the case in many less developed areas and in an emergency, dressings are often improvised as needed. This can consist of anything, including clothing or spare material, which will fulfil some of the basic tenets of a dressing —usually stemming bleeding and absorbing exudate.

Applying and changing dressings is one common task in nursing.

An "ideal" wound dressing is one that is sterile, breathable, and encourages a moist healing environment. This will then reduce the risk of infection, help the wound heal more quickly, and reduce scarring.

SUTURE

A suture is a medical device that doctors, embalmers, and surgeons use to hold skin, internal organs, blood vessels and all other tissues of the human body together after they have been severed by injury, incision or surgery. They must be strong so that they do not break, non-toxic, hypoallergenic (to avoid adverse reactions in the body), and flexible (so they can be tied and knotted easily). In addition, they must lack the so called "wick effect", which means that sutures must not allow fluids to penetrate the body through them from outside, which could easily cause infections.

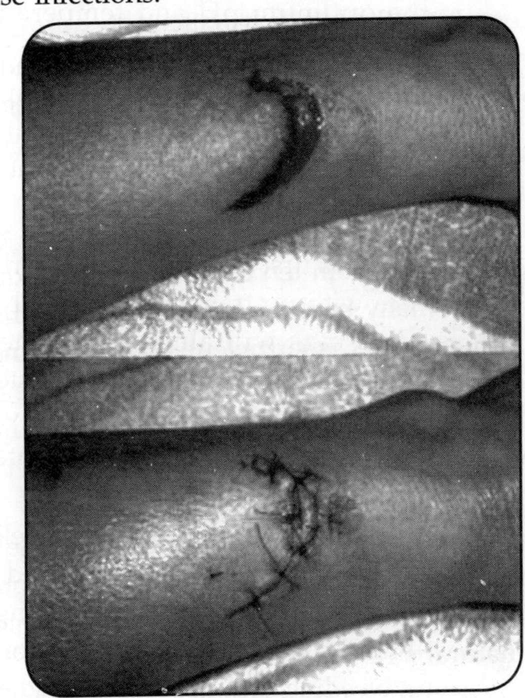

Fig. 28.4: Suture

TYPES OF SUTURES

Sutures (also known as stitches) are divided into two kinds:

- those which are ***absorbable*** and will break down harmlessly in the body over time without intervention, and
- those which are ***non-absorbable*** and must be manually removed if they are not left indefinitely. The type of suture used varies on the operation, with the major criteria being the demands of the location and environment.

Sutures to be placed internally would require re-opening if they were to be removed. Sutures which lie on the exterior of the body can be removed within minutes, and without re-opening the wound. As a result, absorbable sutures are often used internally; non-absorbable externally.

Sutures to be placed in a stressful environment, for example the heart (constant pressure and movement) or the bladder (adverse chemical presence) may require specialized or stronger materials to perform their role; usually such sutures are either specially treated, or made of special materials, and are often non-absorbable to reduce the risk of premature degradation.

1. Absorbable Sutures

Absorbable sutures are made of materials which are broken down in tissue after a given period of time, which depending on the material can be from ten days to eight weeks. They are used therefore in many of the internal tissues of the body. In most cases, three weeks is sufficient for the wound to close firmly. The suture is not needed any more, and the fact that it disappears is an advantage, as there is no foreign material left inside the body and no need for the patient to have the sutures removed.

Absorbable sutures were originally made of the intestines of sheep, the so called catgut. The manufacturing process was similar to that of natural musical strings for violins and guitar, and also of natural strings for tennis racquets. The inventor, a 10th century surgeon named *al-Zahrawi* reportedly discovered the dissolving nature of catgut when his lute's strings were eaten by a monkey. Today, gut sutures are made of specially prepared beef and sheep intestine, and may be untreated (plain gut), tanned with chromium salts to increase their persistence in the body (chromic gut), or heat-treated to give more rapid absorption (fast gut). However, the majority of absorbable sutures are now made of synthetic polymer fibre s, which may be braided or monofilament; these offer numerous advantages over gut sutures, notably ease of handling, low cost, low tissue reaction, consistent performance and guaranteed non-toxicity. In Europe and Japan, gut sutures have been banned due to concerns over bovine spongiform encephalopathy (mad-cow disease), although the herds from which gut is harvested are certified BSE-free. Each major suture manufacturer has its own proprietary formulations for its brands of synthetic absorbable sutures; various blends of polyglycolic acid (Biovek for example), polylactic acid or caprolactone are common.

Occasionally, absorbable sutures can cause inflammation and be rejected by the body rather than absorbed.

2. Non-absorbable Sutures

Non-absorbable sutures are made of materials which are not metabolized by the body, and are used therefore either on skin wound closure, where the sutures can be removed after a few weeks, or in some inner tissues in which absorbable sutures are not adequate. This is the case, for example, in the heart and in blood vessels, whose rhythmic movement requires a suture which stays longer than three weeks, to give the wound enough time to close. Other organs, like the bladder, contain fluids which make absorbable sutures disappear in only a few days, too early for the wound to heal. Inflammation caused by the foreign protein in some absorbable sutures can amplify scarring, so if other types of suture are less antigenic (i.e., do not provoke as much of an immune response) it would represent a way to reduce scarring.

There are several materials used for non-absorbable sutures. The most common is a natural fibre , silk, which undergoes a special manufacturing process to make it adequate for its use in surgery. Other non-absorbable sutures are made of artificial fibres, like polypropylene, polyester or nylon; these may or may not have coatings to enhance their performance characteristics. Finally, stainless steel wires are commonly used in orthopedic surgery and for sternal closure in cardiac surgery.

Surgical Needles for Use with Sutures

Traumatic needles are needles with holes or eyes which are supplied to the hospital separate from their suture thread. The suture must be threaded on site, as is done when sewing at home. Atraumatic needles with sutures comprise an eyeless needle attached to a specific length of suture thread. The suture manufacturer swages the suture thread to the eyeless atraumatic needle at the factory. There are several advantages to having the needle pre-mounted on the suture. The doctor or the nurse or ODP (Out Door Patient)does not have to spend time threading the suture on the needle. More importantly, the suture end of a swaged needle is smaller than the needle body. In traumatic needles with eyes, the thread comes out of the needle's hole on both sides. When passing through the tissues, this type of suture rips the tissue to a certain extent, thus the name traumatic. Nearly all modern sutures feature swaged atraumatic needles.

There are several shapes of surgical needles, including—

- straight.
- half curved or ski.
- 1/4 circle.
- 3/8 circle.
- 1/2 circle.
- 5/8 circle.
- compound curve.

Needles may also be classified by their point geometry; examples include:

- taper (needle body is round and tapers smoothly to a point).
- cutting (needle body is triangular and has a sharpened cutting edge on the inside).
- reverse cutting (cutting edge on the outside).
- tapercut (needle body is round and tapered, but ends in a small triangular cutting point).
- blunt points for sewing friable tissues.
- side cutting or spatula points (flat on top and bottom with a cutting edge along the front to one side) for eye surgery.

Finally, atraumatic needles may be permanently swaged to the suture or may be designed to come off the suture with a sharp straight tug. These "pop-offs" are commonly used for interrupted sutures, where each suture is only passed once and then tied.

SIZES OF SUTURES

Suture sizes are defined by the United States Pharma-copeia (U.S.P.). Sutures were originally manufactured ranging in size from #1 to #6, with #1 being the smallest. A #4 suture would be roughly the diameter of a tennis racquet string. The manufacturing techniques, derived at the beginning from the production of musical strings, did not allow thinner diameters. As the procedures improved, #0 was added to the suture diameters, and later, thinner and thinner threads were manufactured, which were identified as #00 (#2-0 or #2/0) to #000000 (#6-0 or #6/0).

Modern sutures range from #5 (heavy braided suture for orthopedics) to #11-0 (fine monofilament suture for ophthalmics). Atraumatic needles are manufactured in all shapes for most sizes. The actual diameter of thread for a given U.S.P. size differs depending on the suture material class.

SUTURE TECHNIQUES

Common suture stitching techniques include:

- Simple Interrupted Stitch.
- Running Stitch.
- Mattress.
- Horizontal mattress.
- Chest drain suture.
- Vertical mattress.
- Figure 8.
- Continuous locking.
- Subcuticular.

REMOVAL OF SUTURES

While some sutures are intended to be permanent, and others in specialized cases may be kept in place for an extended period of many weeks, as a rule sutures are a short term device to allow healing of a trauma or wound.

Different parts of the body heal at different intervals. Common time to remove stitches will vary: facial wounds 3–5 days; scalp wound 7–10 days; limbs 10–14 days; joints 14 days; trunk of the body 7–10 days.

Not all stitches must be removed. If a small area remains unhealed, notify the health care practitioner. Then if ordered, remove sutures from the healed area only.

ANTIMICROBIAL SUTURES

Another recent development in wound closure involves the use of sutures coated with antimicrobial substances to reduce the chances of wound infection. While long-term studies are not yet available, preliminary results indicate that these sutures are effective at inhibiting bacterial growth in wounds.

STUDY QUESTIONS

1. Write short notes on the following:
   (a) Surgical dressing;
   (b) Suture; and
   (c) Fibre.
2. Explain the different types of suture.
3. How to remove suture?

■■■

29

CHAPTER

GROSS ANATOMICAL STUDIES OF SELECTED PLANTS

SENNA

MORPHOLOGY

Senna consists of dried leaves of *Cassia angustifolia* (Family *Leguminosae*); a small shrub, 60-75 cm high, found throughout the year, cultivated largely in Southern India, especially in districts of Tinnevelly, Madurai and Tiruchirapally and has also been introduced in Mysore; fully grown, thick bluish colour leaves stripped off by hand, collected and dried in shade for 7-10 days, till assume a yellowish-green colour; graded and then packed into large bales.

SYNONYMS

Eng. : Indian senna, Tinnevelly senna

Guj. : Mindhiaval, Sonamukhi

Hindi : Sanaya, Hindisana

MACROSCOPIC STRUCTURE

Leaflets, 2.5-6 cm long and 7-15 mm wide at center, pale yellowish-green, elongated lanceolate, slightly asymmetric at base; margins entire, flat, apex acute with a sharp spine; both surfaces smooth with sparce trichomes; odour, faint but distinctive; taste, mucilaginous and disagreeable but not distinctly bitter.

Transverse section of leaflet through midrib shows an isobilateral structure; epidermal cells, straight walled, containing mucilage; both surfaces bear scattered, unicellular hair, often conical, curved near base, thick-walled, non-lignified; warty cuticle; stomata, paracytic, numerous on both surfaces; mesophyll consists of upper and lower palisade layers with spongy layer in between; palisade cells of upper surface longer than those of lower surface, the latter having wavy anticlinal walls; prismatic crystals of calcium oxalate present in larger veins, and clusters of calcium oxalate crystal distributed throughout the palisade and spongy tissues; midrib biconvex; bundles of midrib and larger veins, incompletely surrounded by a zone pericyclic fibres and a crystal sheath of parenchymatous cells, containing prismatic crystals of calcium oxalate.

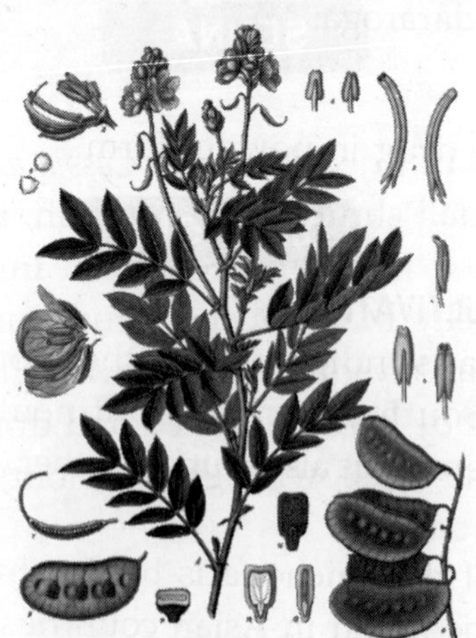

Fig. 29.1: Cassia-angustifolia

IDENTITY PURITY AND STRENGTH

Foreign matter	—	Not more than 1 percent
Total ash	—	Not more than 15 percent
Acid-insoluble ash	—	Not more than 21 percent
Alcohol soluble extractive	—	Not less than 3 per cent
Water-soluble extractive	—	Not less than 25 per cent

CONSTITUENTS

Anthraquinone, glocoside, flavonoids, steroids and resin.

PROPERTIES AND ACTION

Rasa : Katu, Tikta, Kasaya
Guna : Laghu, Ruksa, Tiksna
Virya : Usna
Vipaka : Katu
Karma : Recana

IMPORTANT FORMULATIONS

Pancasakara curna, sarivadyasava

THERAPEUTIC USES

Vibandha, Udararoga.

DOSE

0.5-2 g of the drug in powder form.

CINCHONA

HABITAT AND CULTIVATION

The cinchona is indigenous to the mountainous tropical regions of the South American continent, particularly the tropical area of Peru – it is also found in other countries in tropical South America.

Cultivation of the cinchona is big business, and cinchona plantations can be found in Asian countries such as India and Indonesia - mainly Java. Cinchona is also cultivated in many parts of Africa. In these areas, the cultivation of the cinchona is intensive and carried out on large commercial tree farms. Propagation of the cinchona trees is done from cutting late in the spring season.

Harvest of the product consists of the removal of trunk bark and bark from the branches and the root. The *bark* is normally only removed from six to eight year old trees, and the collected bark is then subjected to drying in the sun on mats. Annually, approximately 8,000 tons of the bark is harvested from such farms.

Shrubs or small, medium-sized to tall canopy trees; raphides absent; axillary thorns absent. Stipules interpetiolar, free at base or interpetiolar, connate at base, broadly triangular, obovate, oblong or ligulate, subcaducous or readily caducous.

Leaves opposite, long- to short-petiolate; blades ovate, elliptic, obovate, broadly obovate, oblong, orbicular, chartaceous, stiffly chartaceous, papyraceous, thinly to thickly coriaceous; foliar pellucid glands absent; domatia sparse tufts or dense tufts of hair or absent. Inflorescence terminal, frondose or not frondose, paniculate, densely or sparsely branched. Flowers bisexual, protandrous.

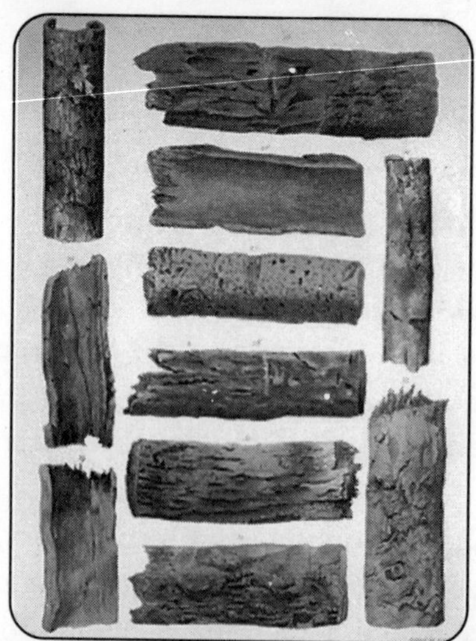

Fig. 29.2: Cinchona bark

Calyx cup-shaped, with small lobes, campanulate or short tubular, persistent; lobes 4 to 6, deltoid or narrowly to broadly triangular, oblong, elliptic or ovate, minute or small, or absent. Calycophylls absent.

Corolla hypocrateriform, actinomorphic, white to cream-white, pinkish-white, reddish-white, pink, red, violet to purple; tube externally minutely puberulent, puberulent, pubescent or hirtellous, internally puberulent, pubescent or hirtellous, without a pubescent ring inside; orifice annular thickening absent; lobes 4 to 6, valvate, narrowly triangular, lanceolate, linear-lanceolate, margin entire, acute at apex.

Stamens alternate to the corolla lobes, included or partially exserted (only tips exserted); anthers narrowly elliptic, elongate or linear, round at base, round at apex, dehiscing by longitudinal slits, dorsifixed near the base; filaments attached at the lower part of the corolla tube, free at base, slender, long, shorter than corolla tube, equal, glabrous.

Pollen colporate, three apertures, exine surface foveolate or perforate, released as monads.

Style exserted just beyond the corolla or included, terete throughout, not fleshy, glabrous; two lobes, ovate, elliptic or oblong.

Ovary inferior, 2-locular, obconical, narrowly obconical or ovoid; placentation axile, placenta peltate to the entire lenght of the septum, ovules many per locule.

Fruit a septicidal capsule, dehiscing acropetally (rarely basipetally), thinly woody. Seeds ascendingly imbricate, laterally compressed; wings bipolar, margin nearly entire, dentate or fimbriate.

IPECACUANHA

MORPHOLOGY

Shape. The ipecacuanha root, is *cylindrical* and tortuous.

Size. 15 cm in length or 5 mm in thickness.

Colour. The colour varies from dark brick-red to dark brown.

Characteristic. Very characteristic of the root is the *annulated* appearance that it presents, the bark of typical pieces being constricted at short intervals so as to resemble a number of discs somewhat irregularly strung together; the constrictions are sometimes quite shallow, but sometimes they penetrate nearly to the wood.

Fracture. The root is hard and breaks with a very short fracture. The transverse section exhibits a thick, dark grey bark which is usually horny, but sometimes starchy, and a small wood in which no distinct pores or pith can be discerned when examined with a lens.

Bark. The bark, when examined under the microscope, is found to contain abundance of starch grains that are mostly compound and, in addition, acicular crystals of calcium oxalate; the wood is free from vessels.

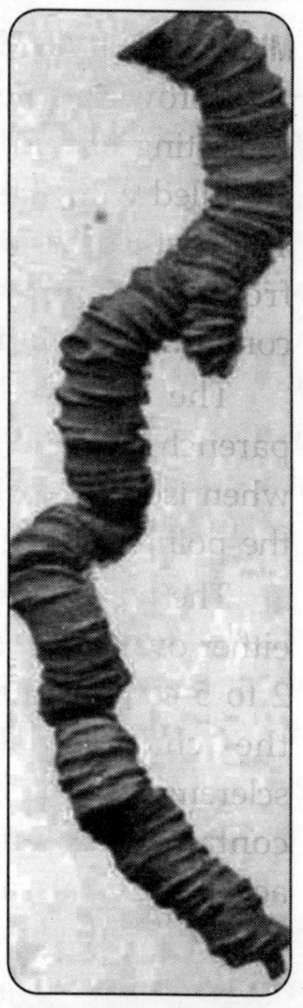

Fig. 29.3: Roots of Ipecacuanha

Odour: The drug has a *slight* odour which to many persons is particularly unpleasant.

Taste: The taste is *slightly bitter*. The powder is often very irritating to the throat and nostrils, producing violent coughing and sneezing.

CONSTITUENTS

Ipecacuanha root contains three alkaloids; two of which, emetine and cephaeline, have been more closely examined, whilst the third, psychotrine, which occurs in much smaller quantity, awaits further investigation. These alkaloids exist in good root to the extent of from 2 to 3 per cent, and are contained chiefly in the bark, the wood yielding only about 1 per cent. The alkaloids ipecamine and hydroipecamine have also been reported as present.

MICROSCOPICAL CHARACTERS

Below the narrow *cork* is a largely developed *cortex* consisting of thin-walled parenchymatous cells most of which are filled with starch, but a few contain acicular *calcium oxalate*. The bast ring is narrow, and both this and the cortex are free from sclerenchymatous cells and fibres and from cells containing colouring matter.

The wood is composed of tracheids, wood fibres, and parenchyma and is free from typical vessels. The tracheids, when isolated, exhibit moderately thick walls, and often near the pointed extremities a large perforation.

The powder is characterised by the starch grains which are either oval or rounded (not over 15μ) or compound with from 2 to 5 constituent grains, by the acicular calcium oxalate, by the characteristic tracheids and by the absence of sclerenchymatous cells, spiral vessels (ipecacuanha stem), cells containing colouring water, calcium oxalate in other than acicular crystals, and typical sclerenchymatous fibres or vessels.

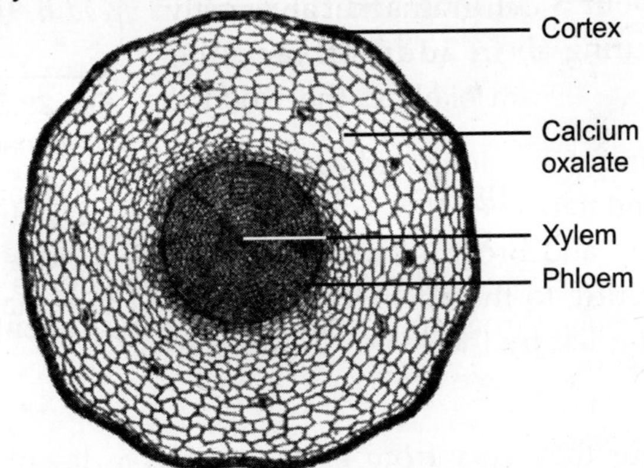

Fig. 29.4: Ipecacuanha. Transverse section, showing dense wood.

USES

Ipecacuanha is largely used as an expectorant and emetic; it also possesses diaphoretic and cholagogue properties. One of its most important uses is as a remedy for dysentery, for which purpose large doses are given (30 to 90 grains). In such cases a remarkable tolerance of the drug is often readily established, or the drug deprived of its alkaloids is administered.

NUX VOMICA

Botanical Name	:	*Strychnos Nux Vomica*
Family	:	Loganiaceae
Parts Used	:	Bark, Leaves, Seeds
Common Name	:	Nux-vomica, Poison Nut, Snake-wood

HABITAT

It is found throughout india in deciduous forests.

MORPHOLOGY

These very beautiful seeds are remarkable for the long plumose awn of white silky hairs that is attached to them.

The integuments of the seed are prolonged at the apex to a slender brittle extension, which is terminated by a feathery tuft of hairs about 5 cm long and the same in *breadth*, the entire seed measuring about 10 cm in *length*.

SHAPE

They are of an elongated oval shape, acuminate towards the apex, and narrowed towards the base, which is obtuse. They are flattened and provided on one side with a ridge running from the centre to the apex of the seed, and terminating in a broken point left by the removal of the awn.

COLOUR

In colour they vary from greyish green to fawn; they are covered with satiny appressed hairs that impart to them a conspicuous sheen.

SEEDS

The seeds have the shape of small discs, 20 to 25 mm in diameter and about 4 mm. thick, of an ash-grey or greenish grey colour, and possessing a distinct sheen.

They are usually not quite flat, being a little depressed on one side and arched on the other, or sometimes irregularly bent.

They are covered with numerous, closely appressed hairs, radiating from the centre to the circumference, to which the satiny sheen of the seeds is due.

The edge of the seed is sometimes rounded, sometimes acute, according to the variety; at one point on the margin there is a distinct prominence (micropyle) from which a raised line passes to the centre of the seed. This line does not exist in the fresh seed, but makes its appearance during the drying; it has frequently been mistaken for the raphe. The hilum is in the centre of either the raised or depressed surface, and may be recognised by the scar left by the funicle.

The dry seed is hard and horny, but softens when soaked in water; it can then easily be split into two thinner discs, exhibiting the small embryo, consisting of a radicle and two leafy cotyledons, embedded in a copious, grey, translucent, horny endosperm.

The seeds are almost *odourless*, but have a persistent, intensely bitter taste.

TRANSVERSE SECTION

The seeds break easily; the transverse section exhibits a white oily *kernel* consisting of two straight cotyledons surrounded by a narrow *endosperm*. Moistened with 80 per cent, sulphuric acid the section assumes, at least in the endosperm but sometimes in the *cotyledons* also, a deep emerald green colour. The same reaction is afforded by the kernels from which the *seed-coats* have been removed after soaking in water.

The seed-coats thus separated, warmed on a slide with a little saturated aqueous solution of choral hydrate and examined under the microscope, are seen to contain not more than an occasional crystal of calcium oxalate. The odour of the crushed seed is characteristic, though not very powerful; the taste is intensely bitter.

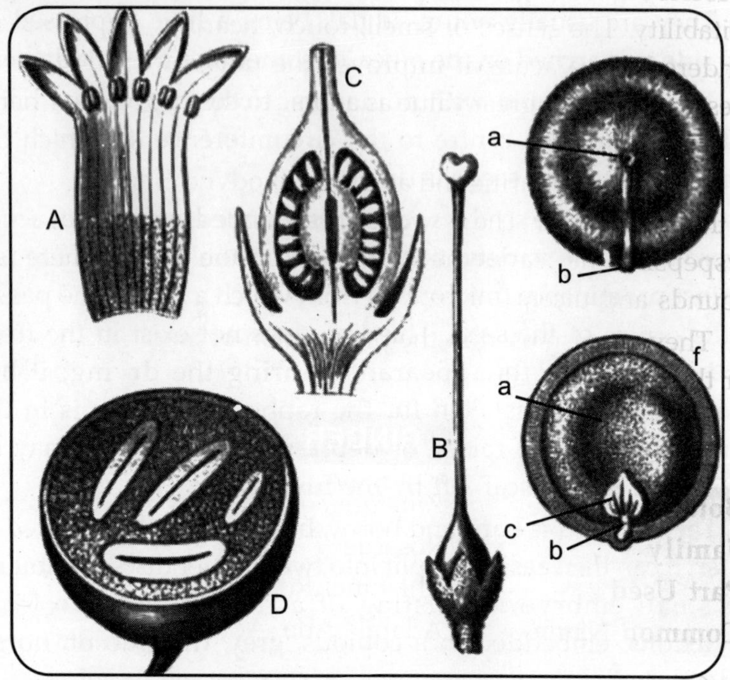

Fig. 29.5: *Nux Vomica.* (A) *corolla* opened, magnified. (B) *ovary* with style, magnified. (C) *ovary* cut longitudinally, more highly magnified. (D) *ripe fruit*, cut transversely, showing seeds; reduced to about one-half. (E) *seed*, entire, natural size: (a) *hilum*; (b) *micropyle*. (F) the same, cut vertically: (a) *endosperm*; (b) *radicle*; (c) *cotyledon*.

(a) The colour of the seed and the satiny hairs.

(b) The straight cotyledons and narrow endosperm.

(c) The green reaction with sulphuric acid.

USES

Strychnos nux vomica is recommended for upset stomach, vomiting, abdominal pain, constipation, intestinal irritation, hangovers, heartburn, insomnia, certain heart diseases, circulatory problems, eye diseases, depression, migraine headaches, nervous conditions, problems related to menopause, and respiratory diseases in the elderly.

In *folk medicine*, it is used as a healing tonic and appetite stimulant. Nux vomica is a common homeopathic medicine prescribed for digestive problems, sensitivity to cold, and irritability. The senses of smell, touch, hearing and vision are rendered more acute, it improves the pulse and raises blood pressure and is of great value as a tonic to the circulatory system in cardiac failure.

It is used in pruritis and as a local anodyne in inflammations of the external ear. The powdered seeds are employed in atonic dyspepsia. The leaves are applied as a poultice on sloughing wounds and ulcers.

They are also used in the preparation of medicated product for the hair and scalp.

GINGER

Botanical Name	:	*Zingiber officinale*
Family	:	Rosacae
Part Used	:	Rhizome, Roots
Common Name	:	Adarak, Ada, Adak

Ginger is the dried *rhizome* of *Zingiber officinale, Rosacae,* a reed-like plant producing leafy stems a metre high, springing from branching rhizomes.

HABITAT

It is a native of Asia, but is cultivated in many tropical countries, notably in the West Indies, in India, Africa, and Japan.

There can be little doubt that ginger was well known in India as a spice from the earliest times. The Greeks and Romans were well acquainted with it, and its use spread in the ninth and tenth centuries through Europe to England. It was introduced by the Spaniards into the West Indies and Jamaica.

CULTIVATED

In Jamaica the plant is largely cultivated. It is propagated by dividing the rhizome into 'fingers', each of which contains a bud, and planting these about a foot apart. They grow rapidly and flower in the autumn. When the aerial stems wither the rhizomes are dug up, freed from the roots, and washed. They are then peeled with a narrow-bladed knife, by which the layer of cork and part of the parenchyma of the cortex are removed, after which they are again washed, and dried in the sun. The product is known as unbleached *Jamaica ginger*.

DESCRIPTION

Much ginger is found in commerce from which the cork layer has not been removed, or which has been deprived of it on the flatter sides only. Such ginger is known as coated' or '*unscraped*', whilst that which has been completely peeled is called '*scraped*'. Sometimes, too, the rhizomes are treated with sulphurous acid or chlorine, or they are dusted over with calcium sulphate or carbonate which imparts to them a whitish appearance; ginger that has been treated so is termed 'bleache' or 'limed' ginger. In addition therefore to being obtained from different countries, ginger may vary in appearance according to the way in which it has been prepared for the market. As with nutmegs, limed ginger is undoubtedly less susceptible to the attacks of insect pests.

Unbleached Jamaica ginger, which is the official variety and the one that is most esteemed, occurs in flattened branched pieces technically termed 'races' or 'hands'.

These vary in length, but average about 7 to 10 cm. From the upper surface of the main rhizome, which is usually straight, numerous branches about 3 cm. in length appear to arise and take an upward course; they are often slightly compressed laterally, enlarged near the *rhizome*, and, tapering abruptly, terminate in the remains of an undeveloped bud or a small depressed scar indicating the point of attachment of an aerial stem.

The *branches* themselves also produce lateral branchlets. All these branches and branchlets arise from buds on the under surface of the rhizome in the axils of cataphyllary leaves. When the growth of the main axis is terminated by the production of an aerial shoot, one of these buds develops, curves upwards, and itself in due time produces an aerial shoot and develops a lateral branch. Each piece of the drug or 'hand' is therefore a sympodial branch system.

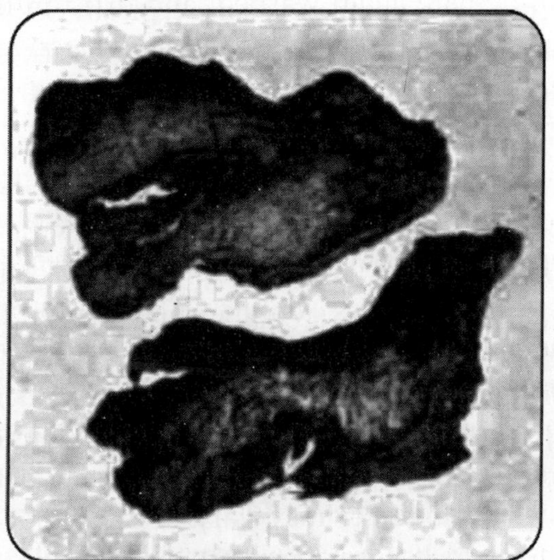

Fig. 29.6: Ginger

The *colour* of the drug is usually pale yellowish buff; the surface is strongly striated or even fibrous, the fibres being the leaf-traces passing through the cortex to the leaves, and laid bare by the peeling of the rhizome. It breaks with a short, mealy or sometimes resinous fracture, short scattered fibres usually protruding from the fractured surface; these are the fibro-vascular bundles in the stele and cortex.

The smoothed transverse section exhibits a large stele which is sharply delimited by a fine yellow line from a narrow cortex, both stele and cortex containing numerous yellow oil-cells. No cork layer is to be discerned. Ginger has an agreeable aromatic odour and a strong pungent taste.

MICROSCOPICAL CHARACTERS

The transverse section exhibits a large stele and a cortex free from cork. The parenchymatous cells, which are very abundant, have very thin walls; some contain yellow oleo-resin, but most are filled with starch. The fibro-vascular bundles in the stele contain a few reticulated vessels supported by sclerenchymatous fibres, which have rather thin walls and large cavities; abutting on the vessels are small cells filled with a dark brown secretion. The starch grains are typically Scitaminaceous; they are simple, 12μ, to 30μ long, ovoid or sack-shaped and fiat, the hilum being at the extreme, pointed end.

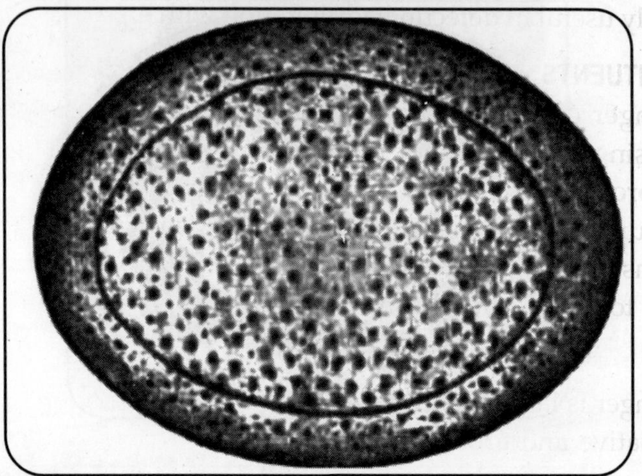

Fig. 29.7: *Ginger* transverse section through the rhizome.

Powdered ginger is characterised by the abundant typical starch, by the very thin walls of the parenchymatous cells, by the characteristic sclerenchymatous fibres, and by the oleo-resin

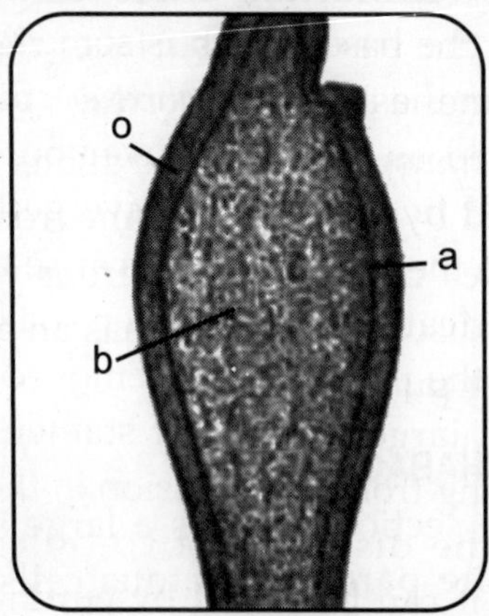

Fig. 29.8: Longitudinal section through a branch, natural size. o, cortex; v, endo-dermis; b, stele.

cells; the latter are mostly broken, but the suberised walls are always to be found. It should contain no cork, no isodiametric sclerenchymatous cells, and no hairs. It should yield about 7 per cent of extract to 90 per cent alcohol, from 12 to 15 per cent to cold water, not more than 6 per cent of ash, and not less than 1.5 per cent of ash soluble in hot water. The last two data are specially useful in detecting adulteration with exhausted ginger.

CONSTITUENTS

Ginger contains from 0.25 to 3 per cent of a volatile oil possessing the aroma but not the pungency of the drug. The latter property is due to a yellowish oily body, gingerol, which is odourless, but has an intensely pungent taste. The drug contains in addition resin and abundance of starch. It yields from 3 to 5 per cent. of ash.

USES

Ginger is largely used as a condiment, and medicinally as a carminative and aromatic stimulant.

CLOVES

DESCRIPTION

The cloves are the *dried flower-buds* of the tree. Each of them consists of a nearly cylindrical, dark reddish-brown portion, slightly tapering at the base, which is sometimes regarded as a gynophore, sometimes as a fleshy *calyxtube*, but is perhaps most correctly interpreted as the solid lower portion of the ovary (Tschirch), crowned by four, thick, divergent calyx-teeth of a similar colour, from the centre of which arise four, paler, brown, unexpanded, imbricated petals. After soaking in water for twenty-four hours the petals can be removed, and they will be found to enclose a large number of stamens bending over a stiff erect style arising from a depression in the centre of a small disc. Just below the disc is the two-celled ovary with its numerous ovules; it can be found by cutting the clove either *longitudinally* or *transversely*.

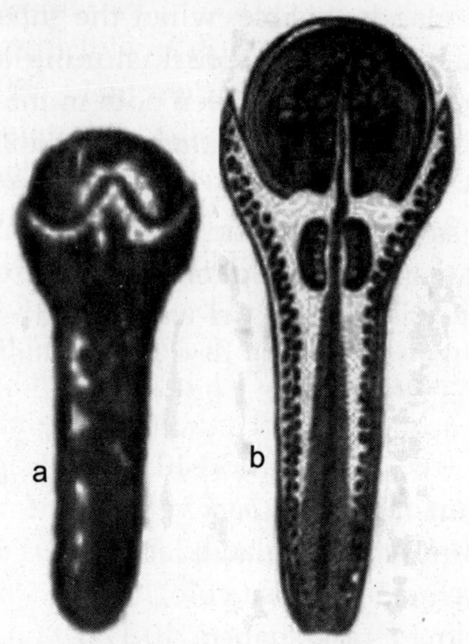

Fig. 29.8: Cloves: (a) natural size; (b) longitudinal section magnified.

The lower part of the ovary is solid and fleshy, spongy near the centre. It contains, especially near the periphery, a large

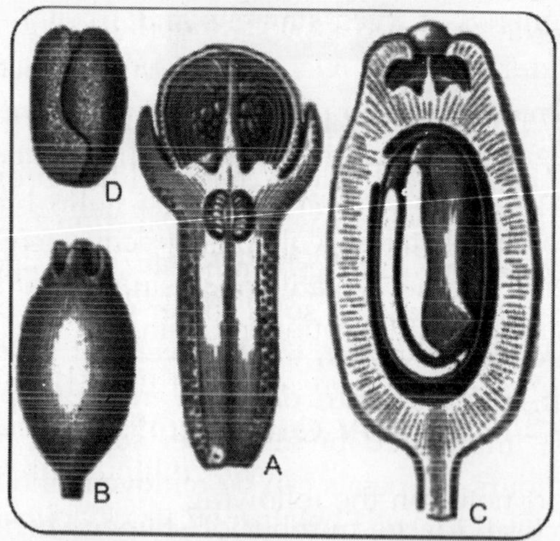

Fig. 29.9: Clove (Eugenia caryophyllata).
(A) clove cut vertically, showing calyx, corolla, stamens, pistil, and ovules; near the margin oil-glands; magnified. (B) fruit (mother clove), natural size. (C) the same, cut vertically and magnified. (D) embryo, natural size. (Luerssen).

number of oil-glands, visible, when the *transverse section* is examined under the lens, as dark shining points or small cavities. Similar glands can be seen both in the calyx-teeth and petals; in the latter they appear as translucent dots by transmitted light.

Cloves are strongly aromatic and have a pungent aromatic taste. Good cloves should be plump and heavy, have a bright, reddish-brown colour, sink in water, and exude oil when indented with the finger-nail.

MORPHOLOGY

Evergreen tree, 9-12 M. (30-40°) high, much branched, forming a pyramidal crown; *bark* yellowish; *leaves* 10 cm long, 5 cm wide, entire, smooth, glandular, parallel veins to midrib, petiolate; *flowers* 15-20, rose-color, cymes; *fruit* berry-like. Flower-*buds* (clove), tack-shaped, 10-17.5 Mm. (2/5-3/4) long, dark brown, consisting of a stem-like, solid, inferior *ovary*, obscurely 4-angled, terminated by 4 *calyx* teeth, and surmounted by a nearly globular head, consisting of 4 *petals* enclosing numerous curved stamens and 1 *style*.

Powder, dark brown; *microscopically* - cellular fragments with large oil reservoirs, spiral tracheae, few fusiform bast-fibres, rosette aggregates of calcium oxalate, many tetrahedral pollen grains; presence of stems show stone cells of large lumina with yellowish-brown substance; volatile extractive soluble in ether 10 p. c. Solvents: alcohol (volatile oil, resin); water (odor part of volatile oil but none of the pungent resin).

STUDY QUESTIONS

Write short notes on the following:

(a) Senna;

(b) Ipecacuanha;

(d) Nux Vomica; and

(e) Cloves.

■■■

INDEX

NOTES